Introduction to Toxicology

As with the previous editions, *Introduction to Toxicology,* Fourth Edition, continues to chart the evolution of the field of toxicology, from the use of natural toxins by ancient tribes through the developments established by Paracelsus, and progresses through to the current topics of public interest. For centuries, the study of toxicology has fascinated students. The book begins with basic toxicological principles, including an historical summary, dose-response relationships (NEW chapter), exposure-response relationships (NEW chapter), disposition, and metabolism of xenobiotic toxic substances. Other important new chapters include target organ toxicity, toxicity of carcinogenic agents and new and updated concepts in toxicity testing, and antidotes and treatment of poisonings. In all, nine new or expanded chapters from the third edition are included.

Current concerns about the effects of therapeutic drugs, carcinogens, industrial toxins, pesticides, and herbicides on human health, animal welfare, and the stability and maintenance of the ecosystem continue to highlight toxicology as an important and growing scientific discipline.

Key features:

- Comprehensive coverage of the field of toxicology which illustrates its importance to and impact on society;
- Uses pertinent examples, tables, and diagrams to aid understanding with learning objectives, summaries, questions, and answers for each chapter;
- Clearly and concisely written and presented concepts for easy comprehension by toxicology, biomedical, health science students and chemistry;
- Examines the complex interactions associated with toxicological events;
- Covers the effect of toxins on biological and physiological systems.

This book successfully condenses the diffuse literature in the field into an accessible and readable text, made easier with the insertion of many tables and figures. It introduces fundamental concepts and builds upon these using topical and relevant historical examples. Its improved format includes learning objectives and summaries of each chapter, as well as questions and answers suitable for self-assessment.

This latest edition is an invaluable resource for undergraduate and graduate toxicology students, as well as an introductory text for other health care students and professionals. The book also functions as a comprehensive introductory reference text for environmental scientists, medical biologists and chemists, chemical engineers, and regulatory agencies, with interests in toxicologically related areas.

Introduction to Toxicology

Fourth Edition

John Timbrell and Frank A. Barile

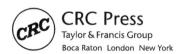

CRC Press
Taylor & Francis Group
Boca Raton London New York

CRC Press is an imprint of the
Taylor & Francis Group, an **informa** business

Designed cover image: Cover photo courtesy of John Trimbell

Fourth edition published 2023
by CRC Press
6000 Broken Sound Parkway NW, Suite 300, Boca Raton, FL 33487-2742

and by CRC Press
4 Park Square, Milton Park, Abingdon, Oxon, OX14 4RN

CRC Press is an imprint of Taylor & Francis Group, LLC

© 2023 John Timbrell and Frank A. Barile

First edition published by Taylor & Francis 1989
Third edition published by Taylor & Francis 2002

Library of Congress Cataloging-in-Publication Data
Names: Timbrell, John A., author. | Barile, Frank A, author.
Title: Introduction to toxicology / John Timbrell, Frank A. Barile.
Description: Fourth edition. | Boca Raton, FL : CRC Press, 2023. |
Revised edition of: Introduction to toxicology / John Timbrell. Third edition. 2001. |
Includes bibliographical references and index.
Identifiers: LCCN 2022038922 (print) | LCCN 2022038923 (ebook)
Subjects: LCSH: Toxicology.
Classification: LCC RA1211 .T56 2023 (print) | LCC RA1211 (ebook) |
DDC 615.9—dc23/eng/20220831
LC record available at https://lccn.loc.gov/2022038922
LC ebook record available at https://lccn.loc.gov/2022038923

ISBN: 978-1-032-03699-1 (hbk)
ISBN: 978-1-032-03692-2 (pbk)
ISBN: 978-1-003-18857-5 (ebk)

DOI: 10.1201/9781003188575

Typeset in Century Old Style
by codeMantra

Contents

AUTHORS   XIII
PREFACE TO THE FOURTH EDITION   XV
ACKNOWLEDGMENTS   XVII

1   Introduction   **1**
    Chapter Outline   1
    1.1   Introduction   1
    1.2   Historical Aspects   3
    1.3   Classification of Toxic Substances   7
          1.3.1   Pharmaceutical and Therapeutic Agents   8
          1.3.2   Food Additives   8
          1.3.3   Industrial Chemicals   8
          1.3.4   Environmental Pollutants   9
          1.3.5   Naturally Occurring Toxins   9
          1.3.6   Household Poisons   9
    1.4   Classification of Exposure   10
          1.4.1   Intentional Ingestion   10
          1.4.2   Occupational Exposure   10
          1.4.3   Environmental Exposure   10
          1.4.4   Unintentional, Accidental Poisoning   11
          1.4.5   Selective Toxicity   11
    1.5   Summary and Learning Objectives   12
    Notes   12
    Bibliography   12
    Suggested Readings   13

2   Dose-Response Relationship   **15**
    Chapter Outline   15
    2.1   Basic Principles of the Dose-Response Relationship   15
    2.2   Receptors   21

CONTENTS

2.3   Synergy and Potentiation   22
2.4   Threshold Dose and NOAEL   23
2.5   Summary and Learning Objectives   23
Review Questions   24
      Short Answer Questions   25
Notes   25
Bibliography   25

3   Exposure-Response Relationship   27
Chapter Outline   27
3.1   Types of Exposure   27
      3.1.1   Acute Exposure   28
      3.1.2   Chronic Exposure   28
      3.1.3   Continuous/Intermittent Exposure   28
3.2   Route of Exposure   28
3.3   Types of Toxic Response   29
      3.3.1   Biochemical Lesions   30
      3.3.2   Pharmacological and Physiological Effects   30
      3.3.3   Immunotoxicity   30
      3.3.4   Teratogenicity   33
      3.3.5   Genetic Toxicity   34
      3.3.6   Carcinogenicity   35
3.4   Biomarkers   36
3.5   Summary and Learning Objectives   37
Review Questions   39
      Short Answer Questions   39
Notes   39
Bibliography   40

4   Disposition of Toxic Compounds   41
Chapter Outline   41
4.1   Absorption of Toxic Compounds   42
4.2   Sites of Absorption   45
      4.2.1   Skin   45
      4.2.2   Lungs   46
      4.2.3   Gastrointestinal Tract   48
4.3   Distribution of Toxic Compounds   51
4.4   Elimination   56
      4.4.1   Urinary Elimination   56

	4.4.2	Biliary Elimination	58
	4.4.3	Pulmonary Elimination	60
	4.4.4	Other Routes of Elimination	60
4.5		Summary and Learning Objectives	60
Review Questions			62
		Short Answer Questions	62
Notes			62
Bibliography			63

5 Metabolism of Xenobiotic Compounds **65**

Chapter Outline — 65

5.1		Objectives of Metabolism	66
5.2		Phase I Reactions	68
	5.2.1	Oxidation Reactions	68
		5.2.1.1 Cytochrome P450	69
	5.2.2	Types of Oxidation Reactions	70
	5.2.3	Reduction Reactions	71
		5.2.3.1 Hydrolysis	72
		5.2.3.2 Hydration	73
5.3		Phase II Reactions	74
	5.3.1	Sulfation	74
	5.3.2	Glucuronidation	74
	5.3.3	Glutathione Conjugation	75
	5.3.4	Acetylation	76
	5.3.5	Amino Acid Conjugation	77
	5.3.6	Methylation	77
5.4		Toxification versus Detoxification	78
5.5		Factors Affecting Toxic Responses	78
	5.5.1	Species	79
	5.5.2	Strain of Animal	79
	5.5.3	Gender Differences	80
	5.5.4	Genetic Factors and Human Variability in Response	80
	5.5.5	Environmental Factors	81
	5.5.6	Pathological State	82
5.6		Summary and Learning Objectives	82
Review Questions			83
		Short Answer Questions	84
Notes			84
Bibliography			84

CONTENTS

6 Target Organ Toxicity **87**
Chapter Outline 87
6.1 Introduction 87
6.2 Liver Toxicity 88
6.3 Kidney Toxicity 89
6.4 Cardiac Toxicity 89
6.5 Toxicity of the Nervous System 91
6.6 Pulmonary Toxicity 92
6.7 Direct Toxic Action: Tissue Lesions 92
6.8 Summary and Learning Objectives 93
Review Questions 93
Short Answer Question 94
Note 94
Bibliography 94

7 Carcinogenic and Mutagenic Compounds **95**
Chapter Outline 95
7.1 Introduction 95
7.2 Mechanisms of Chemical Carcinogenesis and Mutagenesis 96
7.3 DNA Repair Mechanisms 98
7.4 Multistage Carcinogenesis 98
7.5 Chemical Carcinogens 99
7.6 Cancer Chemopreventive Agents 100
7.7 Summary and Learning Objectives 101
Review Questions 101
Notes 102
Bibliography 102
Review Articles 103
Suggested Readings 105

8 Drugs as Toxic Substances **107**
Chapter Outline 107
8.1 Types of Drug Toxicity 108
8.2 Acetaminophen (Paracetamol in UK, EU) 108
8.3 Aspirin (Acetylsalicylic Acid, Acetylsalicylate, ASA) 110
8.4 Hydralazine 113
8.5 Halothane 115
8.6 Debrisoquine 116
8.7 Thalidomide 117

8.8   Drug Interactions   118

8.9   Altered Responsiveness: Glucose-6-Phosphate
Dehydrogenase Deficiency   119

8.10   Summary and Learning Objectives   120

Review Questions   121

     Short Answer Question   121

Notes   121

Bibliography   122

Suggested Readings   122

9   Industrial Toxicology   123

Chapter Outline   123

9.1   Occupational and Commercial Use of Industrial Chemicals   123

9.2   Means of Exposure   124

9.3   Toxic Effects   124

9.4   Examples of Hazardous Industrial Chemicals   126

9.5   Regulatory Legislation   130

9.6   Summary and Learning Objectives   131

Review Questions   132

     Short Answer Question   132

Notes   132

Bibliography   133

10   Food Additives and Contaminants   135

Chapter Outline   135

10.1   Introduction   135

10.2   Tartrazine   138

10.3   Saccharin   139

10.4   Food Contaminants   140

     10.4.1   Botulinum Toxin   141

     10.4.2   Aflatoxin   141

     10.4.3   Ginger Jake   142

     10.4.4   The Toxic Oil (Spanish Oil) Syndrome   142

10.5   Summary and Learning Objectives   143

Review Questions   144

     Short Answer Question   145

Notes   145

Bibliography   146

Suggested Readings   146

CONTENTS

11   Pesticides and Herbicides   **147**
      Chapter Outline   147
      11.1 Introduction and Types of Pesticides and Herbicides   147
      11.2 Dichloro-diphenyltrichloroethane   149
      11.3 Organophosphorus Compounds   153
      11.4 Paraquat   156
      11.5 Fluoroacetate   158
      11.6 Summary and Learning Objectives   159
      Review Questions   160
            Short Answer Questions   160
      Notes   160
      Bibliography   160
      Suggested Readings   162

12   Environmental Pollutants   **163**
      Chapter Outline   163
      12.1 Introduction   163
      12.2 Air Pollution   165
      12.3 Particulate Matter   167
      12.4 Acid Rain   168
      12.5 Metals   170
            12.5.1 Lead Pollution   170
            12.5.2 Arsenic   172
            12.5.3 Mercury and Methylmercury   174
      12.6 Water Pollution   177
      12.7 Food Chains   178
      12.8 Endocrine Disruptors   180
      12.9 Summary and Learning Objectives   184
      Review Questions   185
            Short Answer Question   185
      Notes   186
      Bibliography   186
      Suggested Readings   188

13   Natural Products   **189**
      Chapter Outline   189
      13.1 Introduction   190
      13.1 Plant Toxins   190
            13.1.1 Pyrrolizidine Alkaloids   190
                  13.1.1.1 Case Study   190

13.1.2	Pennyroyal Oil	191
13.1.3	Ricin	192
13.1.4	Bracken	192
13.2	Animal Toxins	193
13.2.1	Snake Venoms	195
13.2.2	Tetrodotoxin	195
13.3	Fungal Toxins	196
13.3.1	Death Cap Mushroom	196
13.3.2	Aflatoxins	197
13.4	Microbial Toxins	197
13.4.1	Botulism and Botulinum Toxin	197
13.4.2	*E. coli* Infections and Exotoxins	197
13.5	Summary and Learning Objectives	198
	Review Questions	199
	Short Answer Questions	199
	Notes	199
	Bibliography	199
	Suggested Readings	200

14 Commercial and Domestic Products — **201**
Chapter Outline		201
14.1	Introduction	201
14.2	Carbon Monoxide	202
14.3	Ethylene Glycol (Antifreeze)	204
14.4	Cyanide	206
14.5	Alcohol (Ethanol, Ethyl Alcohol)	208
14.6	Glue Sniffing and Solvent Abuse (Hydrocarbons)	208
14.7	Summary and Learning Objectives	209
	Review Questions	210
	Short Answer Questions	210
	Notes	210
	Bibliography	211

15 Fundamentals of Toxicity Testing — **213**
Chapter Outline		213
15.1	Introduction	213
15.2	Evaluation of Toxicity	214
15.3	Epidemiological Studies	215
15.4	Animal Welfare	216
15.5	Considerations for Experimental Testing	217
15.5.1	Acute Toxicity Tests	219

CONTENTS

15.5.2 Sub-chronic Toxicity Tests   220
15.5.3 Chronic Toxicity Tests   221
15.6 *In Vitro Testing* as Alternatives to Animals   223
15.7 Summary and Learning Objectives   225
Review Questions   225
    Short Answer Questions   225
Notes   226
Bibliography   226

16   Risk Assessment   229
Chapter Outline   229
16.1 Introduction   229
16.2 Risk Assessment and Interpretation of Toxicological Data   230
    16.2.1 Risk Assessment   230
        16.2.1.1 Hazard Identification   231
        16.2.1.2 Dose-Response Assessment   232
        16.2.1.3 Exposure Assessment   235
        16.2.1.4 Risk Characterization   236
16.3 Biomarkers in Risk Assessment   238
16.4 Summary and Learning Objectives   239
Review Questions   240
    Short Answer Questions   240
Notes   240
Bibliography   240

17   Antidotes and Treatment of Poisoning   243
Chapter Outline   243
17.1 Introduction   243
17.2 Poison Control Centers   244
17.3 General Supportive Measures   244
17.4 Specific Antidotes   246
17.5 Toxicology Laboratories   247
17.6 Summary and Learning Objectives   247
Review Questions   248
    Short Answer Questions   248
Bibliography   248

ANSWERS TO CHAPTER QUESTIONS   251
GLOSSARY   271
INDEX   283

Authors

John Timbrell DSc is Emeritus Professor of Biochemical Toxicology, King's College London, UK. He received his BSc in Biochemistry from the University of Bath and Ph.D. in drug metabolism from St. Mary's Medical School, University of London, UK after which he spent 2 years as a research fellow in the Department of Chemical Pharmacology, NHLBI, NIH, Bethesda, Md, USA. After that time he worked in the University of London at the Royal Postgraduate Medical School, then School of Pharmacy and finally Kings' College London, Dr. Timbrell is the founding editor of the publication *Biomarkers* and has served on the editorial boards of several toxicology related journals and served on the UK Government Commitee on Toxicity. He is a Fellow of the Royal Society of Chemistry and was the recipient of the Young Scientist award of the European Society of Toxicology. His main topics of interest included the role of taurine in detoxication/protection, toxicology of the liver, mechanisms of toxicity of compounds especially hydrazines, and biomarkers of chemical-induced dysfunction. He has published 137 original scientific papers, reviews and book chapters and is also the author of *Study Toxicology through Questions, Principles of Biochemical Toxicology, Fourth Edition, Introduction to Toxicology, Third Edition* and *The Poison Paradox*.

Frank A. Barile, Ph.D., is a Professor in the Toxicology Division (retired), and past Chairman of the Department of Pharmaceutical Sciences, St. John's University College of Pharmacy and Health Sciences, New York.

Dr. Barile received his B.S. in Pharmacy, M.S. in Pharmacology, and Ph.D. in Toxicology at St. John's University. After completing a post-doctoral fellowship in Pulmonary Pediatrics at the Albert Einstein College of Medicine, Bronx, NY, he moved to the Department of Pathology, Columbia University, St. Luke's Roosevelt Hospital, NY, as a Research Associate. In these positions, he investigated the role of pulmonary toxicants on collagen metabolism in cultured lung cells. In 1984, he was appointed as Assistant Professor in the Department of Health Sciences at City University of NY. Sixteen years later, he rejoined St. John's University in the Department of Pharmaceutical Sciences in the College of Pharmacy.

Dr. Barile holds memberships in several professional associations, including the U.S. Society of Toxicology (U.S. SOT), American Association of University Professors, American Association for the Advancement of Science, American Society of Hospital Pharmacists, New York City Pharmacists Society, New York Academy of Sciences, and New York State Council of Health System Pharmacists. He is past President of the *In Vitro* and Alternative Methods (IVAM) Specialty Section of the U.S. SOT and a former member of the Scientific Advisory Committee for Alternative Toxicological Methods (SACATM), NIEHS, U.S. National Institutes of Health (U.S. NIH). He is past Editor of *Toxicology in Vitro* and *Journal of Pharmacological & Toxicological Methods*, Elsevier Ltd. Publishers.

Dr. Barile is the recipient of Public Health Service research grants from the National Institute of General Medical Sciences (NIGMS, NIH) and from private foundations dedicated to animal husbandry. He has authored and co-authored approximately 120 original research manuscripts, review articles, research abstracts, and conference proceedings in peer-reviewed toxicology and biomedical journals. He has also published several books and has related chapters in the field. He contributed original *in vitro* toxicology data to the international *Multicenter Evaluation for In Vitro Cytotoxicity* (MEIC) program. He has lectured regularly to pharmacy and toxicology undergraduate and graduate students in clinical and basic pharmaceutical and toxicological sciences and was awarded "Professor of the Year" for the College of Pharmacy by the St. John's University Student Government Association (2003).

Dr. Barile has served on several U.S. government advisory committees, including Toxicology Assessment Peer Review Committee, U.S. EPA, OPPT (2013); Scientific Advisory Committee on Alternative Toxicological Methods (SACATM), and the National Toxicology Program Interagency Center for the Evaluation of Alternative Toxicological Methods (NICEATM) (2005–2009); U.S. FDA, National Center for Toxicology Research (NCTR), Systems Biology Subcommittee (2016); National Institute of Occupational Safety & Health (NIOSH) & Oak Ridge Associated Universities (ORAU), NIOSH SK Profiles Review Group (2014); and U.S. FDA advisory committee on alternative toxicological methods (ACATM) (2013).

Dr. Barile received the Faculty Recognition Award, Am. Association of University Professors (AAUP)-Faculty Association, St. John's University, 2002–2003, 2004–2005, 2013–2014, and 2015–2016, and received the prestigious Public Health Service Medallion from the Director of the NIEHS, Dr. Linda Birnbaum, for contributions to SACATM (2009).

Dr. Barile continues as Science Advisor for the Humane Society of the U.S. to encourage development, incorporation, and substitution of *in vitro* alternative methods for the reduction, refinement, and replacement to animal experimentation and toxicology testing.

Preface to the Fourth Edition

It is my pleasure to collaborate with Dr. John Timbrell on the fourth edition of *Introduction to Toxicology*. Since the publication of the third edition in 2002, the discipline of toxicology has journeyed through a rapidly changing planet that traditionally did not present fast-moving developments. Unlike other evolving technological fields, such as computer engineering and mobile devices, toxicology has not been a prime mover in the applied sciences, and even slower in many parts of the world. Also, in comparison to other biomedical applications, advances in toxicology are also not as rapid as those encountered within genetic, stem cell, or immunologic therapeutics. However, the crosstalk among these areas involving the basic tenets of toxicology has enabled the latter to express a variety of new applications and knowledge within the last generation, advances which reflect the problems and issues encountered by society. The topics reflect increasing societal concerns such as those seen with the environment, endocrine-disrupting chemicals (endocrine disruptors, ED), and chemical and biological threats to public health. In particular, the basic science of toxicology has shifted consistently toward applied realms, including understanding the fundamentals of poisons and their mechanisms, notwithstanding the features, causes, and pathologies. Consequently, this fourth edition retains its previous commitment to, and is primarily concerned with, the basic underlying principles of toxicology at the introductory level.

The fourth edition presents the field of toxicology as a thought-provoking update. To students in the health and biomedical sciences and to established health professionals, the arena of toxicology is inspiring and is important for overall knowledge of biomedical systems. The reviews, criticisms, and suggestions garnered over the last 20 years, since the presentation of the last edition has enabled the production of an updated, applied, and mechanistic text. Each chapter has been revised to include topical information, as well as clearer illustrations and explanatory tables, while several new chapters are inserted. In addition, some chapters have been rewritten and updated with biochemical formulas, chemical structures, and toxicological mechanisms.

The fourth edition also highlights new fields of toxic exposure, such as dose-response relationships, target organ toxicity, teratogenic and mutagenic compounds, and risk assessment.

In general, and as with previous versions, the book examines the complex interactions associated with toxicological events because of intentional or inadvertent chemical and drug exposure. Special emphasis is placed on pharmacological and toxicological mechanisms of action, **toxicokinetics**, and detection and identification of chemicals in physiological compartments. Other contemporary issues in toxicology, including various means of possible exposure to therapeutic and non-therapeutic agents, an overview of protocols for therapeutic management of various toxic administrations, and the remedies associated with their pathology, are conveyed. Lastly, chapter summaries, learning objectives, study questions, and references are updated.

It is hoped that this edition inspires a greater respect among toxicology and health professional students as they strive to understand the consequences of exposure to the multitude of chemicals. As our society becomes more scientifically adept at many levels, its thirst for information about chemical exposure increases. Accordingly, students and established scientists in the field will develop a greater awareness and appreciation for the costs of exposure to chemical compounds, of the risk from biological threats, or of the adverse effects of environmental pollutants. As a generation becomes more knowledgeable, its preparedness is stronger and its response to threats is more formidable.

FAB, December 2022

Acknowledgments

My appreciation is extended to Dr. John Timbrell for my participation in revising the fourth edition of *Introduction to Toxicology*. I am most appreciative to the editorial staff at CRC Press, particularly Stephen Zollo, Editor for Toxicology Group, for coordinating this collaboration, Ms. Laura P., Editorial Assistant and Ms. Assunta P., Project Manager. Their patience and focus were of great sustenance in the completion of this project.

I am continuously indebted to my wife Pauline, whose encouragement, inspiration, and reassurance have sustained my efforts by believing in my abilities, in the force of my dedication, and in the value of my contributions.

Chapter 1

Introduction

Chapter Outline

This chapter introduces historical highlights and basic principles of toxicology:

1.1	Introduction	1
1.2	Historical Aspects	3
1.3	Classification of Toxic Substances	7
	1.3.1 Pharmaceutical and Therapeutic Agents	8
	1.3.2 Food Additives	8
	1.3.3 Industrial Chemicals	8
	1.3.4 Environmental Pollutants	9
	1.3.5 Naturally Occurring Toxins	9
	1.3.6 Household Poisons	9
1.4	Classification of Exposure	10
	1.4.1 Intentional Ingestion	10
	1.4.2 Occupational Exposure	10
	1.4.3 Environmental Exposure	10
	1.4.4 Unintentional, Accidental Poisoning	11
	1.4.5 Selective Toxicity	11
1.5	Summary and Learning Objectives	12
	Notes	12
	Bibliography	12
	Suggested Readings	13

1.1 Introduction

Toxicology is the study of interactions between chemicals or drugs,[1] and biological systems. Humans, mammals, and environmental entities on the planet are increasingly exposed to chemicals of an enormous variety. These substances range from

DOI: 10.1201/9781003188575-1

metals and inorganic chemicals to large complex organic molecules, yet all possess the potential to induce toxicity. Accordingly, toxicology is multidisciplinary which encompasses the study of pathological, biochemical, and physiological effects of such substances within interacting species. Thus, the challenge in this field refers to the application of basic chemistry, biochemistry, physiology, and pathology, along with experimental observation, to gain an understanding of how and why substances cause disruption in biological systems, which lead to toxic effects.

Approximately 100,000 chemicals, plastics, gases, metals, and therapeutic drugs are produced yearly in the United States, up to 10,000 of which are newly synthesized. This escalation in chemical production renders our environment and inhabitants vulnerable to their effects (Figure 1.1), compelling the toxicology community to pursue and understand the causes and mechanisms of the untoward effects and to accurately monitor, carefully analyze, and predict risk for science and public health.

In recent years, the problem of human and animal exposure to potentially toxic chemicals in the environment was brought to the attention of the public through the publication of *Silent Spring* (Rachel Carson, 1962). The book describes the devastating effects of **pesticides** on the flora and fauna of the North American environment. The discussion of the issue was continued in *The Apocalyptics: Cancer and the Big Lie* (Edith Efron, Simon & Schuster Pub., 1984), declaring that Carson and other scientists probably exaggerated the dangers of chemicals. However, today few would contest the importance of awareness and

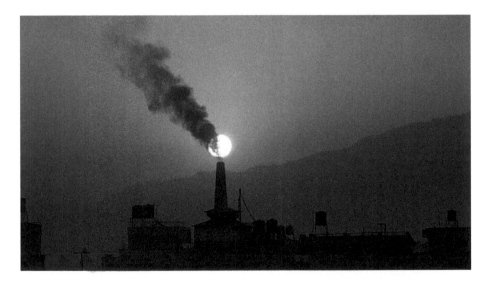

Figure 1.1 Toxicology is concerned with the exposure of living systems in the environment to toxic substances from a variety of sources. (Air pollution by brick factories at Mahalaxmi municipality, Lalitpur, Nepal. Janak Bhatta, https://commons.wikimedia.org/wiki/File:Air_pollution3.jpg, Creative Commons CC0 1.0 Universal Public Domain Dedication.)

knowledge of the potential toxicity posed to humans from synthetic chemicals spilled into the environment. Thus, the field of toxicology in general, and environmental toxicity in particular, has spawned another dimension: the social, moral, and legal aspects of exposure of human and animal populations to chemicals of unknown or uncertain threats, of which hazard and risk assessments and value judgments have emerged. The regulatory toxicologist, whose unique role has recently blossomed in our society, is often asked to make such decisions.

1.2 Historical Aspects

In the public arena, toxicology has been referred to as 'the study of poisons', which begs the question 'what is a poison?' Poisons span a wide range of sources and chemical forms, from naturally occurring plant alkaloids to synthetic nerve gases. Thus, a poison is a substance that has harmful effects on living systems; in addition, designation of a substance as a poison depends on its application, dose, and concentration. For example, historically, arsenic has been considered a poison for humans; however, it has also been used and is currently approved as a therapeutic drug. The apparent conflicting aspects of such a notorious chemical will be further explained in later sections as our concept of toxicology evolves.

Recently the study of poisons has become a justifiable scientific pursuit. At one time, however, it was mainly a practical art utilized for malevolent intentions. Poisons have also played an important part in human history as subtle and silent military weapons.

Prehistoric humans were aware that liquids extracted from animals and plants contained natural poisons which were used on their weapons. For instance, early hunters dipped arrowheads into liquids containing poisonous concoctions (thus the origin of the term *toxikon*) and propelled on an arrow from a bow. Subsequent study and categorization of poisons probably started by 1500 BCE, evidenced in part by the *Ebers papyrus*, the earliest collection of medical records, containing many references and recipes for poisons. Ancient Egyptians were able to distill prussic acid from peach kernels; arsenic, aconite, and opium were also known in Hindu medicine as recorded in the *Vedas*, around 900 BCE, and the ancient Chinese used **aconite** as an arrow poison. In his writings, Hippocrates (400 BCE) documented the ancient Greek's professional awareness of poisons and the principles of toxicology; in particular, they demonstrated advanced knowledge of principles regarding the treatment of poisoning by the influence absorption and the development of antidotes. For example, Nicander of Colophon (185–135 BCE), physician to Attalus, King of Pergamon, experimented with poisons using condemned criminals as subjects. His studies produced treatises like *Theriaca and Alexipharmica,* documents on antidotes to poisonous reptiles and substances. The document mentions 22 specific poisons including ceruse (white lead), litharge (lead oxide), aconite (wolfsbane), cantharides (blistering agent), conium (hemlock), hyoscyamus (henbane), and opium (narcotic). He also recommended linseed tea to induce vomiting and suggested that extracting the venom from the bite of a venomous animal be used as treatment. Similarly, Mithridates

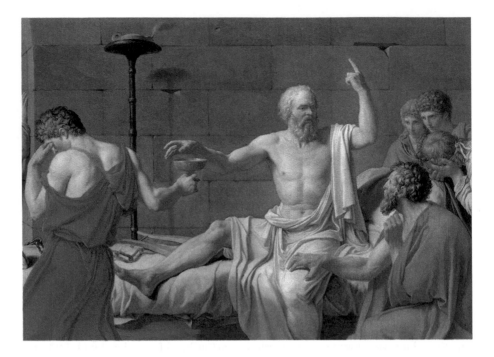

Figure 1.2 Painting depicting the death of Socrates in prison about to drink hemlock given by his executioner, Jacques-Louis David. (Metropolitan Museum of Art, New York City, USA. https://commons.wikimedia.org/wiki/File:David_-_The_Death_of_Socrates_-_detail2.jpg. https://www.metmuseum.org/collection/the-collection-online/search/436105. Creative Commons CC0 1.0 Universal Public Domain Dedication.)

(132–36 BCE), King of Pontus (Asia Minor, modern-day eastern Black Sea Region of Turkey), used incarcerated criminals to identify antidotes to venom and poisonous substances and regularly protected himself with a mixture of 50 different antidotes (*Mithridatum*[2]).

The first documented law against poisoning was issued in Rome by Sulla in 82 BCE to protect against careless dispensing. The Greek physician Dioscorides (50 AD) made a particularly significant contribution to toxicology by classifying poisons as animal, plant, or mineral and recognized the value of emetics in the treatment of poisoning. His treatise on *Materia Medica* was a major work on the underlying principles of poisons and their antidotes, establishing this text as common knowledge for fifteen centuries.

The use of poisons in society for murder, suicide, and political assassination is also well documented in the origins of toxicology. For example, in 399 BCE Socrates committed suicide by drinking from the executioner's cup of poisonous hemlock (Figure 1.2). Claudius, Emperor of Rome (41–54 AD), was purportedly poisoned with arsenic by his wife Agrippina (and niece). Nero, Claudius' successor, employed a professional to poison Claudius' son, Britannicus, who dissolved arsenic in the water used to cool the banquet soup, thus avoiding the suspicions of the Emperor's taster.

The abundant use of poisons and the difficulty in detecting them in food or specimens made it necessary for treatments to be devised, and one of the first documents known on treatments for poisoning was written by Maimonides (1135–1204) in *Treatise on Poisons and Their Antidotes,* that detailed some of the treatments thought to be effective.

In the Middle Ages, the art of poisoning for political ends developed into a cult. In the ancient Italian republics, the Borgias were infamous during the fifteenth and sixteenth centuries. In seventeenth-century Italy, a woman by the name of Toffana prepared cosmetics containing arsenic (Aqua Toffana) which were used to remove unwanted rivals, husbands, and enemies! Similarly, Catherine de Medici prepared poisons and tested them on the poor and sick of France, noting all the clinical signs and symptoms.

One of the most important concepts in toxicology was espoused in the sixteenth century by the scientist Paracelsus. He was born Philippus Theophrastus Aureolus Bombastus von Hohenheim near Zurich in 1493, to a physician who was interested in chemistry and biology and an expert in occupational medicine. Paracelsus was a free thinker who disagreed with the dogma current at the time and was espoused by Galen. Paracelsus thought observation was crucial and understood the importance of chemistry in medicine. He believed that 'like cures like', contrary to Galen who taught that diseases of a particular intensity would be cured by a medicine of opposite intensity. Consequently in Paracelsus's understanding, 'a poison in the body would be cured by a similar poison – but the dosage is very important.' He advocated for the use of inorganic chemicals, such as salts, as treatments. Although these salts were believed to be too poisonous by contemporaries, he emphasized that the dose was very important in establishing cures. Paracelsus summarized this concept in a renowned statement: 'All substances are poisons; there is none that is not a poison. The right dose differentiates a poison from a remedy.'

This perception is especially crucial for the safe use of drugs but also important for proper handling of other chemicals (see below). It underlies the basis of risk assessment of chemicals which is founded on the assessment of threshold doses as well as in establishing safe and non-toxic levels. Even seemingly innocuous substances such as common table salt (sodium chloride) could be poisonous given the optimum circumstances.

Paracelsus also believed that diseases were localized to particular organs and that poisons could damage particular organs (target organs), a concept that has been generally proven to be correct. His contribution to medicine and toxicology is significant although not recognized until after his death in 1541.

Another significant figure in toxicology was Orfila, a Spanish physician (1787–1853) who recognized it as a separate discipline. He contributed to the specialized field of forensic toxicology by devising means of detecting poisonous substances, with the intention of substantiating that the act of poisoning had taken place. Since then toxicology developed in a more systematic scientific style

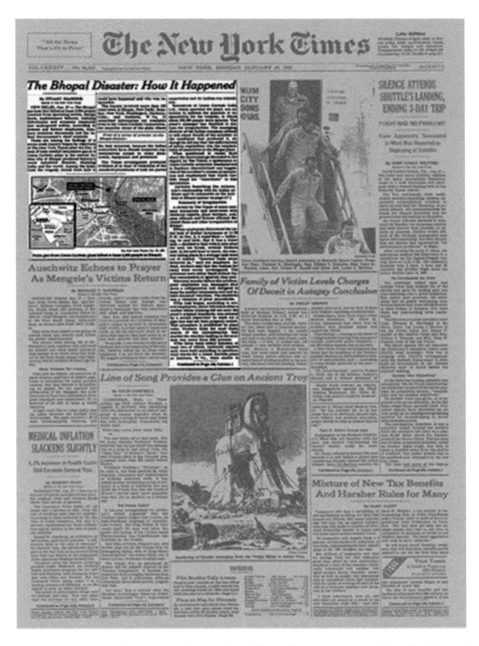

Figure 1.3 From The New York Times headline of January 28, 1984: "The Bhopal Disaster: How It Happened". (https://www.nytimes.com/1985/01/28/world/the-bhopal-disaster-how-it-happened.html.)

and began to include the study of the mechanism of action of poisons; that is, the molecular basis for how drugs and chemicals interact with the organs, tissues, and cells. Indeed, Claude Bernard (1813–1878) believed that the study of the effects of substances on biological systems could not only shed light on the mechanism of the poison but also enhance the understanding of those systems with which it interacted. For instance, he was the first to identify the site of action of curare, a neuromuscular blocking muscle relaxant, as either the nerve ending or the neuromuscular junction.

More recently, in 1945, Sir Rudolph Peters studied the mechanism of action of arsenical war gases. He was able to devise the effective **antidote**, British Anti-Lewisite (BAL) used for the treatment of military personnel exposed to these gases. Other examples of toxic chemicals have been studied at the mechanistic level and have benefited our understanding of basic biochemistry, including cyanide and fluorocitrate. Cyanide inhibits the mitochondrial electron transport chain, while fluorocitrate inhibits aconitase, a critical enzyme of the Krebs cycle.

In the 20th century, some industrial chemical disasters have occurred which have highlighted the need not only for understanding the toxicity of compounds, drugs, and food additives used in industry but also created the need for the organized study of toxic substances by the industries manufacturing them and for government legislation to control them. This has resulted in the establishment of government regulatory agencies to implement administrative action.

For example, in 1984 one of the worst industrial disasters occurred in Bhopal, India where a factory manufacturing the insecticide, carbaryl, leaked a large amount of an intermediate reaction chemical gas, the extremely noxious compound methyl isocyanate (Figure 1.3). The leak 'that killed at least 2,000 people resulted from operating errors, design flaws, maintenance failures, training deficiencies and economy measures that endangered safety, according to present and former employees, company technical documents and the Indian Government's chief scientist' (New York Times, January 1984).

At the time, since little was known of the toxicity of this compound, treatment of the victims was uncertain and inadequate.

Another major reason for testing chemicals in toxicity studies is to allow the substances to for classification according to hazard categories such as toxic, explosive, or flammable. This enables enactment of regulatory decisions about marketing, distribution, transport, storage, and labeling, among other uses. The categories thus established encompass almost all chemicals that are encountered in the environment. With this in consideration, the question becomes 'are all chemicals toxic?' The following common knowledge phrase perhaps provides an answer: 'there are no safe chemicals, only safe ways of using them.'

1.3 Classification of Toxic Substances

Toxic substances are classified according to their use or exposure: pharmaceutical agents (*drugs*), food additives, pesticides, herbicides, occupational (industrial) chemicals, environmental pollutants, naturally occurring toxins, and commercially available (household) chemical products. These categories are individually discussed in greater detail in later chapters but are briefly introduced here.

1.3.1 Pharmaceutical and Therapeutic Agents

As pharmacologically active agents, 'drugs and chemicals are our friends'. Their benefit to society has enabled humans to improve their quality of life as well as their lifespan.[3] However, they have generally been designed to be highly potent in biological systems, making them potentially toxic. Thus, drug toxicity may be a consequence of an overdose, a rare untoward (**idiosyncratic**) effect, an adverse reaction (*side effect*), or an accumulation of the compound in the biological system (see Chapter 5 for details).

Drugs vary enormously in chemical structure and possess a wide variety of biological activities. They are the only foreign substances with known biological activity that humans ingest intentionally, including alcohol, the active principles in cigarettes, and mood-enhancing drugs. Drugs used in veterinary practice are also considered and included here since humans consume the products from animals treated with these substances.

1.3.2 Food Additives

Food additives are xenobiotic (external) substances usually of low biological activity which are also ingested. Many different additives are combined with food-processing systems to alter the flavor or color, prevent spoilage, or chemically change the nature of the foodstuff. There are also several potentially toxic substances that are regarded as contaminants occurring naturally in food, resulting from cooking, storage, or processing. Most of these substances, both natural and artificial, are present in food in undetectable amounts, but for the majority, little is known of their chronic or cumulative toxicity. In many cases, they are ingested daily for perhaps decades, exposing a tremendous number of people. Public awareness of this has influenced the preparation and manufacture of foodstuffs, such as additive-free nutrients available for consumption.

1.3.3 Industrial Chemicals

Industrial chemicals contribute to environmental pollution and are a direct or indirect hazard in the workplace where they are handled, formulated, or manufactured. There is a vast range of chemical types, and many different industries involve the handling or manufacture of hazardous chemicals. In general, industrial exposure includes exposure to chemical solvents used as a basis for chemical reactions. Although government regulations are set to limits of exposure and safety practices in the workplace, actual exposure levels still prove to be hazardous chronically and acute exposure due to accidents occurs. The time between the development of diseases such as cancer, which is often diagnosed later in life, often makes it difficult to determine if a chemical is the cause, until and unless sufficient numbers of persons in the workforce have presented with the disease in order to establish an association with the toxic compound.

1.3.4 Environmental Pollutants

There are several chemical sources of environmental pollution including industrial processes, such as the manufacture of chemicals, the spreading of commercial chemical products, such as pesticides and herbicides, and the release of chemical waste into the environment. Environmental pollutants are released into the atmosphere, waterways, oceans, or discarded on land.[4]

Commercial pesticides, including insecticides and rodenticides, as well as herbicides, are purposely sprayed onto agricultural land and on household lawns with the potential for human exposure either via the crop itself or through contamination of drinking water or air. A major problem with the release of pesticides is their **persistence** in the environment with a corresponding increase in concentration during passage through the **food chain**.

1.3.5 Naturally Occurring Toxins

Many plants and animals produce toxic substances for both defensive and offensive purposes. Naturally occurring toxins of animal, plant, and microbiological origins comprise a wide variety of chemical types, result in a variety of toxic effects, and are a significant cause of human poisonings. The concept currently expounded by some individuals that 'natural (organic) is safer' is not entirely accurate since some of the most toxic substances on the planet are of natural origin. Natural toxins feature in poisoning via contamination of food, by accidental exposure to poisonous plants or animals, and by insect or animal vectors (stinging or biting).

1.3.6 Household Poisons

Household poisons include some of the substances in the previous categories such as pesticides, drugs, and solvents. Exposure to these types of compounds is usually acute rather than chronic. Many household substances used for cleaning, disinfecting, and elimination of indoor pests are irritants and corrosive. Consequently, they cause severe skin and eye lesions upon exposure. If swallowed in significant quantities or if highly concentrated solutions are ingested, household materials such as bleach and baking soda cause severe tissue damage to the nose, throat, esophagus, and stomach. Some drugs and pesticides are widely available and consequently are often found in the home and are also hazardous. For example, the herbicide paraquat and the analgesic drug acetaminophen are toxic and have both contributed significantly to human poisoning deaths.

1.4 Classification of Exposure

In some cases, the pathway to exposure is determined by the nature of the toxic substance. For example, gases and vapors from volatile solvents lead to inhalation exposure, whereas non-volatile liquids are associated with skin contact. Many industrial chemicals are often linked to chronic effects due to long-term occupational exposure, whereas household substances are usually involved in acute poisoning following a single episode of accidental exposure.

Types of exposure are briefly discussed at this introductory stage, but the topic is further explored in later chapters.

1.4.1 Intentional Ingestion

Therapeutic drugs, food additives, and nutritional supplements are consumed daily by many, often for long periods of time. Exposure to these compounds, especially repeated or chronic exposure, is eventually associated with some adverse responses such as **allergic reactions** or **tolerance**. Alcohol, smoking, and drug consumption are ubiquitous social habits, often on a chronic basis, ultimately responsible for chronic toxic effects.

It is important to note that illicit, illegal acts of violence, such as suicide and homicide, are not uncommon and involve acute or chronic poisons. Both illicit and prescribed drugs are often employed, although household products are easily available and readily administered in opportunistic circumstances.

1.4.2 Occupational Exposure

Occupational exposure is encountered in an industrial setting or in private commercial businesses, such as in manufacturing settings or with commercial contractors. Toxicity is predominantly chronic and continuous; the route toward exposure is either via inhalation or dermal. Consequently, pulmonary **irritation** and dermatitis are common occupational illnesses. Acute exposure occurs in the event of an accident such as a fire, explosion, spillage, leakage, or as a result of poor working practices. For example, cleaning reactor vessels that store contained solvents leads to acute toxicity resulting from excessive contact with the chemical or its vapors.

1.4.3 Environmental Exposure

Gaseous or liquid effluents from manufacturing briefly or continuously contaminate the immediate environment as well as more distant atmospheric or aquatic targets. This form of exposure is usually chronic, but isolated accidents at factories have occurred where acute exposure of humans outside the factory has resulted in severe toxicity.[5] Chronic exposure to gases, such as sulfur dioxide, nitrogen oxides, and carbon monoxide, occurs in industrial areas and regions of heavy traffic and results in acute irritation; chronic toxic effects, however, are largely unknown.

Environmental exposure is also important in relation to pesticides capable of contaminating air, water, and food. Large-scale spraying potentially exposes communities to chemicals or their residues both within their food and via the air.

1.4.4 Unintentional, Accidental Poisoning

Unintentional, accidental poisoning is usually acute rather than chronic. Drugs, pesticides, household products, and natural products are involved in this type of exposure; children and the elderly are the most common victims. Erroneous unintentional ingestion of a poisonous herbal or vegetable product, cleaning fluid, or pharmaceutical agent is responsible for toxicity seen in this category as does accidental ingestion of an excessive dose of a drug. Inhalation of fumes from heaters, ovens, gas burners, and fires is also an important cause of accidental poisoning.

1.4.5 Selective Toxicity

An important concept in toxicology, selective toxicity, encompasses the differences in susceptibility to toxic effects between different species of animal or plant, or between different cells in the body, such as the susceptibility of tumor cells versus normal cells.

In many cases, selective toxicity is a useful attribute which is incorporated in the design of antibacterial drugs, pesticides, or chemotherapeutic agents (anticancer drugs); that is, it is the basis of having selective toxic action at those targets while sparing normal cells. It is also of relevance to the prediction of risk in humans based on studies in other species.

The explanations for selective toxicity vary but are divided into those due to differences in absorption, distribution, metabolism, and excretion of a chemical (toxicokinetics) or those due to biochemical differences affecting the presence of a receptor or target molecule (**toxicodynamics**). For example, insects are more susceptible to the toxicity of DDT than mammalian organisms for two reasons: (1) DDT penetrates insect cuticles more readily than mammalian skin, and (2) insects have greater surface area to volume ratio and therefore absorb relatively more of the insecticide. Insects are also more susceptible to some organophosphorus insecticides because the compounds are metabolized by oxidative desulphuration which produces a product that inhibits acetylcholinesterase; in mammals, however, this enzymatic hydrolysis produces a metabolite that is more readily excreted and does not inhibit acetylcholinesterase.

The rodenticide norbormide is active against rodents because they possess a receptor in smooth muscle, whereas humans, cats, and dogs do not. Other rodenticides take advantage of the feature that rodents do not have a vomit reflex, unlike many other mammals. Therefore, with oral ingestion of a poisonous chemical, the rat is unable to rid itself of the substance by vomiting.

In therapeutics, the antibiotic penicillin is active against a variety of bacteria because the drug interferes with synthesis of the cell wall as the bacteria multiply. Since mammalian cells do not have cell walls, they are not affected by the action of the antibiotic.

1.5 Summary and Learning Objectives

This chapter presents the *origins* of toxicology in antiquity, sometimes in relation to intentional poisoning. Some notable figures were mentioned especially Maimonides, Paracelsus, Orfila, and Bernard, individuals who all helped develop toxicology from an art to a science. The breadth and scope of toxicology are illustrated by the variety of types of toxic substances to which humans and animals are exposed, ranging from drugs, food additives, industrial chemicals, environmental pollutants, household poisons, to naturally occurring toxins.

The types of exposure, such as occupational, accidental, or intentional, are outlined, while toxicity is selective, affecting different cell types uniquely (tumor vs. normal) or species (mammalian vs. microorganism). This concept is used for the design of anticancer drugs, antibiotics, and pesticides.

One of the most important concepts that underlie toxicology is the dose-response relationship. First formulated by Paracelsus (in his famous phrase 'All substances are poisons, there is none that is not; the right dose distinguishes a poison from a remedy') establishes the relationship between the dose of a toxicant and the effect it produces or the toxic response.

Notes

1. For convenience, the term "chemicals" include organic, inorganic, synthetic, naturally-occurring agents and compounds, and therapeutic and non-therapeutic drugs.
2. *Mithradatic effect* refers to immunity against the action of a poison produced by small and gradually increasing doses of the same. The King supposedly was unsuccessful in committing suicide by poison because of his ingestion of repeated small doses taken to become invulnerable to assassination by poison.
3. In less than a century, in the western world, the advent of modern pharmaceuticals has universally has contributed to the increase in human lifespan to an average of over 80 years.
4. Smoke from factories and car exhaust fumes contain several known toxic constituents and constitute a major source of air pollution.
5. See Bhopal.

Bibliography

Aleksunes, L.M. and Eaton, D.L., Chapter 2. Principles of toxicology, in: *Casarett and Doull's Toxicology: The Basic Science of Poisons*, (pp. 25–64), Klaassen, C.D. (Ed.), 9th edition, McGraw-Hill, New York, 2018.

Ballantyne, B., Marrs, T. and Syversen, T. L. M. Basic elements of toxicology, in: *General and Applied Toxicology*, (pp. 3–56), Ballantyne, B., Marrs, T. and Syversen, T. L. M. (Eds.), 3rd edition, John Wiley & Sons, Ltd, Hoboken, NJ, 2009.

Barile, F.A. Chapter 1. Introduction, in: *Barile's Clinical Toxicology: Principles and Mechanisms*, 3rd edition. CRC Press, Taylor & Francis, Boca Raton, FL, 2019.

Deichmann, W.B., Henschler, D., Holmstedt, B. and Keil, G., What is there that is not a poison: A study of the Third Defence by Paracelsus, *Archives of Toxicology*, 58, 207, 1986.

Hayes, A.W., Wang, T. and Dixon, D., *Loomis's Essentials of Toxicology*, 5th edition, Academic Press, Elsevier, Amsterdam, 2019.

Hodgson, E., *A Textbook of Modern Toxicology*, John Wiley & Sons, New York, 2010.

Koeman, J.H., Chapter 1. Toxicology: History and scope of the field, in *Toxicology: Principles and Applications*, (pp. 2–15), Niesink, R.J.M., de Vries, J. and Hollinger, M.A. (Eds.), CRC Press, Taylor & Francis, Boca Raton, FL, 1996.

Lane, R.W., Chapter 1. The Wissenschaften of toxicology: Harming and helping through time, in: *Principles and Methods of Toxicology*, (pp. 3–34), Hayes, A.W. and Kruger, C.L. (Eds.), 6th edition, CRC Press, Taylor & Francis, Boca Raton, FL, 2014.

Lee, B.M., Kacew, S. and Kim, H.S. *Lu's Basic Toxicology*, 7th edition, CRC Press, Taylor & Francis, Boca Raton, FL, 2017.

Rim, K.T. Adverse outcome pathways for chemical toxicity and their applications to workers' health: A literature review. *Toxicology Environmental Health Sciences*, 1–10, 2020. Doi: 10.1007/s13530-020-00053-7.

Shaw, I.C. and Chadwick, J., *Principles of Environmental Toxicology*, CRC Press, Taylor & Francis, Boca Raton, FL, 1998.

Walker, C.H., Sibly, R.M., Hopkin, S.P. and Peakall, D.B., *Principles of Ecotoxicology*, 4th edition, CRC Press, Taylor & Francis, Boca Raton, FL, 2012.

Wexler, P. and Hayes, A.N., Chapter 1. The evolving journey of toxicology: A historical glimpse, in: *Casarett and Doull's Toxicology, The Basic Science of Poisons*, (pp. 3–24), Klaassen, C. D. (Ed.), 9th edition, McGraw-Hill, New York, 2018.

World Health Organisation, Chemical safety, https://www.who.int/health-topics/chemical-safety#tab=tab_1. Last accessed April 2022.

World Health Organisation, Environmental health, https://www.who.int/health-topics/environmental-health#tab=tab_1. Last accessed April 2022.

Suggested Readings

Blum, D., *The Poisoner's Handbook: Murder and the Birth of Forensic Medicine in Jazz Age* Penguin Books, New York, 2011.

Carson, R. *Silent Spring*, Chapman & Hall, London, 1965.

Mann, J., *Murder, Magic and Medicine*, Oxford University Press, London, 1994.

Munter, S. (Ed.), *Treatise on Poisons and Their Antidotes, vol. II of the Medical Writings of Moses Maimonides*, J. P. Lippincott, Philadelphia, PA, 1966.

Thompson, C.J.S. *Poisons and Poisoners*, H. Shaylor, London, 1931.

Timbrell, J.A. *The Poison Paradox*, Oxford University Press, Oxford, 2005.

Chapter 2

Dose-Response Relationship

Chapter Outline

In this chapter, the disposition of chemicals in biological systems is discussed:

2.1	Basic Principles of the Dose-Response Relationship	15
2.2	Receptors	21
2.3	Synergy and Potentiation	22
2.4	Threshold Dose and NOAEL	23
2.5	Summary and Learning Objectives	23
Review Questions		24
	Short Answer Questions	25
Notes		25
Bibliography		25

2.1 Basic Principles of the Dose-Response Relationship

> All substances are poisons; there is none which is not a poison. The
> right dose differentiates a poison and a remedy.
>
> Paracelsus (1493–1541)

Paracelsus was first to recognize the concept that toxicity is a relative phenomenon and that it depends not only on the toxic properties but on the dose of the compound administered.[1] This relationship between the dose of a compound and the response it elicits is a fundamental concept in toxicology. However, the nature of the response must first be considered. The toxic response that is humblest to observe is death, but this is a crude measurable parameter. A better indicator of a toxic response is the presence of a pathological lesion such as organ damage. And a more precise, predictive, and readily measured response is a biochemical, pharmacological, or chemical change.

All-or-none (absolute) responses, such as death, and graded (percent of 100) responses, such as the inhibition of an enzyme or the level of a marker of physiological damage, are distinguishable. Both all-or-none and graded responses show a typical dose-response relation. In both cases, there is a lower dose at which there is no measurable effect and an upper dose where there is a maximal response. Very often in a toxicity study, either in whole animals or in isolated cells, lethality is the first parameter of toxicity applied but this offers little information about the underlying mechanism of toxicity. However, it is often important to understand the limits of dosing in practical terms. Although it is not always necessary to determine the lethal dose, it is important to calculate whether toxicity occurs at one dose or a multiple of the dose encountered. However, in certain situations, it is extremely difficult to predict the most probable human dose. Similarly, extrapolating the possible effects on humans from the available data is daunting (refer to Chapter 16, Risk Assessment for further discussion of this concept).

It should be noted that dose refers to the total amount of a substance administered to an organism orally or parenterally, whereas dosage includes a characteristic reference to size of the organism, typically according to body weight or surface area, as well as the rate of administration. Dosage is more precise, therefore, and can be related to other organisms, as concentration of substance per kg of body weight.

Figure 2.1 illustrates a dose-response plot for percent of maximum response at 100% versus log of the concentration (or dosage). The graph represents either an all-or-none or a graded response. A standard method to determine the dose-response relationship is to calculate the percentage of test subjects at a specific concentration that expresses the desired response. This effect is then plotted against the concentration resulting in a typical sigmoid-shaped curve (Figure 2.1).

Furthermore, interpretation of the dose-response or concentration-effect relationship is based on the following assumptions:

- The response is usually proportional to the concentration at the target site.[2]
- The concentration at the target site is related to the dose.
- The response is causally related to the structure or class of the compound administered.

Some dose-response effects, such as liver necrosis caused by the analgesic acetaminophen or the solvent carbon tetrachloride, can be demonstrated; however, the drug-receptor interaction which underlies the response is not as readily observed. Thus, carbon tetrachloride is toxic because of a variety of specific liver effects including damage to membranes and inhibition of enzymes.

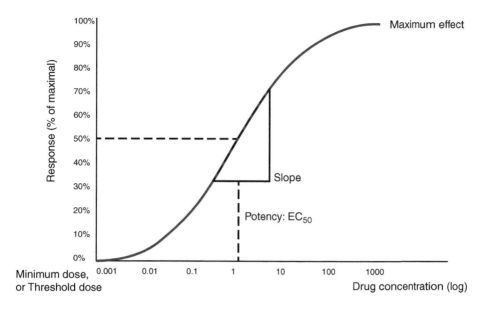

Figure 2.1 Typical dose-response curve. Percent of maximum response (100%) is plotted against the log of drug concentration (in wt. of substance/unit vol.) or dosage (wt. of substance/body wt.). The slope of the curve is a parameter used to measure the relative toxicity of the chemical and the range of safety between dosages. The effective concentration at 50% (EC_{50}) is extrapolated from the 50% response (Y-axis), which equals about 1.5–2.0. (From: Stack overflow, Public Network. https://chemistry.stackexchange.com/questions/141850/what-is-the-meaning-of-the-slope-in-a-graded-dose-response-curve.)

There are well-known areas in toxicology where receptors are critically involved. As noted above, the biological effects of the herbicide dioxin and related compounds have well-characterized receptor target sites. Interaction of dioxin with the **Ah receptor** directly leads to increased synthesis of cytochrome P450 thus leading to a series of reactions with resulting metabolic disturbances. Another well-documented example of a receptor interaction occurs with the peroxisome proliferators, which interact with the **peroxisome proliferator-activated receptor (PPAR)**.[3]

Although a toxic response is observed after exposure to a substance at known doses, it is usual to demonstrate responses within a range of doses of the compound, assuming a relationship exists between doses within the range and the magnitude of the response.

The shape of the dose-response curve depends on the type of toxic effect measured, the concentration at the target site, and the underlying mechanism. For example, when HCN reacts with cytochrome aa3, it binds irreversibly and limits the function of the electron transport chain in the **mitochondria** a function

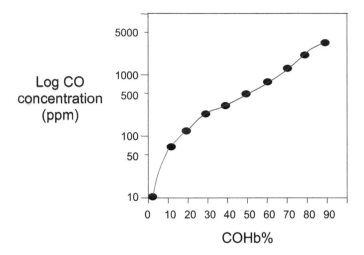

Figure 2.2 Dose-response curve for carbon monoxide concentration (CO, ppm) versus carboxyhemoglobin levels in blood (%). As the concentration of CO in air (log ppm, dose) rises, the percent of CO bound to hemoglobin (COHb%, response) increases proportionately as a typical dose-response sigmoidal-shaped curve. Toxic effects also depend on time of exposure and rate of inhalation. Important to note that exposure to 1,500–2,000 ppm CO for 1 hour is immediately dangerous to life or health (IDLH, NIOSH). (National Institute for Occupational Safety and Health (NIOSH), Centers for Disease Control and Prevention (U.S.), https://www.cdc.gov/niosh/idlh/; and, Agency for Toxic Substances and Disease Registry (U.S.), 2012.)

vital to the viability of the cell. Thus, the dose-response curve for lethality is very steep and the toxic range of doses for cyanide is narrow. Alternatively, the toxicity of carbon monoxide (CO) depends on its concentration in the ambient, inspired air. Figure 2.2 illustrates the concentration (dose) of CO in air (log ppm) versus the percent of CO bound to hemoglobin (COHb%, response). As the concentration increases, the amount bound to Hb increases proportionately as a typical dose response.

The dose-response relationship provides for determination of several parameters. When lethality is the endpoint, the LD_{50} is calculated—defined as the dosage of a substance which is lethal for 50% of animals in the exposed group.[4] The LD_{50} value varies for the same compound between different groups of the same species of animal. The value itself is only of use in a comparative sense, allowing to establish a basis for toxicity of a compound relative to its dosage ranges (Figure 2.3) as well as to other substances (Table 2.1, Figure 2.4). It also enables comparison of toxicity using various routes of administration (Table 2.2) or in different species (Table 2.3), as well as for classification purposes, such as hazard warnings. Consequently, significant protocols have been validated and have replaced the routine use of the LD_{50} with the development of alternative models to animal testing.

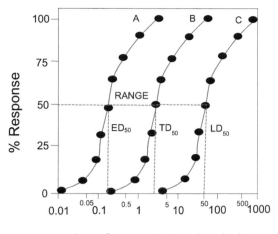

Figure 2.3 Comparison of dose-response curves for (a) efficacy, (b) toxicity, (c) lethality. The relationship between the effective (**ED$_{50}$**), toxic (**TD$_{50}$**), and lethal doses (**LD$_{50}$**) for 50% of the test subjects within the groups is computed by extrapolation of the lines drawn from the 50% level, at about 0.2, 3.0, and 50 mg/kg, respectively. The range between the ED$_{50}$ and TD$_{50}$, between 0.2 and 3.0 mg/kg, specifies the margin of safety of the compound.

The ED$_{50}$ (effective dose 50%) and the TD$_{50}$ (toxic dose 50%) are similarly calculated as with the LD$_{50}$. They are derived from the dose-response curves where the pharmacological or toxic effect is plotted against dosage, respectively.

Table 2.1 Approximate LD$_{50}$ Values for Several Diverse Substances in Order of Toxicity (Most to Least Toxic) and According to Species

Substance	Species	LD$_{50}$ mg/kg
Fentanyl	Monkey	.030
2,3,7,8-Tetrachlorodibenzo-p-dioxin	Rat	.02
(TCDD, in agent orange)	Rat	1.0
Mercury (II) chloride	Human	1–2
Strychnine		
Arsenic trioxide	Rat	14
Caffeine	Rat	192
Methanol	Human	810
Delta-9-tetrahydrocannabinol (δ-9-THC)	Rat	1,270
Ethanol	Rat	7,060
Vitamin C (ascorbic acid)	Rat	11,900

Source: From https://en.wikipedia.org/wiki/Median_lethal_dose#References; last accessed April 2022.Route of administration is oral for all chemicals.

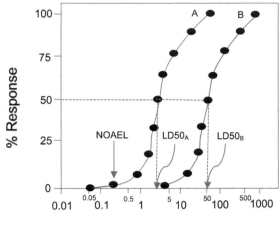

Log Concentration (mg/kg)

Figure 2.4 Comparison of dose-response curves for two compounds A and B. For compound A, there is a threshold level dose below which there is no-observed adverse-effect level (NOAEL, about 0.2 mg/kg). The LD50 for each compound is determined by extrapolation as shown. This shows compound B is less toxic than A (as LD50$_A$ is smaller than LD50$_B$) but is toxic at a lower dose (no threshold).

Table 2.2 Effect of Route of Administration on LD$_{50}$ Calculation (mg/kg) of Various Compounds in Rodent (Rat)

Route	Ricin	Aspirin	Pentobarbital	Morphine	Ethanol
Oral	29	200–1,600	280	900	12,500
Subcutaneous	-	600–1,800 (m)	130	109	-
Intraperitoneal	.029	-	130	100	-
Intravenous	.00750	-	80	50	-
Inhalation	-	-	-	-	20,000 (ppm)

Source: From He et al. (2010); and, Agency for Toxic Substances and Disease Registry, Toxic Substances Portal | ATSDR (cdc.gov).
Note: m = mouse.

The graph is plotted as a graded response, such as the inhibition of a biochemical marker. Thus, the effect is expressed as a proportion of the measured response.

Table 2.3 Species Differences in Toxicity to Metals (Oral LD_{50})

Metal salts	Oral LD_{50} (mg/kg)	
	Rat	Mouse
Dibutyltin Cl_2	150	35
$CuCl_2$	140–584	190
$ZnCl_2$	350–1,100	350
$PdCl_2$	200–2,704	>1,000
$SnCl_2$	700	1,200

Source: From Egorova and Ananikov (2017).

Similarly, as with the ED_{50} and TD_{50}, the IC_{50} is the concentration of a chemical agent necessary to inhibit 50% of the measurable parameter, which is any indicator of cellular or biochemical function. The IC_{50} is then calculated based on the slope and linearity of the straight line, which is plotted according to percent loss of the indicator versus concentration.

An important parameter in relation to drugs is the **therapeutic index**, determined from the ratio of the LD_{50} (or TD_{50}) to the ED_{50}:

$$\frac{LD_{50}}{ED_{50}} \text{ or } \frac{TD_{50}}{ED_{50}}$$

In general, the greater the ratio, the wider the margin of safety between the toxic dose and the pharmacologically effective dose. However, the therapeutic index does not suggest the nature of the shape of the dose-response curve and therefore potential for overlap between toxicity and therapeutic effect is possible. However, comparison of the dose-response curves will yield this information (Figure 2.3) which for different compounds illustrates comparative hazard potential (Figure 2.4).

2.2 Receptors

Receptors play an important part in both pharmacological and toxicological responses. Several well-understood receptor-compound interactions include the binding of the aryl hydrocarbon receptor (AhR) to aromatic compounds (dioxin, 2,3,7,8-tetrachlorodibenzo-ρ-dioxin [TCDD]), and the opioid receptors located throughout the body to their target molecules (opioids). While initial actions of agents involve their corresponding receptors, many toxic responses do not necessarily involve direct interactions with the same specific receptors, where toxic effects result from disturbances in enzyme function and metabolic pathways related to the pharmacological response. Thus, the target site is related to the receptor where the dose-response relationship relies on the pharmacological effects. That is, the receptor must be occupied and bound by the chemical agent in order for a response to occur. There is also a critical concentration at which all the receptors are occupied, thus producing the maximum response.

For example, hydrogen cyanide (HCN) and CO interact with, and disturb the function of, important proteins, such as cellular cytochrome aa_3 and red blood cell hemoglobin, respectively. The toxic effects of these compounds are a direct result of interaction with their target sites and the magnitude of the effects depends on the number of molecules of toxicant bound to the protein. Thus, the more sites on the protein occupied by the chemical, the greater is the toxic effect. There is a concentration of HCN and CO at which all the sites are occupied,[5] yielding the classical dose-response curve (Figures 2.1 and 2.2).

2.3 Synergy and Potentiation

In many cases, exposure to chemicals occurs not to a single substance but to mixtures of substances, particularly applicable with polypharmacy therapeutics, where patients are treated simultaneously with several drugs.[6] Similarly, exposure to environmental pollutants and industrial chemicals produces exposure to many chemicals simultaneously.

The effects of such mixtures are different from those of each constituent separately and consequently are less predictable. The simplest situation is when compounds from the same class have similar effects and the overall toxicity of the mixture is the sum of the individual toxic effects, thus described as **additive**. However, two or more substances also combine to produce a response greater than the sum of the individual responses (**synergistic** effect). For example, carbon tetrachloride and alcohols together are more toxic to the liver than expected from the sum of the two individual effects. **Potentiation** provides a similar outcome, except only one of the compounds produces pathology. For example, the therapeutic drug disulphiram,[7] used in the treatment of alcohol addiction, is nontoxic at therapeutic doses. However, it potentiates the toxicity of alcohol when administered together. The drug, which is targeted to deter further drinking, inhibits the enzyme aldehyde dehydrogenase (ADH) and allows for an accumulation of acetaldehyde, a metabolic product of ethanol, resulting in unpleasant physiological effects.

The opposite result is also observed as a decreased response from a mixture compared with the individual constituents, referred to as **antagonism**. Several therapeutic modalities rely on this receptor antagonism by blocking the action of the toxicological agent, such as the intervention of opioid overdose with naloxone. Finally, tolerance to a substance is precipitated after repeated exposure; the response decreases despite continuous dosage administration. The mechanism is theorized to be a result of enzyme induction, increased metabolism, or competition for receptors.

2.4 Threshold Dose and NOAEL

In the calculation of lethal or toxic doses, many compounds present with doses below which no adverse effect or response is measurable (threshold dose or no-observed-adverse-effect level [NOAEL]). This is adequately demonstrated for **quantal responses** such as lethality, the presence or absence of a pathological lesion, or a teratogenic effect. Thus, the threshold dose is the level at which the anticipated response does NOT occur in the population (Figure 2.4). Alternatively, the concept is also applied to variable responses such as marker inhibition, which is measured with increasing concentrations of the compound.

The concept of a threshold dose for toxic effects is an important one in toxicology because it implies that there is a level of safety for the chemical. While this is generally accepted for most types of responses, it is not necessarily valid for chemical carcinogenesis mediated via a **genotoxic** mechanism. In the case of carcinogens, the dose-response curve, when extrapolated in reference to NOAEL, crosses the x-axis at the origin rather than at some positive value or dosage level (Compound B, Figure 2.4), suggesting that there is a response at all exposure levels tested above the NOAEL. Within limits of the analytical techniques available, there is no safe exposure level which can be set with confidence.

No-observed-adverse-effect level is also important for setting exposure limits, as with the **acceptable daily intake (ADI)**. This factor is used to determine the safe intake of food additives, vitamins, minerals, and permissible amounts of contaminants such as pesticides and residues of veterinary drugs, to establish the presence of safe levels of by-products.

In the industrial and manufacturing fields, exposure is similarly regulated and set as the **threshold limit value (TLV**, U.S.) or **maximum exposure limit (MEL**, U.K.). While these values are based on human exposure for an eight-hour working day, NOAEL calculation is derived from animal toxicity studies using the most sensitive species and the best selective tests.

2.5 Summary and Learning Objectives

One of the most important concepts that underlie toxicology is the dose-response relationship. First formulated by Paracelsus (in his famous phrase 'All substances are poisons, there is none that is not; the right dose distinguishes a poison from a remedy') establishes the relationship between the dose of a toxicant and the effect it produces or the toxic response. The relationship is based on three premises: the response is proportional to the concentration of the chemical at the target site; the concentration is proportional to the dose; and, the response is causally related to the toxicant. The target site may be a receptor with a specific function (e.g. Ah receptor) or an enzyme (e.g. cytochrome aa_3) or a protein (e.g. hemoglobin); however, receptors are not always involved in toxic reactions.

Several important parameters are calculated from the dose-response curve – the NOAEL, which is determined from the bottom of the curve; the maximal effect; and, the dose resulting in a 50% effect or which affects 50% of the animals exposed to the agent. The consequence is due to a biochemical or pharmacological effect (ED_{50}), a toxic (TD_{50}), or a lethal effect (LD_{50}). The therapeutic index (TD_{50}/ED_{50}) and the margin of safety (TD_{50}/ED_{50}) are determined from these ratios. The NOAEL can also be used to compute the ADI or tolerable daily intake (TDI) that is involved in the risk assessment of food additives or food contaminants, respectively.

The **plasma level** reflects the concentration of the chemical at the target site; it is governed by distribution, which is restricted by binding to plasma proteins, is usually non-covalent (ionic, **hydrophobic**, hydrogen, Van der Waals' forces), saturated or subject to displacement by other compounds. The plasma level is used to derive kinetic parameters such as **half-life, area under the curve (AUC)** and **volume of distribution (V_D)**. Chemicals are sequestered and accumulate in tissue compartments (e.g. adipose tissue) depending on physicochemical characteristics, such as **lipid solubility**.

Chemicals accumulate after repeated exposure if the frequency of dosing is greater than the half-life or elimination.

Review Questions

Select one choice which best answers the question.

1. A dose of a chemical A is toxic to animals *in vivo*. Chemical B is not toxic even when given at doses several orders of magnitude higher than the dose of A. When A and B are administered together at the same dose, the toxic response is greater than that of the dose of A alone.
   This an example of: (a) antagonism; (b) synergism; (c) additive; (d) potentiation; (e) none of the above.
2. Which information is gained from an acute toxicity study? (a) No Effect Level; (b) LD_{50} (c) the therapeutic index; (d) the target organ; (e) all of the above.
3. The therapeutic index is defined as: (a) TD_{50}/LD_{50}; (b) ED_{50}/LD_{50}; (c) LD_{50}/ED_{50} (d) ED_{50}/TD_{50}; (e) LD_1/ED_{99}
4. Oil/water partition coefficient of a chemical is an indication of: (a) carcinogenicity; (b) long half-life; (c) potential for bioaccumulation; (d) low apparent volume of distribution (e) chronic toxicity.
5. Absorption of which of the following is facilitated by the pH in the stomach?: (a) weak organic bases; (b) strong acids; (c) weak organic acids; (d) strong bases; (e) none of the above.
6. The apparent 'volume of distribution' (V_D) for a chemical *in vivo* is: (a) equal to the water solubility of the chemical; (b) sometimes larger than the total body volume; (c) equal to the volume of total body water; (d) smaller than the total body water if highly bound in tissues; (e) none of the above.
7. The half-life of a drug in the blood is determined by: (a) metabolism of the compound; (b) volume of distribution; (c) plasma protein binding; (d) urinary pH; (e) total body clearance.
8. The term **'first-pass phenomenon'** refers to which of the following?: (a) the drug is eliminated unchanged; (b) the drug is mostly metabolized by

the liver before reaching the systemic circulation; (c) the drug is completely absorbed from the GI tract; (d) the drug is completely eliminated by the kidneys; (e) none of the above.

9. Select (a) if 1, 2 and 3 are correct, select (b) if 1 and 3 are correct, select (c) if 2 and 4 are correct, select (d) if only 4 is correct, select (e) if all four are correct. Which features of a chemical favor accumulation in biological systems? (a) binding to plasma proteins; (b) lipophilicity; (c) low volume of distribution; (d) resistance to metabolism.

10. Answer A. if the statement is true or B. if the statement is false. The binding of drugs to proteins in systemic circulation involves the formation of covalent bonds.

Short Answer Questions

11. Describe the following topics as applied to toxicological principles: (a) volume of distribution; (b) binding of drugs to plasma proteins; (c) first-pass phenomenon; (d) Fick's law of diffusion.

12. Describe the following as they apply to toxicological principles: (a) pH partition theory; (b) plasma half-life; (c) plasma clearance; (d) enterohepatic recirculation.

Notes

1. Dose-response and concentration-effect are often used interchangeably, where the latter is a more precise measurement at the target site.

2. Target site refers to a specific or non-specific receptor located at the organ affected (see Receptors below).

3. PPAR family of nuclear receptors plays a major regulatory role in energy homeostasis and metabolic function.

4. Arguably an antiquated and inaccurate measurement for predicting human or mammalian toxicity, it is controversial as to its usefulness and necessity in toxicology. Recently, its regulatory requirement for toxicity testing in animals has changed (U.S. FDA).

5. Saturation point.

6. Polypharmacy.

7. Used in the treatment for alcohol addiction and abuse.

Bibliography

Agathokleous, E., Kitao, M. and Calabrese, E.J., Environmental hormesis and its fundamental biological basis: Rewriting the history of toxicology. *Environmental Research*, 165, 274–278, 2018. Doi: 10.1016/j.envres.2018.04.034.

Barile, F.A. Chapter 7. Dose-response, in: *Barile's Clinical Toxicology: Principles and Mechanisms*, (pp. 91–98), 3rd edition, CRC Press, Boca Raton, FL, 2019.

Clark, B. and Smith, D.A. *An Introduction to Pharmacokinetics*, 2nd edition; Wiley-Blackwell, London, 1991.

Egorova, K.S. and Ananikov, V.P. Toxicity of metal compounds: Knowledge and myths, *Organometallics*, 36(21), 4071–4090, 2017. Doi: 10.1021/acs.organomet.7b00605.

He, X., McMahon, S., Henderson, T.D. II, Griffey, S.M. and Cheng, L.W. Ricin toxicokinetics and its sensitive detection in mouse sera or feces using immuno-PCR. *PLoS One*, 5(9), e12858, 2010. Doi: 10.1371/journal.pone.0012858

Krishnan, K., Chapter 7, Toxicokinetics, in: *Casarett and Doull's Toxicology. The Basic Science of Poisons*, (pp. 401–430), Klaassen, C.D. (Ed.), 9th edition, McGraw Hill, New York, 2019.

Pratt, W.B. and Taylor, P. (Eds.), *Principles of Drug Action: The Basis of Pharmacology*, 3rd edition; Churchill Livingstone, New York, 1990.

Timbrell, J.A. *Principles of Biochemical Toxicology*, 4th edition, Informa Healthcare, New York, 2009.

Wilbur, S., Williams, M., Williams, R., Scinicariello, F., Klotzbach, J.M. Diamond, G.L. and Citra, M. Toxicological profile for carbon monoxide. *Agency for Toxic Substances and Disease Registry (ATSDR, Atlanta, GA, U.S.)*, 2012. https://wwwn.cdc.gov/TSP/ToxProfiles/ToxProfiles.aspx?id=1145&tid=253. Last accessed November 2022).

Zbinden, G., Biopharmaceutical studies, a key to better toxicology. *Xenobiotica*, 18(1), 9, 1988.

Chapter 3

Exposure-Response Relationship

Chapter Outline

This chapter considers exposure of biological systems to chemicals and drugs and their pathological consequences.

3.1	Types of Exposure	27
	3.1.1 Acute Exposure	28
	3.1.2 Chronic Exposure	28
	3.1.3 Continuous/Intermittent Exposure	28
3.2	Route of Exposure	28
3.3	Types of Toxic Response	29
	3.3.1 Biochemical Lesions	30
	3.3.2 Pharmacological and Physiological Effects	30
	3.3.3 Immunotoxicity	30
	3.3.4 Teratogenicity	33
	3.3.5 Genetic Toxicity	34
	3.3.6 Carcinogenicity	35
3.4	Biomarkers	36
3.5	Summary and Learning Objectives	37
	Review Questions	39
	Short Answer Questions	39
	Notes	39
	Bibliography	40

3.1 Types of Exposure

There are several basic exposure conditions for toxic compounds, of which three are considered here: **acute**, **chronic**, and continuous/intermittent exposure. Overall, acute and chronic exposures are relative terms intended for comparative purposes.

DOI: 10.1201/9781003188575-3

3.1.1 Acute Exposure

Acute exposure applies to a single episode or a short time period where a particular amount of a substance enters the organism (e.g. overdose of a drug).

In general, an exposure of less than 24 hours is also regarded as acute. Exposure to most toxic gases requires less than 24 hours for toxicity (carbon monoxide and hydrogen cyanide). In addition, a single intravenous (IV) injection of a chemical is certainly classified as an acute exposure.

3.1.2 Chronic Exposure

Chronic exposure is a relative period for which continuous, or repeated, exposure is required beyond the acute phase for the same chemical to induce a toxic response. Chronic exposure applies to repeated exposure to a substance which then accumulates or causes a cumulative toxic effect. Thus, the terms are flexible adaptations to define the onset of chemical intoxication. In addition, there is some considerable overlap in judgment when assigning labels to exposure periods.

3.1.3 Continuous/Intermittent Exposure

Frequency of administration considers a single or repeated administration of a dose of the drug or toxin during the exposure period. Although not exclusive, single-dose exposures are essentially associated with acute duration and are the most frequent and convenient methods of experimental drug administration. Most complications, however, are usually associated with *continuous* or *intermittent*-repeated contact with a chemical or dose of a drug beyond the accepted acute frequency, within the time defined as chronic. Examples of *continuous*-repeated exposure parallel therapeutic protocols such as with IV infusions, delayed release oral or parenteral dosage forms, administration of volatile drugs using an uninterrupted inhalation apparatus, or transdermal cutaneous delivery systems, as well as industrial or occupational contact with ambient toxins, such as with the toxic substances released during the 9/11 events in New York City (September 11, 2001). Thus, chronic toxicity can apply to an event which occurs over many weeks, months, or years after exposure to intermittent, repeated doses or after an acute exposure to a particular toxic substance.

3.2 Route of Exposure

Briefly, there are several routes of exposure to which a chemical accesses the physiological compartments of the body (routes of exposure are discussed in greater detail and incorporated into the topics in Chapter 4).

Exposure via the gastrointestinal tract is the most common route for most drugs, food additives and contaminants, natural products, and other potentially toxic substances. Inhalation is particularly important in an industrial environment while pesticides are also inhaled in commercial, occupational, and household settings, especially during spraying. Absorption via the skin is also important in an industrial and agricultural setting, as chemical solutions contact the dermal layers.

The site and route of absorption are also important:

1. Route influences the eventual **systemic toxicity** (see Chapter 4).
2. Site of absorption affects **local toxicity**.

For example, irritant substances cause inflammation at the site of absorption; toxicity depends on the conditions at this site. As particles such as asbestos are inhaled, they damage cells of the lung by contact, but will not particularly damage the skin. Skin is more resistant to asbestos because of the outer (epidermal and dermal) layers of keratinized cells and its poor absorptive properties.

Drugs also gain access to the body by other routes. In particular, IV, subcutaneous (SC), and intramuscular (IM) injections are employed in clinical medicine, while **intraperitoneal (IP)** administration is commonly used in experimental animals. IV and IP injections allow for *rapid distribution* to most parts of the body, whereas SC and IM permit *slow absorption*.

3.3 Types of Toxic Response

Biological systems respond in many ways to toxic compounds. Many toxic responses have a biochemical basis, yet the expression of those responses is very different. For example, the biochemical interaction between a toxic compound and a nucleic acid leads to tumors, but in a developing embryo, a birth defect could be the result. Alternatively, an interaction with a receptor causes major physiological effects such as loss of blood pressure or inhibition of an enzyme, resulting in sufficient biochemical perturbation to lead to tissue damage and **necrosis**. Toxic responses are divided into seven categories based on the result:

1. direct toxic action: tissue lesions;
2. biochemical lesions;
3. pharmacological or physiological effects;
4. immunotoxicity;
5. teratogenicity;
6. genetic toxicity;
7. carcinogenicity.

There is significant overlap among these toxic responses, and some chemicals cause more than one type of effect.

For example, in many cases, biochemical effects underlie the toxicity and lead to tissue damage or other pathological lesions (see the "Acetaminophen" section, Chapter 8 and the "Animal toxins" section, Chapter 13). However, some biochemical effects of drugs or chemicals do not lead to detectable pathological lesions but to morbidity or mortality of the organism through biochemical or physiological dysfunction (see the "Acetylsalicylate" section, Chapter 8).

3.3.1 Biochemical Lesions

Biochemical lesions are often associated with the development of pathological changes, such as cell degeneration, but also cause the death of the whole organism by interfering with vital functions, such as respiration. For example, cyanide toxicity results in cell death by interfering with the electron transport chain in the mitochondria such that oxygen cannot be incorporated. The net effect is death of cells in vital organs such as the heart and brain. Some biochemical effects are reversible, such as the binding of carbon monoxide to hemoglobin that is not at a sufficiently high level to cause death of the organism. Carbon monoxide exposure does not normally result in significant pathology, except at high levels from which the damage be irreversible (see the "Carbon monoxide" section, Chapter 14).

A common toxic response in the liver resulting from a disturbance of normal intermediary metabolism of lipids is fatty liver. A more specific type of derangement is phospholipidosis where **phospholipids** accumulate in several tissues, particularly the lungs and adrenal glands. The appetite suppressant chlorphentermine and cardiovascular drug amiodarone are known to cause phospholipidosis. Biochemical lesions are also responsible for death by organ failure. For example, aspirin overdose leads to biochemical and physiological derangements, such as ATP depletion, **acidosis**, and hyperthermia, resulting in organ failure (see below). Fluoroacetate, a natural product used as a rodenticide, blocks the Krebs' cycle. This rapidly progresses to the death of the animals that have ingested it, usually due to heart failure.

3.3.2 Pharmacological and Physiological Effects

Physiological responses to pharmacological agents are characterized by the overriding effects of drugs on normal body functions. For example, some compounds cause changes in blood pressure by affecting β-**adrenoceptors** or by interfering with vascular dilation or constriction. Although normally used therapeutically to ameliorate cardiovascular diseases, this class of drugs causes toxicity if ingested in excess amounts. Alternatively, a decrease in blood pressure is sufficient to initiate a successive development such as ischemic tissue damage due to insufficient blood flow.

3.3.3 Immunotoxicity

Toxic reactions involving the immune system are manifested in several ways: as hypersensitivity or allergic reactions; autoimmunity where a physiological component is attacked by the immune system, categorized as indirect immunotoxicity; and, immunosuppression and immunostimulation, labeled as direct immunotoxicity. Hypersensitivity occurs when the immune system is stimulated after individuals are exposed to chemicals which bind to or alter a

Table 3.1 Classification of Immunological Hypersensitivity Reactions

Immunological type	Antigen (AN)	Antibody (AB)	Immunological reaction	Example
Type I Hypersensitivity reaction	Unrecognized, free AN	IgE fixed to mast cell	Degranulation, release of mediators	Allergic reactions, asthma, some drugs
Type II Antibody-mediated cytotoxic reaction	AN associated with altered cell membrane determinants	IgG, IgM, and IgA	Complement-mediated cytotoxic reaction	Drug induced
Type III Immune complex reaction	Microorganisms AN-AB immune complex	IgG	Complement-mediated AB	Serum sickness, infection-associated
Type IV Delayed-type hypersensitivity – cell-mediated immunity	AN-specific T-cell activation	T_H1 memory cells	Cytokine release, granulocytes	Contact hypersensitivity (jewelry, metals, and plants)

macromolecule, commonly a protein. The protein must be large enough and have sufficient molecules attached where it is recognized as external by immune surveillance, consequently producing an **antigen**. Most commonly the chemical acts as a **hapten** – that is, the molecule reacts with and becomes attached to an **endogenous** protein, which renders the entire molecule as extraneous. Allergic reactions develop at the site of exposure, such as within the lungs or on contact with skin or cause a systemic reaction. For example, the industrial chemical toluene diisocyanate causes allergic-type reactions because of exposure of the lungs.

Immune reactions appear in several forms, including stimulation of a physiological response, such as **bronchoconstriction**, or cellular destruction by complement components of the immune system. The hepatotoxicity of halothane, an anesthetic, and the adverse effects of hydralazine, an arterial vasodilator, are examples of drugs that illicit autoimmune reactions. Responses generated from halothane and hydralazine represent idiosyncratic immune-mediated reactions.[1] The antibiotic penicillin is most associated with allergic reactions, producing several different forms ranging from innocuous skin rashes to severe and fatal anaphylactic shock.

Table 3.1 outlines the four types of hypersensitivity reactions. Type I antibody-mediated (hypersensitivity) reactions occur as three phases. The initial *sensitization phase* is triggered by contact with a previously unrecognized antigen.

This reaction entails binding of the antigen to immunoglobulin E (IgE) present on the surface of mast cells and basophils. The second *activation phase* follows an additional dermal or mucosal challenge with the same antigen. The third *effector phase* stimulates degranulation of neutrophils and eosinophils. Antigens involved in type I reactions are generally airborne pollens, including mold spores and ragweed, as well as food ingredients. Ambient factors, such as heat and cold, drugs (opioids and antibiotics), and metals (silver and gold), precipitate chemical allergies of the type I nature.

Type II antibody-mediated cytotoxic reactions differ from type I in the nature of antigen, the cytotoxic character of the antigen-antibody reaction, and the type of antibody formed (IgM or IgG). In general, antibodies are formed against target antigens that are *altered cell membrane determinants*. Examples of type II reactions include transfusion reactions, Rh incompatibility, autoimmune, and drug-induced reactions, the last of which is of greater interest in clinical toxicology.

As with type I reactions, drug-induced type II cytotoxicity requires that the agent behaves as a hapten. The chemical binds to the target cell membrane and proceeds to operate as an altered cell membrane determinant that changes the conformational appearance of a component of the cell membrane. Examples of drugs that traditionally induce type II reactions include penicillin and toluene diisocyanate.[2]

Type III immune complex reactions are localized responses mediated by antigen-antibody immune complexes. Type III reactions are stimulated by microorganisms and involve activation of complement.

Type IV (delayed-type) hypersensitivity cell-mediated immunity involves antigen-specific T-cell activation. The reaction starts with an intradermal or mucosal challenge (*sensitization stage*) which requires prolonged local contact with the agent, usually for at least 2 weeks. A subsequent repeat challenge stage induces differentiated T_H1 (memory) cells to release cytokines. Contact hypersensitivity resulting from prolonged exposure to plant resins, jewelry, and industrial metals (occupational hazard in metal industries; nickel, cadmium), for example, is caused by the **lipophilicity** of the chemical in oily skin secretions, thus acting as a hapten.

Immunosuppression is the result of a direct effect on the immune system, resulting in an inadequate immunological function. A compound that produces immunosuppression alters the immune components such as the thymus that produces T-lymphocytes (T-cells), or the bone marrow, which is responsible for the production of B-lymphocytes (antibody-producing plasma cells). The industrial and environmental contaminant dioxin [2,3,7,8-tetrachlorodibenzo-ρ-dioxin (TCDD)] is an immunosuppressant capable of impairing the function of the thymus and interfering with production of lymphocytes.

Immunostimulation is associated with the immune system's response to an administered protein, which although it is recognized of human origin, is identified as antigenic. Novel peptide drugs, such as those derived from recombinant deoxyribonucleic acid/ribonucleic acid (DNA/RNA), and vaccines, are produced through immune stimulation.

3.3.4 Teratogenicity

Teratogenicity is characterized by an altered developmental response whereby the embryo or fetus is affected, leading to a functional and/or structural abnormality. Normal neonatal and adult development of the human or animal is of consequence. Although some cytotoxic compounds are teratogenic, in many cases the malformations are the result of a perturbation in the development of the organism rather than direct damage to the embryo or fetus, as the latter usually results in death and spontaneous miscarriage.

Teratogens are often relatively non-toxic to the mother but interfere with the development or growth of any of the stages of the embryo. Timing of the exposure or dosing with a **teratogen,** relative to the stages of pregnancy, is crucial (Figure 3.1).

The embryo and fetus are especially sensitive to chemical exposure, mainly because the sequence of events in embryogenesis and fetal development is easily disturbed. There are several characteristics of teratogenesis:

- Teratogens are generally selective for the developing organism rather than the maternal physiology.

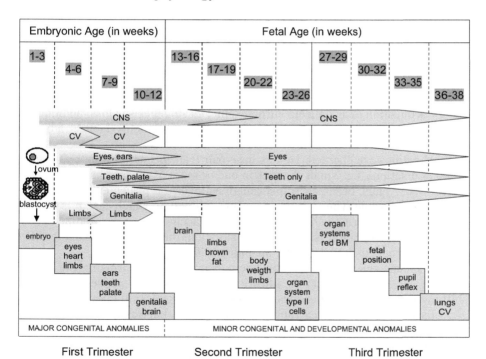

Figure 3.1 Timeline of fetal development and teratogenic susceptibility. CNS, central nervous system; CV, cardiovascular; BM, bone marrow. (From: Chintalapati and Barile, 2019.)

- Susceptibility of the embryo or fetus varies depending on the embryonic stage in relation to exposure, i.e., first, second, or third trimesters.
- Abnormalities detected are as specific to the stages of exposure as to the chemical.

In general, outcomes of exposure of a developing organism take the form of malformations, growth retardation, functional disorders, and spontaneous miscarriage or death.

Mechanisms underlying teratogenesis are well documented such that interference in cellular function explains the pathologic consequences. Teratogenic effects develop and are observable during maturation of the offspring whereas mutagenic disturbances are more likely to occur during the gestational periods. For example, diethylstilbestrol (DES), a therapeutic drug once prescribed as a sedative during pregnancy, was eventually understood to be associated with development of vaginal cancer in the female offspring of the mothers exposed to the drug. This outcome was delayed and observable in the girls at puberty, at least 12 years after their birth and original exposure.

3.3.5 Genetic Toxicity

Mutations that result from interactions between chemicals and genetic material involve alterations in coding or non-coding regions of the chromosomes, and potentially transfer heritable changes in genotype to the subsequent generations.

These interactions of chemicals with genetic material are divided into three types: aneuploidization, clastogenesis, and mutagenesis. Aneuploidy refers to loss or acquisition of a complete chromosome; clastogenesis is loss, addition, or rearrangement of parts of chromosomes; mutagenesis denotes the loss, addition or alteration of a small number of base pairs.

Mutations are characterized as base-pair transformations, base-pair additions, or deletions, i.e., small changes in one or more of the four bases that constitute DNA. Thus, base-pair transformations involve replacement of a base by another of the same type (i.e., purine or pyrimidine), in which case it is a base-pair transition. Alternatively, a purine base replacement by a pyrimidine is designated base-pair transversion. In either situation, the transcriptional alteration results in erroneous translation for an amino acid.

The consequence of base-pair deletions or additions, involving the loss or addition of base pairs, effect a modification of the entire base-pair sequence and a shift in the reading of the genetic code, resulting in frameshift mutations.

Large deletions and rearrangements follow breakage and erroneous reconstitution of DNA molecules. Similarly, large segments of the chromosome become inverted (clastogenesis). These types of changes inevitably lead to major adverse consequences in the cell because of the number of genes potentially affected.

Naturally occurring vinca alkaloids, used therapeutically as chemotherapeutic drugs, interfere with the process of mitosis or meiosis and disturb the separation of chromosomes during mitosis (aneuploidization) leading to non-disjunction or unequal partition. The drugs interfere with spindle formation during cell division, compromising cell viability, with potential tissue damage and cell death.

There are numerous ways in which compounds cause mutations. Chemically reactive compounds, such as the chemotherapeutic alkylating agents, interact directly with DNA in the cell nucleus; bromouracil, which is incorporated into DNA during cell replication, triggers errors in newly synthesized DNA. In mammals, mutations in germ cells are a prime generator of birth defects; in somatic cells, mutations are also understood to underlie development of cancer in many instances.

3.3.6 Carcinogenicity

Several human and animal cancers are caused by chemical carcinogens, the evidence of which is found in both clinical human prospective and retrospective studies and with experimental animals.

Chemical carcinogenesis is a specific toxic effect that leads to uncontrolled proliferation of cells of a tissue or organ, differing in malignancy and type of tissue affected. Many chemically-induced cancers are the result of mutations in somatic cells. Thus, carcinogens interfere with genetic control of cellular processes via mutation.

Cancer is a multi-stage process, requiring **initiation** followed by **promotion** and progression. Exposure to a carcinogen, such as chemically reactive alkylating agents, vinyl chloride, and aflatoxins, initiates an event, followed by several exposures to a promoter substance. Experimental evidence indicates that the initiating event produces an irreversible change, such as damage to DNA, and precedes the promotion stage. For example, tumors of mouse skin are induced by application of an initiator such as benzo(a)pyrene, a polycyclic hydrocarbon, followed by a phorbol ester (promoter). Several exposures to an initiator result in tumors in the absence of a promoter. Initiation typically involves interaction between DNA and a reactive chemical, while promotion encompasses alterations in genetic expression and clonal growth[3] from the original initiated cell.

During progression, neoplastic (cancerous) cells change **phenotype** and become malignant tumors involving increased growth and invasion of healthy tissue. However, not all carcinogens are **mutagenic**, such as ethionine and asbestos. Therefore, mechanisms that do not involve mutagenic events (**epigenetic mechanisms**) explain cancers caused by such compounds. Furthermore, not all mutagens are carcinogens, although correlation between mutagenicity and carcinogenicity, for the purpose of mutagenicity tests, is well documented and regarded as predictive of potential carcinogenicity. Mutagenicity tests are used for prediction of germ cell defects and heritable genetic damage.

Peroxisome proliferators are examples of classes of chemical carcinogens that are not mutagenic. This class of carcinogens has been extensively studied, in association with drugs and industrial occupational chemicals. Compounds such as the cholesterol-lowering drug clofibrate and plasticizers, such as phthalate esters, produce liver tumors in rodents after repeated exposures. The mechanism is purported to be associated with peroxisome proliferation, an intracellular **organelle**, as well as an increase in the number of enzymes located in the peroxisome. The net effect is an increase in liver size due to hyperplasia. Interestingly, the carcinogenic effect with clofibrate and other compounds has only been demonstrated in rodents. It appears that the phenomenon of peroxisome proliferation requires a cellular receptor and only those species that possess a functional receptor are responsive to these chemicals. Humans, it appears, do not possess fully functional peroxisome proliferator-activated receptors (PPAR[4]).

The mechanism underlying carcinogenicity of peroxisome proliferators involves a combination of increased oxidative stress, due to amplified production of hydrogen peroxide in the peroxisome and enhanced cell proliferation. **Peroxisomal proliferator** chemicals show a distinct dose threshold for both the peroxisomal effects and tumor induction thus allowing for calculated prediction of human and animal risk assessment.

3.4 Biomarkers

Determination of significant exposure to a chemical substance, the response of the organism to that chemical, and its potential susceptibility to toxic effects are all crucial parameters in toxicology. **Biomarkers** are tools that facilitate measurement of these indicators.

To date, several types of biomarkers are useful in predictive toxicology as well as indicators for toxicological responses. Biomarkers have been developed for measuring exposure, response, and susceptibility of organisms to toxic substances. Exposure is determined by measuring the dose administered, subject to toxicokinetic parameters. However, with some chemicals, more precise estimates of exposure are blood levels, which approximate the concentration in organs, particularly those that are targets for toxicity.[5] However, a metabolite might also be responsible for the harmfulness and therefore measuring the parent chemical may not be an appropriate biomarker. Consequently, measurement of the metabolite in blood or urine, as well as the parent chemical, is of value. Unlike biomarkers of exposure, which are relatively few for chemicals, there are many biomarkers of response, which are amenable to detection. These include increased levels and activity of enzymes, which appear in blood when an organ is damaged, stress proteins (via induction), urinary constituents, and pathological changes detected at observable, apparent, microscopic, and subcellular levels. Thus, biomarker detection is a valid indicator of altered structure or function.

Recently novel biomarkers have been identified that reflect changes in genes (genomics) or expression (epigenetics), changes in proteins expressed from genes (proteomics), and changes in metabolites resulting from the proteins (metabonomics).

Finally, biomarkers of susceptibility are generally determined in individual members of a population. Susceptibility markers reflect genetic deficiencies in enzymes involved in detoxification or xenobiotic metabolism such as CYP 2D6 or N-acetyltransferase. Less common are susceptibility markers of increased

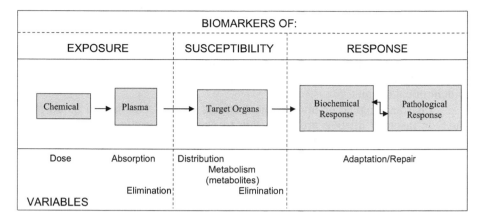

Figure 3.2 Three types of biomarkers and their interactions with variables. Panels represent the three stages from initial exposure of the organism (absorption into plasma), susceptibility of target organs including influence of distribution and metabolism, and biochemical and pathological responses. Biomarkers measure activity at any point (shaded boxes) and reflect activity in the variables below. (Adapted from Waterfield and Timbrell 1999b).

responsiveness of a receptor or resulting from a metabolic disorder, such as glucose 6-phosphate dehydrogenase deficiency, leading to increased vulnerability. Figure 3.2 illustrates the relationship of biomarker pathways and the variables that affect detection.

3.5 Summary and Learning Objectives

Exposure to chemicals is either **acute** or **chronic** as are the corresponding responses. Routes of exposure affect type and location of the response which are local or systemic. Biological systems respond in many ways ranging from simple irritation to complex immunological reactions. The major types of toxic responses observed are direct toxic action, tissue lesions, biochemical lesions, pharmacological or physiological effects, immunotoxicity, teratogenicity, genetic toxicity, and carcinogenicity.

Certain organs are *targets* for toxicity, such as the *liver*, due to its structure, role in metabolism, and function. Hepatocytes are metabolically active cells. Liver pathology as a result of chemical trauma includes **steatosis**,[6] necrosis, and damage to the biliary system. Kidney is also a target due to its high metabolic activity and role in elimination of waste products. Toxic effects in organs and tissues involve primary (e.g. lipid peroxidation), secondary (e.g. damage to specific proteins or DNA), and tertiary (e.g. necrosis) events.

Direct tissue damage and subsequent pathology result from *local corrosion* or *systemic effects* leading to liver necrosis. Direct damage is often due to interaction with macromolecules or as a result of **apoptosis**.

Biochemical lesions occur when chemicals or drugs interfere with specific enzymes or pathways which lead to cell dysfunction. Some effects are reversible such as the interaction of carbon monoxide with hemoglobin. Recovery is generally complete with no apparent effects when reversible. Pathological lesions such as steatosis and phospholipidosis also result from biochemical lesions.

Pharmacological or physiological effects such as changes in blood pressure or vascular dilation are often due to acute or chronic administration of drugs. However, effects such as bronchoconstriction and production of excessive amounts of secretions also occur with chemicals, such as organophosphate pesticides.

Immunotoxicity manifests as allergic reactions, autoimmune reactions, immunosuppression, or hypersensitivity. Allergic reactions require the production of an antigenic protein. Immune stimulation is divided into four immunologically based reactions (Types I–IV), including antibody, complement, and cell-mediated reactions (e.g. as with hydralazine and halothane). Autoimmune reactions result in self-destruction of body constituents (e.g. halothane). Immunosuppression directly affects components of the immune system, such as lymphocytes or B-cell-producing bone marrow (e.g. dioxin).

Teratogenesis comprises interference with the development of the embryo or fetus resulting in structural or functional abnormalities. These are manifested as spontaneous miscarriages, malformations, growth hindrance, or functional disorders (e.g. thalidomide). Teratogens are selective, specific for the embryo/fetus, and often show steep dose-response relationships. Malformations that result depend on the stage of development during exposure.

Genetic toxicity requires interference with the genetic material of the cell resulting in heritable changes in the genotype. Three types of interaction are notable: aneuploidization (loss or acquisition of complete chromosomes); clastogenesis (loss, addition, or rearrangement of parts of chromosomes); and, mutagenesis (loss, addition, or alteration of base pairs). Aneuploidy and clastogenesis result in major cellular effects. Base-pair changes lead to consequences, such as frameshift mutations, which predispose the organism to tumor formation.

Carcinogenesis involves the production of tumors, resulting from uncontrolled proliferation of cells, in part as a response to chemical exposure (e.g. vinyl chloride, arsenic, and aflatoxin). However, carcinogens are not necessarily mutagens, especially when epigenetic mechanisms insert more complex pathways (e.g. peroxisome proliferators). The *multi-step process* of carcinogenesis encompasses initiation, promotion, and progression, usually in order. Initiation is characterized by irreversible changes in DNA, followed by promotion, alteration of gene expression, and growth of clonal cells. During progression, cells undergo phenotypic changes where cells transform into malignant tumors.

Determination of exposure, detection of responses, and resolution of susceptibility to chemicals involves the characterization of *biomarkers*, corresponding to *exposure*, *response*, and *susceptibility* to chemicals. Biomarkers of exposure include metabolites and adducts with proteins signifying internal exposure, whereas biomarkers of response vary from increases in serum enzymes to regulation of gene expression. Lastly, biomarkers for susceptibility are limited to individual indicators such as the presence or absence of enzymes or isozymes.

Review Questions

Select one choice that best answers the question.

1. Which of the following is the *most important* factor in determining the extent of toxicity of a chemical? (a) dose; (b) metabolism; (c) elimination; (d) absorption; (e) all of the above.
2. Which of the following is (are) not considered one of the four general types of toxic effects involving the immune system? (a) anaphylaxis; (b) immunosuppression; (c) skin sensitization; (d) autoimmune reaction; (e) bronchoconstriction.
3. Chemicals that are active during the first week of pregnancy after fertilization of the egg are most likely to cause which effect in the embryo? (a) death; (b) malformations; (c) functional abnormalities; (d) growth retardation; (e) sterility.
4. Which of the following statements mostly accurately describes the function of biomarkers? (a) they are useful as indicators of exposure; (b) used to detect changes in genes; (c) useful to measure stress proteins; (d) functional as indicators of exposure, response, or susceptibility; (e) can detect mutagenesis.

Short Answer Questions

5. List the types of toxic responses that a living system undergoes because of exposure to (a) chemical. Give an example of each type.
6. List the four different types of immune hypersensitivity reactions. Use examples to support your answer.

Notes

1. Idiosyncratic refers to rare responses to drugs, the reaction of which is of unknown origin.
2. Because of their small molecular weight, most drugs and chemicals, as single entities, generally circulate undetected by immune surveillance systems.
3. In cancerous growth, clonal replication refers to unrestricted formation of mutated copies of original cells.
4. In the field of molecular biology, the peroxisome proliferator-activated receptors (PPARs) are a group of nuclear receptor proteins that function as transcription factors regulating the expression of genes.

5. Blood levels for some rapid acting chemicals, such as CN, are reliable for monitoring pathology.
6. Accumulation of lipids in the liver.

Bibliography

Aldridge, W.N., *Mechanisms and Concepts in Toxicology*, Taylor & Francis, London, 1996.

Allison, M. R. and Sarraf, C. E. *Understanding Cancer. From Basic Science to Clinical Practice*, Cambridge University Press, Cambridge, 1997.

Chintalapati, A. J. and Barile, F. A. (Ed.), Chapter 32. Reproductive and Developmental Toxicity, in: *Barile's Clinical Toxicology: Principles and Mechanisms*, 3rd edition, CRC Press, Boca Raton, FL, 2019.

Hodgson, E. and Levi, P.E. (Eds.) *Introduction to Biochemical Toxicology*, 2nd edition, Appleton and Lange, Norwalk, CT, 1994.

Krishnan K., Chapter 7, Toxicokinetics, in: *Casarett and Doull's Toxicology. The Basic Science of Poisons*, Klaassen, C.D. (Ed.) 9th edition; McGraw Hill, New York, 401–430, 2019.

Parham, P., *The Immune System*, 5th Edition, W.W. Norton & Co., New York, London, 2021.

Strimbu, K., and Tavel, J.A, What are Biomarkers? *Current Opinions HIV AIDS*, 5(6), 463–466, 2010. Doi: 10.1097/COH.0b013e32833ed177.

Timbrell, J. A., Biomarkers in toxicology. *Toxicology*, 129, 1–12, 1998.

Timbrell, J. A., *Principles of Biochemical Toxicology*, 4th edition, Taylor & Francis Ltd. London, 2009.

Waterfield, C.J., Biomarkers of response, Chapter 85; In: *General and Applied Toxicology*, Ballantyne, B., Marrs, T. and Syversen, T.L.M. (Eds.), 2nd edition, Macmillan & Co., Basingstoke, 1999a.

Waterfield, C. J. and Timbrell, J. A., Biomarkers – An overview, in: *General and Applied Toxicology*, 2nd edition, Ballantyne, B., Marrs, T.C. and Syversen, T.L.M., (Eds.), Macmillan & Co., Basingstoke, 1999b.

Chapter 4

Disposition of Toxic Compounds

Chapter Outline

This chapter discusses the disposition of chemicals and drugs in biological systems. The fate of toxic substances in biological systems is divided into four interrelated phases: (1) absorption; (2) distribution; (3) metabolism (discussed in Chapter 5); and (4) elimination.

4.1	Absorption of Toxic Compounds	42
4.2	Sites of Absorption	45
	4.2.1 Skin	45
	4.2.2 Lungs	46
	4.2.3 Gastrointestinal Tract	48
4.3	Distribution of Toxic Compounds	51
4.4	Elimination	56
	4.4.1 Urinary Elimination	56
	4.4.2 Biliary Elimination	58
	4.4.3 Pulmonary Elimination	60
	4.4.4 Other Routes of Elimination	60
4.5	Summary and Learning Objectives	60
Review Questions		62
	Short Answer Questions	62
Notes		62
Bibliography		63

DOI: 10.1201/9781003188575-4

4.1 Absorption of Toxic Compounds

Absorption of toxic compounds into biological systems involves transport of toxicants through cell membranes, occurs through sites of absorption – skin, lungs, and gastrointestinal tract (GIT), and is influenced by factors affecting absorption.

Before a substance exerts its effect, it enters biological compartments. The rate and site of absorption are important factors affecting entry into these spaces. There are several sites for first contact between a toxic compound and a biological system, but absorption necessarily involves passage across cell membranes. Consequently, it is important to consider the structure and characteristics of biological membranes in order to understand the passage of substances across them.

Membranes are composed mainly of phospholipids and proteins arranged as a fluid bilayer (Figure 4.1). The proteins and phospholipids vary in structure and composition depending on the cell type in which the membrane is located. However, proteins are structural, such as those that anchor cells to other tissues, or they present with specific functions, as carriers for membrane transport. Phospholipids have polar head groups (Figures 4.1 and 4.2) and the **fatty acid** nonpolar chains (tails) are saturated, **unsaturated**, or a mixture. The degree of saturation influences fluidity of the membrane, i.e. the greater the saturation of the fatty acid chains, the more rigidity and less fluidity rendered to the membrane. Cholesterol esters and carbohydrates also provide unique features to specific membranes within their corresponding tissues.

The structure of biological membranes determines their function and characteristics. One of the most important features is that they are selectively permeable, which allows certain substances to pass through them, depending on the following physicochemical characteristics: (1) lipid solubility, (2) similarity to endogenous molecules, and (3) polarity or charge across the membrane.

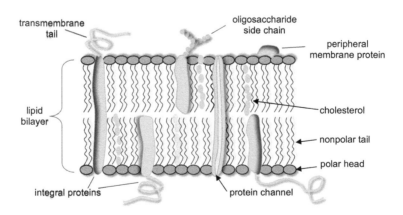

Figure 4.1 Fluid mosaic model of the mammalian lipid bilayer cell membrane.

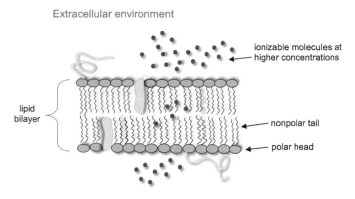

Extracellular environment

ionizable molecules at
higher concentrations

lipid
bilayer

nonpolar tail

polar head

Intracellular cytoplasmic space

Figure 4.2 Illustration of passive diffusion across a semi-permeable lipid bilayer membrane. Extracellular circulatory flow of fluid and ionization potential create a gradient across the membrane influencing passage of molecules. Other structures are labeled in Figure 4.1.

Lipid solubility of a chemical substance is usually represented by its **partition coefficient**: the oil/water partition coefficient refers to the comparative solubility of the chemical in organic versus aqueous solvents, determined by the ability of a chemical to disperse between an organic (lipid-soluble, oil) solvent and aqueous (water-soluble) buffer. The concentration that dissolves between the organic and aqueous phases is measured. The greater the ratio of oil/water solubility, the greater is the lipid solubility of a compound.

Chemical substances navigate through biological membranes by *diffusion*, defined as the transport of molecules across a semi-permeable membrane. *Diffusion* proceeds according to the following pathways: (1) passive diffusion, (2) active transport, (3) facilitated diffusion, (4) Filtration, and (5) **phagocytosis/pinocytosis**.

1. **Passive diffusion:** The most common movement of a chemical substance (solute) occurs down a concentration gradient, i.e. from an area of higher concentration of the solute to an area of lower concentration. The process is not energy-dependent, and no electrical gradient is generated. Lipophilic molecules, small ions, and electrolytes generally gain access through membrane compartments by passive diffusion since they are not repelled by the phospholipid bilayer of the cell membrane. Most passive diffusion processes, however, are not molecularly selective.
2. **Active transport:** Active transport of compounds across membranes has several important features including:
   a. the requirement for a specific membrane carrier;
   b. metabolic energy is necessary to operate the system;
   c. the process is inhibited by metabolic poisons;

     d. saturation occurs at high substrate concentrations yielding **zero order** kinetics;

     e. transport occurs against a concentration gradient;

     f. similar substrates compete for uptake.

       There are various kinds of active transport systems that involve carrier molecules including **uniporters**, **symporters**, and **antiporters**. The uniporter system transports one molecule in a single direction, while symporters and antiporters transfer two molecules in the same or opposite directions, respectively. These membrane transport arrangements are specific for endogenous and nutrient substances but chemical analogs, similar molecules, and ions are also transported by the carriers. For example, the drug fluorouracil, an analog of uracil, and lead ions are absorbed from the GIT by specific active transport systems.

3. **Facilitated diffusion**: This has the following salient features:

     a. requires a specific membrane carrier;

     b. concentration gradient across the membrane is not necessary;

     c. the process is **saturated** by high substrate concentrations.

       Unlike active transport, no energy expenditure is compulsory. As with active transport, facilitated diffusion applies to endogenous substances and essential nutrients but is also responsible for moving xenobiotics that are structurally similar to endogenous compounds. The transport of glucose from the intestinal tract into the systemic blood circulation involves facilitated diffusion.

4. **Filtration:** Small molecules pass through pores in the membrane formed by proteins, usually according to hydrostatic forces,[1] provided by the pumping action of the heart or gravity. In general, the molecular weight (MW) cut-off for solutes transported along with water is about 100–200 MW units.

       The principles of diffusion are embodied in the **pH-partition theory** – only non-ionized lipid-soluble compounds are absorbed by passive diffusion down a concentration gradient. Furthermore, **Fick's Law** states that the rate of diffusion of a substance across a unit area (such as a surface or membrane) is proportional to the concentration gradient. This rate of diffusion is described by the formula:

$$\text{Rate of diffusion} = KA(C_2 - C_1)$$

where K=constant, A=surface area, C_2=concentration outside, and C_1=concentration inside, the membrane.

       The relationship applies to a system at constant temperature and for diffusion over unit distance. The concentration gradient is represented by $(C_2 - C_1)$. Passive diffusion is a **first-order process**; that is, the rate of diffusion is *proportional* to the concentration (the higher the concentration, the greater the rate of diffusion).

       Figure 4.2 illustrates a typical dynamic biological system where the membrane attempts to maintain equilibrium with the xenobiotic compound on either side, consequently, a concentration gradient across the membrane is continuously generated and ions diffuse from higher to lower concentrations. However, the system is not static since circulatory blood flow and ionization principles alter ionic movement (Figure 4.2). In addition, lipid solubility and ionization[2] affect pH of the extracellular fluid. Lipid-soluble compounds traverse biological membranes by dissolution in the phospholipid components of the membrane, with movement down the concentration gradient. Although ionized compounds require more active transport systems, they are capable of similar movement if in some non-ionized form. The degree of ionization is calculated from the **Henderson–Hasselbalch equation**:

$$pH = pK_a + \frac{\text{Log}\left[A^-\right]}{[HA]}$$

where pK_a=the dissociation constant for an acid, [A-]/HA=the ionized/non-ionized components of the molecule, respectively, and pH refers to the acid/base environment of the solvent solution or fluid environment.

5. **Phagocytosis and pinocytosis:** These processes involve invagination of the membrane to enclose an extracellular particle. These mechanisms, for instance, account for the absorption of insoluble and higher MW substances, such as uranium dioxide and asbestos, into the lungs.

4.2 Sites of Absorption

There are three major sites for the absorption of xenobiotics: skin, lungs, and GIT. Although the GIT is an important site for absorption of xenobiotics[3] in toxicology, responsible for passage of chemicals from the GIT to the systemic circulation, the lungs and skin are also significantly involved in absorption of volatile, airborne compounds and liquids, respectively.

4.2.1 Skin

The skin is constantly exposed to volatile, airborne xenobiotics such as gases, solvents, and solutions, rendering absorption through the dermal layers as a potentially critical route. However, although skin has the largest surface area of any organ, its structure presents a barrier to absorption. The organ is composed of an outer layer of epidermal squamous epithelial cells, concentrated with **keratin** and a limited blood supply (Figure 4.3), thus providing a formidable wall for most xenobiotics.

Absorption through the skin is mainly limited to lipid-soluble compounds such as organic solvents. Fatalities have occurred, however, following penetration of toxic compounds, such as with the insecticide parathion.

Anatomy of the Skin

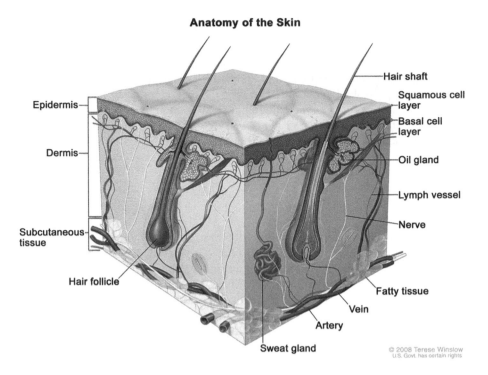

Figure 4.3 Structure of mammalian skin showing epidermis, dermis, and subcutaneous layers. (From PDQ Cancer Information Summaries, U.S. National Center for Biotechnology Information (NCBI), National Institutes of Health (NIH), https://www.ncbi.nlm.nih.gov/books/NBK65824/, ©Terese Winslow, U.S. Govt. public domain 2008; https://www.teresewinslow.com/#/skin/.)

4.2.2 Lungs

The lungs are exposed to a variety of atmospheric substances including gases (carbon monoxide), vapors from volatile solvents (methylene chloride), aerosols, and particulate matter (asbestos). These airborne substances are more concentrated in an industrial or workplace environment. Also, the air in an urban environment contains noxious gases (sulfur dioxide and nitrogen oxides), particulates (fiberglass, pollen), solvent vapors, and aerosols from domestic and commercial products.

Mammalian lungs have a large surface area, approximately 50–100 m2, with an extensive blood supply. The barrier between alveolar air and capillary blood circulation is one cell membrane thick (Figures 4.4a and b). Consequently, absorption from the lungs is rapid and efficient, rivaling the speed of absorption with intravenous (IV) injection. Two factors that affect absorption via the lungs are blood flow and respiratory rate. For compounds with low solubility in the

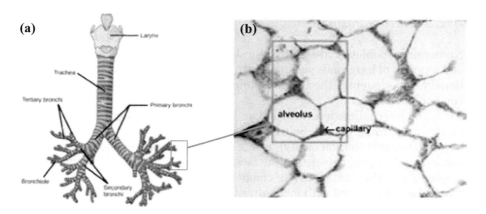

Figure 4.4 (a) Structure of the mammalian respiratory system illustrating the larynx, trachea, bronchi, bronchioles, alveolus, and capillary (in text box). (Licensed under Creative Commons©, CC BY; https://aecbio11.fandom.com/wiki/8.2_The_Mammalian_Respiratory_System.) (b) Enlarged microscopic image of alveolus and capillary showing the vast arrangement of air spaces (clear areas) formed by the thin arrangement of the cellular structure of the alveoli. Molecules of chemical substances that enter the air spaces of the alveoli encounter a large surface area that facilitates absorption and gas exchange. (Licensed under Creative Commons©, CC BY-SA-NC; https://aecbio11.fandom.com/wiki/8.2_The_Mammalian_Respiratory_System.)

plasma compartment of the blood, which is mostly composed of water, absorption is mainly dependent on the rate of blood flow; i.e. as systemic circulation carries more molecules toward the alveolar membrane, the rate of absorption increases. This is in contrast to compounds with high solubility in plasma, where absorption is mainly dependent on respiratory rate, i.e. rapid ventilation eliminates molecules from the lungs, attracting more molecules into the alveolar spaces from the plasma. Interestingly, the rapid rate of blood flow ensures continuous removal of xenobiotics from the absorption site and, therefore, a concentration gradient is replenished.

Molecular, lipid-soluble compounds, such as solvents, are readily absorbed through the alveolus and, for the factors noted above, account for a rapid and efficient route of entry from the lungs to capillaries and the systemic circulation. The size of the particle is a major factor in determining where in the respiratory system it is deposited and whether it is absorbed. Chemicals and particles suspended in solution are processed by pinocytosis and phagocytosis. For example, insoluble uranium dioxide particles are inhaled but eventually result in kidney damage when they reach the systemic circulation. Lead is also absorbed in particulate configuration from the air. Lead particles, 0.25 μm diameter or greater, penetrate alveolar membranes but uranium dioxide particles of more than 3 μm diameter do not permeate.

4.2.3 Gastrointestinal Tract

Numerous xenobiotics are orally ingested through the diet. Oral medications and a variety of hazardous substances are swallowed either accidentally or intentionally. Consequently, the GIT is an important site of absorption for exogenous compounds.

The internal environment of the GIT varies throughout its length, particularly regarding the pH. Substances consumed orally first encounter the lining of the mouth (buccal cavity), where the pH in humans is normally 7.0. The substance then progresses into the stomach where the pH is between 1 and 3, depending on the contents. The compounds remain in the stomach for hours particularly if ingested with food, after which it passes into the small intestine, where the basic environment promotes a pH between 6 and 9. Absorption is facilitated in the small intestine because of its extensive blood supply and large surface area, the latter of which is due to folding of the lining and the presence of villi (Figure 4.5).

Due to changes in pH throughout the length of the GIT, different chemical substances are absorbed depending on their physicochemical characteristics. Lipid-soluble, non-ionized compounds are absorbed along the whole length of the tract, but ionized, charged molecules are generally not absorbed by passive diffusion. In addition, the acid-base nature of the chemical also influences its absorption within the pH of the environment. For instance, the Henderson–Hasselbalch equation calculates the extent of ionization of aniline (a weak base) and benzoic acid (a weak acid) depending on the pH prevailing in the stomach and small intestine. Figure 4.6 illustrates the ionization potentials of weak acids (WA) in the acidic environment of the gastric (stomach) juices. WA substances lean toward greater *non-ionized*, lipid-soluble species in the pH of the stomach where absorption is favorable.

Conversely, weak bases (WB) are *ionized*, water-soluble in the acidic environment of the stomach such that absorption is not favored (Figure 4.6a). In the basic milieu of the small intestine, WB are non-ionized, lipid-soluble molecules which favor their absorption here (Figure 4.6b). However, it is important to note that absorption is favored for almost all molecules in the small intestine due to the influence of extensive blood flow and contact with its large surface area. Although WA exist mainly in the ionized form in the small intestine (Figure 4.6b), the substances pass through the GI membranes and are removed by the flow of the systemic circulation.

These two factors ensure that WA are integrated into the small intestine if they have not been fully absorbed in the stomach.[4]

Another factor that affects absorption from the GIT is the presence of food. Food content in the stomach delays absorption if the compound is preferentially absorbed in the small intestine, as food prolongs gastric emptying time. However, the presence of food material in the stomach facilitates absorption of the chemical substance if it is miscible with fat present in the foodstuff.

When drugs and other xenobiotic compounds are administered, the vehicle used to suspend or dissolve the compounds has a major effect on the eventual toxicity by affecting the rate of absorption and distribution. Thus an organic,

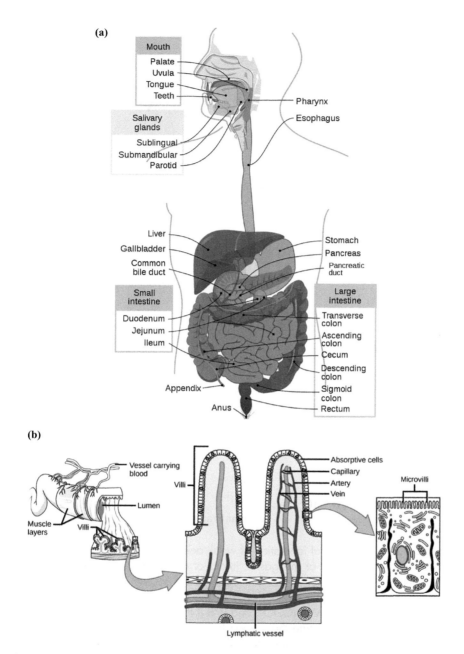

Figure 4.5 (a) Outline of the human gastrointestinal tract (GIT) showing features from the buccal cavity through to the anus. (Licensed under Creative Commons©, CC BY-SA. https://en.wikipedia.org/wiki/Human_digestive_system.) (b) Diagram of microscopic view of the small intestine, the major site of absorption for orally administered compounds. Inner lining of the longitudinal section of the ileum possesses folds lined with villi which increase surface area. Villi contain numerous microvilli (brush border) which facilitate absorption of substances from the lumen. (Licensed under Creative Commons©, CC BY. https://en.wikipedia.org/wiki/Human_digestive_system.)

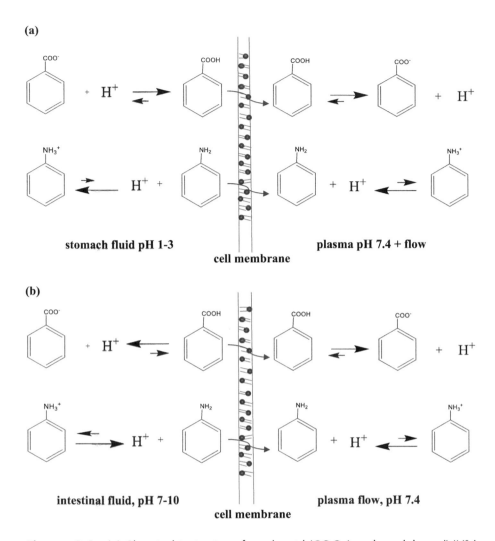

Figure 4.6 (a) Chemical ionization of weak acid (COO⁻) and weak base (NH³⁺) in the acidic environment of the gastric juices of the stomach. Arrows indicate the preponderance of molecules in the non-ionized state for the WA and ionized state for the WB. Equilibrium is always driven to the right during normal plasma flow. (b) Chemical ionization of WA (COO⁻) and WB (NH³⁺) in the basic environment of the small intestine. Arrows indicate the preponderance of molecules in the ionized state for the WA and non-ionized state for the WB. Equilibrium is always driven to the right due to plasma flow.

lipid-soluble solvent enhances the passage of substances through the physiological membranes according to the principles of Henderson–Hasselbalch. Thus the fate of a compound is subject to the conditions of the compartment in which it is present.

Chemicals and drugs are also administered parenterally – direct injection as with IV, intraperitoneal (IP), intramuscular (IM), subcutaneous (SC, subq.), and intradermal (ID).

4.3 Distribution of Toxic Compounds

Distribution of toxic compounds in the body is influenced by: volume of distribution (V_D), plasma concentrations, half-life (t½), area under the curve (AUC), plasma protein binding, site of action, and accumulation.

After xenobiotic chemicals or drugs have been absorbed, they filter into systemic blood circulation. The part of the vascular system into which the compound is absorbed depends on the site of exposure. Absorption through the skin leads to the peripheral blood supply (dermal capillaries), whereas the major pulmonary circulation is involved if the compound is airborne and absorbed into the lungs. For most compounds, oral absorption is followed by entry into the portal vein supplying the liver with blood from the GIT.

After the capillaries, the chemicals enter the major blood vessels of the systemic circulation, then distributed throughout the body. The physicochemical properties of the compound determine its dilution and distribution into tissues and organs. Distribution into specific tissues involves negotiating biological membranes according to the principles of nonionic/ionic absorption (as discussed above). Only the non-ionized form of compounds traverses from the systemic circulation into tissues by passive diffusion. Specific transport systems operate for other compounds, while phagocytic and pinocytic processes transport large molecules, particles, or suspensions of large molecules. The concentration of the compound in the plasma and the plasma level profile (Figure 4.7) reflects the distribution. For example, compounds distributed into all tissues, such as lipid-soluble solvents (carbon tetrachloride), have low plasma concentrations (and higher tissue distribution), whereas substances ionized at the pH of the plasma do not readily distribute into tissues, have proportionately higher plasma concentrations (and lower tissue distribution). This is quantified as the apparent volume of distribution, V_D:

$$V_D(L) = \frac{\text{Dose} \quad (\text{mg})}{\text{Plasma concentration} \quad (\text{mg}/\text{L})}$$

V_D is the total of the compartments of body fluids into which the substance is apparently distributed. The determination is based on the dose of the drug administered versus the plasma concentration. Measurement of the concentration of compound in the plasma compartment is necessary and allows for the calculation of V_D.

Calculation of the V_D also suggests whether an exogenous compound is localized in a specific tissue (or organ) or is confined to the plasma. Thus, if a substance distributes mainly into adipose tissue, the plasma concentration is low and the V_D is larger. The substance is not necessarily evenly distributed in body water however and reaches high concentrations in one tissue or organ.

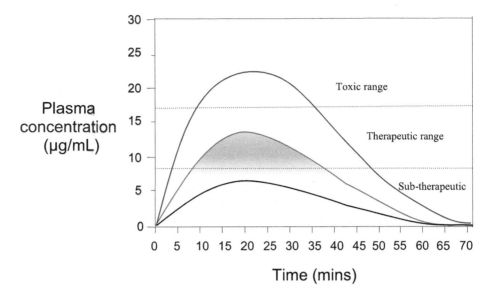

Figure 4.7 Plasma level profile of three different doses of a xenobiotic administered orally. Delay in oral absorption is subject to factors associated with oral administration as well as first-pass metabolism. The area under the curve (AUC) for the therapeutic range represents the target dose (shaded).

The concentration of a chemical in the plasma compartment of the blood and its change over time (Figure 4.7) reflects the absorption and distribution of the chemical, as well as metabolism and elimination. It also determines critical toxic and targets therapeutic ranges. In addition, after a drug is administered orally, the plasma level profile is different from the profile of a drug administered intravenously (IV, Figure 4.8). The plasma level of a chemical and its change over time is important because:

a. plasma level reflects the available concentration of the chemical in the systemic circulation more readily than the dose of the chemical administered;
b. it reflects the available concentration of the chemical at the target site;
c. aides in the calculation of other parameters for chemical distribution such as t½, AUC, and body burden;
d. it designates the type of distribution which the compound is undergoing (i.e. which compartments it is distributed to); and,
e. when plotted versus time, reflects the duration of significant exposure (AUC).

A measure of the overall exposure to a drug or chemical is demonstrated by the body burden, determined by $V_D \times$ plasma concentration.

The t½ of a chemical in the circulation is calculated from the straight line of the plasma log concentration versus time graph (Figure 4.9). Half-life is

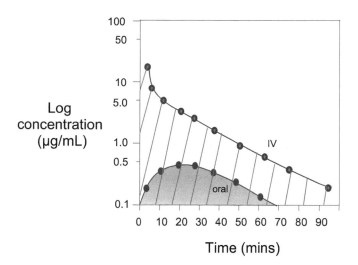

Figure 4.8 Plasma level profile of a xenobiotic compound administered intravenously (IV) and orally. Delay in oral absorption is subject to factors associated with oral administration as well as first-pass metabolism, not apparent in IV administration.

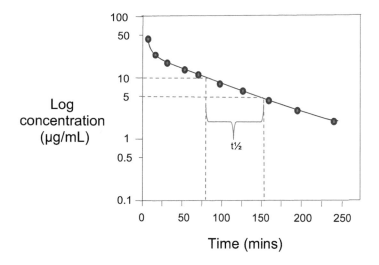

Figure 4.9 Plasma level profile of a xenobiotic administered intravenously (IV). The $t\frac{1}{2}$ is calculated as the time required to decrease the plasma concentration by 50% (from the straight line of this graph, about 75 minutes from 10 to 5 µg/mL).

defined as the time required for the plasma concentration to decrease by 50% on a linear plot and is influenced by its metabolism and elimination. Predictably, a substance with a long half-life is in contact with the biological system for longer than a compound with a shorter half-life and reflects the ability of the substance to accumulate with repeated or chronic dosing. It is normally a constant value, unless the process that determines the decline in plasma level, metabolism, or elimination, is saturable.

Clinically, the plasma level of a drug is important information for the treatment of patients suffering from overdoses of drugs. Thus, it allows the clinical toxicologist to determine a precise exposure sequence rather than estimating an excessive dose based on the patient's signs and symptoms. It is also important for calculating the elimination rate and time of dosing. Experimentally, plasma concentration predicts the absorption profile of the chemical and exposure of organs and tissues. Repeated dose studies are also planned based on the plasma concentration and half-life of the compound.

Figures 4.7 and 4.8 illustrate the ranges of AUC. The AUC available after oral dosing is less than that after IV dosing, principally because steady-state drug plasma levels are influenced by absorption and metabolism in the GIT or liver. This 'first-pass metabolism' is responsible for delaying the appearance of the parent compound in the circulation after oral dosing.

Another indicator of the ability of the mammalian physiology to eliminate the compound is **total body clearance**, calculated as:

$$\frac{\text{dose (unit wt.)}}{\text{AUC}\left(\text{unit wt.}/\text{time}\right)}$$

Distribution is also altered by the interaction of xenobiotic chemical agents with proteins in plasma and macromolecules in other tissues. Many therapeutic drugs bind plasma proteins non-covalently, reducing distribution to target tissues and organs, since the xenobiotic is now attached to a large non-absorbable molecule unable to pass across membranes. Chemicals in plasma often exist in equilibrium between the bound and unbound form and the extent of binding varies among different compounds. Binding to plasma proteins involves ionic forces, hydrogen bonding, hydrophobic bonding, and van der Waals' forces. Exogenous compounds bind most commonly to circulating albumin as well as other plasma lipoproteins.

Distribution of xenobiotic drugs and chemicals to target tissues, that incorporate the site of action, alters the desired (or undesired) effect of the chemical. For example, barbiturates must pass through the **blood-brain barrier (BBB)** of the central nervous system (CNS) in order to exert a pharmacological or toxic effect. The BBB forms a selectively permeable gateway to the CNS, due to the arrangement of the capillaries serving the brain, and the positioning of the surrounding glial cells that do not allow the ready passage of substances. Lipid-soluble compounds such as the barbiturates enter the brain by passive diffusion. An exception is phenobarbital, a weak acid that is amenable to ionization and does not readily permeate the BBB. Formerly, the ionization principle was used to treat barbiturate poisoning by increasing the plasma pH with infusions of sodium bicarbonate, increasing ionization of the barbiturate in plasma, changing the equilibrium, and forcing more non-ionized drug to diffuse out of the brain.

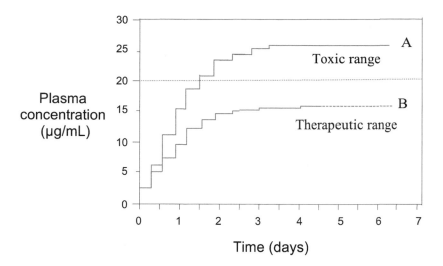

Figure 4.10 Accumulation of two drugs, A and B, following multiple doses. Drug A t½ = 12 hours, Drug B t½ = 7–8 hours. Dosing interval of every 8 hours is equivalent to Drug B.

Today however treatment of barbiturate overdose is symptomatic and follows general guidelines for maintaining the ABCs[5] of emergency management.

Another compound with similar ionic properties, with known toxicity to the central nervous system, is methyl mercury, a lipophilic mercury derivative able to cross the BBB.

Lipophilic xenobiotics localize chiefly in adipose tissue, preventing detection at the plasma level and increasing V_D. For example, polybrominated biphenyls, substances once used extensively in the synthetic chemical industry, are very persistent and highly fat soluble. Their localization in body fat results in extended half-lives, resulting in significant toxicological consequences. The short-acting barbiturate thiopental, used as a pre-surgical anesthetic, is highly lipophilic compared to drugs of the same class and has a rapid onset of action due to its ability to enter the brain quickly.

Potentially noxious xenobiotics that are chronically ingested or exhibit continuous exposure over shorter periods, alter their disposition. If the dosing interval is *shorter* than the half-life the compound accumulates in the plasma (Figure 4.10, toxic range). Blood and tissue levels increase disproportionately with significant consequences. Thus, since the dosing interval of every 8 hours is shorter than the plasma t½ of drug A (12 hours) the plateau level reached in the plasma allows drug A to accumulate to toxic levels, particularly with repeated dosing or chronic exposure, notwithstanding the lower level of each dose. Drug B, however, has a t½ equal to 8 hours, about the same as the desired dosing interval of about every 8 hours.

4.4 Elimination

Elimination[6] of toxic compounds involves:

- urinary elimination;
- biliary elimination;
- elimination via lungs and skin.

Elimination of chemical substances from the body is an important determinant of the extent of their biological effect; rapid elimination reduces the propensity for toxicity and shortens the duration of the toxicologic (or pharmacologic) effect. For some toxic substances, removal of the compound is a goal of treatment.

Elimination of external compounds is reflected in their $t\frac{1}{2}$. The plasma $t\frac{1}{2}$, which echoes metabolism and distribution, reflects the time required for the chemical to decrease to half of its plasma concentration. In contrast, whole-body $t\frac{1}{2}$ is the time required for elimination of half of the compound concentration and consequently reflects total excretion of the compound.

The predominant route for the majority of drugs and chemicals is through the kidneys, with urine as the final destination. Other routes include secretion into the bile, removal of the vaporized chemicals into the expired air from the lungs (reserved for volatile and gaseous compounds), and secretion into the GIT, milk, sweat (through skin), tears, and saliva.

4.4.1 Urinary Elimination

Elimination into the urine from the systemic blood or plasma circulation applies to relatively small, water-soluble molecules that are filtered through the nephrons of the kidneys; larger molecules, such as proteins, do not pass through the intact glomerular membranes of the **nephron**, whereas lipid-soluble molecules, such as bilirubin, are reabsorbed from the proximal renal tubules back into the blood.

Based on cardiac output, the kidneys filter approximately 125 mL of blood per minute and encounter a significant proportion of xenobiotics. Removal into the urine involves three coordinated mechanisms: filtration from the blood through the pores of the **glomerulus**; diffusion from the systemic circulation into the tubules; and active transport into the tubular fluid.

The structure of the kidney facilitates elimination of compounds from the blood circulation (Figure 4.11). Most small molecules dissolved in the plasma are transported to the glomerulus – the primary filtering component of the basic unit of the kidney, the nephron. Aided by large pores in the glomerular capillaries and the hydrostatic pressure of the blood, molecules enter the glomerular capsule (Bowman's capsule) and the proximal tubules, destined for the tubular filtrate. Non-ionized compounds within the pH of the tubular fluid, are reabsorbed from the tubules back into the circulation. Water-soluble molecules that are ionized at the pH of the tubular fluid are not reabsorbed and flow toward the urine.[7] Thus molecules flow through the tubular vessels, into the surrounding extracellular

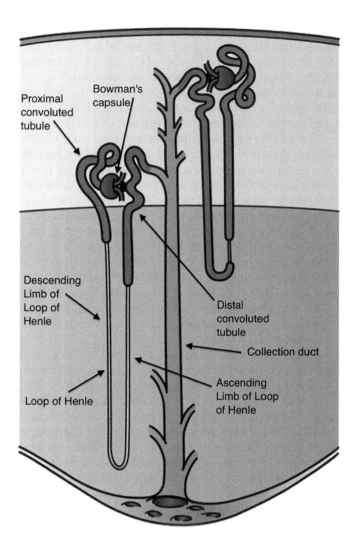

Figure 4.11 Diagram of structural features of the nephron – basic filtering unit of the kidneys. (http://open.umich.edu/education/med/resources/second-look-series/materials. Artwork: Holly Fischer; Creative Commons © CC 3.0. https://commons.wikimedia.org/wiki/Category:Nephron#/media/File:Kidney_Nephron.png.)

fluid (Loop of Henle), and back into the blood circulation, provided there is a concentration gradient in the direction from tubule to blood.

Chemicals, such as ρ-aminohippuric acid, a metabolite of ρ-aminobenzoic acid (PABA), are actively transported from the systemic circulation into the tubules by specific ion transport systems.

The rate of passive diffusion of compounds into the tubules is *proportionate* to the concentration in the systemic circulation, so that the greater the concentration of chemical in the blood, the faster the rate of elimination. However, when elimination is mediated via active transport or facilitated diffusion, which involves the use of specific carriers, the rate of elimination is *constant* and the carrier molecules are saturated by large amounts of compound.

Important toxicological consequences occur when the rate of elimination is *constant* and the dose of a compound is increased, resulting in an elevation of the plasma level, and the risk of accumulation is greater. Conversely, when elimination is via passive diffusion, the rate of elimination increases since it is proportional to the plasma concentration. If elimination is via active transport, however, increasing the dose leads to saturation of renal excretion and toxic levels rise in the plasma and tissues. Continuous intake of ethanol, for instance, beyond the elimination rate, increases plasma levels, accompanied by troublesome effects on the CNS.

The binding of the chemical agent to circulating plasma proteins (plasma protein binding) reduces elimination via passive diffusion especially if a high percentage of the drug or chemical is bound. Only unbound chemicals are able to passively diffuse into the tubules. Protein binding does not affect active transport however and a compound such as p-aminohippuric acid, which is 90% bound to plasma proteins, is cleared in the first pass of blood through the kidney. Other therapeutic drugs, such as the oral **anticoagulant** warfarin, are about 95%–97% protein bound, thus varying elimination rates. Monitoring plasma drug levels of the anticoagulant are critical for proper clinical results.

Urinary pH enhances elimination of a chemical if the drug or its metabolite is ionizable as it enters the tubular fluid. For example, an acidic drug, such as phenobarbital, is ionized at alkaline urinary pH while a basic drug, such as amphetamine, is ionized at an acidic urinary pH. This toxicokinetic feature was applied in the past to enhance renal excretion of the drugs. The concept, however, although theoretically valid, is longer incorporated into the clinical approach to overdose.

The pH of urine is affected by diet – high-protein diet or antacids, for instance, cause urine to become more acidic or basic, respectively. A high rate of blood flow through the kidney, such as with high fluid intake, boosts urine output, which facilitates elimination.

4.4.2 Biliary Elimination

Biliary elimination is an important route for few xenobiotics, especially large **polar** substances. In the liver, hepatocytes secrete bile into the canaliculi, bile duct, and eventually into the intestine (Figure 4.12). Compounds excreted into the bile are usually eliminated in the feces, where MW is an important factor.

As with **renal elimination** via active transport, biliary excretion is saturable – i.e. increasing concentrations of compounds in the liver is a risk. For example, the drug furosemide produces hepatic damage in mice as a result of saturation of the biliary elimination route with a corresponding increased concentration in the liver. Bu et al. (2014) report on the elimination of **polychlorinated biphenyls** (PCBs) and organochlorine pesticides (OCPs) by the Australian population. The data from biomonitoring analysis reveals the intrinsic human elimination half-lives of PCBs and OCPs are 6.4–30 years, principally because of the persistent

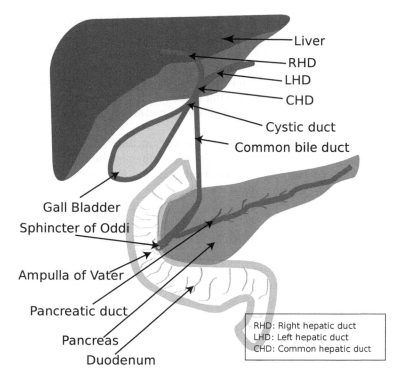

Figure 4.12 Diagram of liver and biliary anatomy. (Biliary system new.svg. Creative Commons © CC 3.0. Derivative work of author: Vishnu 2011. https://commons.wikimedia.org/wiki/File:Biliary_system_new.svg.)

Table 4.1 Comparison of Elimination Half-Lives for PCBs (in Years)

Country	PCB-118	PCB-138	PCB-146	PCB-153	PCB-156
U.K.	9.3	10.8	-	14.4	-
N.A.	5.7	3.7	-	8.4	7.5
Japan	6.3	-	-	-	19
Australia	11	12	21	17	18

Source: Partial data from: Bu et al. (2015).
Abbreviations: U.K., United Kingdom; N.A., North America.

bioaccumulation of the lipid-soluble pollutants and probably enhanced by biliary elimination processes (Table 4.1).

In addition, a compound in the GIT **microflora (normal flora)** is metabolized by bacteria present and converts them to more lipid-soluble substances which are reabsorbed from the intestine through the portal venous blood supply. This **enterohepatic recirculation** pathway leads to cycling of the compounds which increases toxicity (Figure 4.12). If a compound is ingested orally, transported directly to the liver, and extensively excreted into bile, none of the parent compound reaches the systemic circulation. Alternatively, the GI microflora metabolizes the compound to a more toxic metabolite which is reabsorbed resulting in a systemic toxic effect. Compounds ingested orally also directly interact with GI bacteria, bypassing the enterohepatic recirculation. For example, naturally occurring glycosides, such as cycasin, are hydrolyzed to the potent carcinogen methylazoxy methanol by bacteria flora when ingested orally.

Outcomes of biliary elimination, therefore, include: (1) increase in half-life of the compound; (2) production of toxic metabolites in the GIT; (3) increase in hepatic exposure via enterohepatic recirculation; and (4) saturation of liver metabolic capacity and hepatic damage.

4.4.3 Pulmonary Elimination

The pulmonary system is an important route of elimination for volatile compounds and gaseous metabolites of xenobiotics. For example, about 50%–60% of a dose of the aromatic hydrocarbon benzene is eliminated in expired air. Elimination is enhanced by passive diffusion from blood into the alveolus assisted according to concentration gradient equilibrium. This is an efficient route of elimination for lipid-soluble compounds as the capillary and alveolar membranes are thin and in very close proximity to allow for normal gas exchange involved in respiration (Figures 4.4a and b). There is a continuous concentration gradient between the blood and alveolar air as the lungs rapidly remove gas or vapor. This is an important factor in the treatment of poisoning by gases such as the highly toxic carbon monoxide.

4.4.4 Other Routes of Elimination

Elimination into breast milk is a selective route for chemicals that are preferentially lipid-soluble. Newborn animals are particularly at risk from toxic substances secreted into milk. For example, nursing mothers exposed to dichlorodiphenyltrichloroethane (DDT) secrete the pesticide into breast milk, risking a larger dose to the suckling infant than the mother, on a weight basis. Xenobiotics are excreted into other body fluids such as sweat, tears, semen, or saliva principally based on the toxicokinetics.

4.5 Summary and Learning Objectives

This chapter summarizes three of the four phases of disposition of chemicals in biological systems: absorption through membranes; distribution throughout the physiological compartments; and, elimination from the body. The fourth phase, metabolism, the metabolic fate of chemicals, is presented in Chapter 5.

All three phases of disposition require the chemical to cross biological membranes, which consist of phospholipid bilayers with various types of proteins interspersed. Depending on the structure and the physicochemical characteristics of the chemical, passage through a membrane occurs by one of several processes: filtration through pores, for small molecules; passive diffusion, for most lipid-soluble xenobiotics; active transport, for chemicals similar to endogenous substances such as amino acids; facilitated diffusion involving chemicals whose properties are amenable for active transport; and, phagocytosis/pinocytosis, for large molecules and suspended particles.

Passive diffusion is the most common method of transport of xenobiotics across biological membranes. It depends on three critical factors that together form the pH-partition theory: the chemical must form a concentration gradient; it should be lipid-soluble (measured as partition coefficient) and should be non-ionized. The degree of ionization is calculated using the Henderson–Hasselbalch equation.

Fick's Law of Diffusion defines the rate of diffusion of molecules through membranes in proportion to surface area and concentration gradient.

Active transport and facilitated diffusion require carrier proteins are saturable and undergo competitive inhibition. Active transport also requires energy. Absorption occurs from three main sites: skin (large surface area, poorly vascularized, not readily permeable), GIT (major site, well vascularized, variable pH, large surface area, transport processes, presence of food and GIT bacteria), and lungs (large surface area, well vascularized, readily permeable). Chemicals and drugs are also administered parenterally – direct injection as with iv, IP, IM, SC or subq, and ID. The result of the absorptive phase is that the compound enters the systemic circulation. Absorption from the GIT results in first-pass metabolism occurring in the intestinal wall or liver.

Distribution is the phase in which the compound is carried to the tissues by blood or lymph.

The plasma level reflects the concentration at the target site and is governed by distribution. Distribution is restricted by binding to plasma proteins, which is usually non-covalent (ionic, hydrophobic, hydrogen, and van der Waals' forces), saturated, or subject to displacement by other compounds. The blood level of a chemical is used to derive kinetic parameters such as half-life, area AUC and V_D Chemicals are sequestered and accumulate in tissue compartments (e.g., adipose tissue) depending on physicochemical characteristics such as lipid solubility.

Elimination involves the process of removal of a chemical from the organism via the urine, bile, or expired air. Elimination via the kidney into the urine is the major route involving filtration through the glomerulus by passive diffusion, filtration, or active transport from the blood into the nephron. The extent of biliary elimination is influenced by MW of the compound and triggers the enterohepatic recirculation pathway. Removal of substances from expired air in the lungs involves passive diffusion.

Chemicals accumulate after repeated exposure if the *frequency* of dosing is greater than the half-life or time required for elimination.

Review Questions

Choose one answer which is most appropriate.

1. Oil/water partition coefficient of a chemical is an indication of: (a) carcinogenicity; (b) long half-life; (c) potential for bioaccumulation; (d) low apparent volume of distribution; (e) chronic toxicity.
2. Absorption of which of the following is facilitated by the pH in the stomach? (a) weak organic bases; (b) strong acids; (c) weak organic acids; (d) strong bases; (e) none of the above.
3. The apparent 'volume of distribution' (V_D) for a chemical *in vivo* is: (a) equal to the water solubility of the chemical; (b) sometimes larger than the total body volume; (c) equal to the volume of total body water; (d) smaller than the total body water if highly bound in tissues; (e) none of the above.
4. The half-life of a drug in the blood is determined by: (a) metabolism of the compound; (b) volume of distribution; (c) plasma protein binding; (d) urinary pH; (e) total body clearance.
5. The term 'first-pass phenomenon' refers to which of the following?: (a) the drug is eliminated unchanged; (b) the drug is mostly metabolized by the GIT and liver before reaching the systemic circulation; (c) the drug is completely absorbed from the GIT; (d) the drug is completely eliminated by the kidneys; (e) none of the above.
6. Answer (a) if the statement is true or (b) if the statement is false. Absorption of drugs into biological systems by passive diffusion is facilitated by ionization of the compound.

Short Answer Questions

7. Describe the principles of absorption according to the Henderson–Hasselbalch theory.
8. Describe the following topics as applied to toxicological principles: (a) volume of distribution; (b) binding of drugs to plasma proteins; (c) first-pass phenomenon; (d) Fick's law of diffusion.

Notes

1. That is, by water pressures.
2. Non-ionized molecules are in equilibrium with their corresponding acid and base ions as dictated by the formula $HA \leftrightarrow H^+ + A^-$.
3. Originally referred to as "foreign substances", xenobiotics is a more appropriate term that describes non-native, exogenous chemicals that access and permeate biological systems.
4. Although theoretically, chemical ionization predicts absorption of WA/WB in the stomach environment, physiologically the function of the stomach is primarily churning and digestion, and not absorption.

5. Maintain **A**irway, **B**reathing, and **C**irculatory integrity.
6. The terms 'elimination' and 'excretion' have traditionally been used interchangeably, although the former is more appropriate.
7. In contrast, charged electrolytes such as Na^+, Cl^-, and HCO_3^{2-}, are actively reabsorbed into the systemic circulation in order to adjust plasma pH and balance the systemic buffering system.

Bibliography

Barile, F.A. Chapter 10, Toxicokinetics, in: *Barile's Clinical Toxicology: Principles and Mechanisms*, (pp. 111–138), 3rd edition, CRC Press: Taylor & Francis, Boca Raton, FL, 2019.

Bu, Q., MacLeod, M., Wong, F., Toms, L-M.L., Mueller, J.F. and Yu, G., Historical intake and elimination of polychlorinated biphenyls and organochlorine pesticides by the Australian population reconstructed from biomonitoring data. *Environment International* 74, 82–88, 2015. Doi: 10.1016/j.envint.2014.09.014.

He, X., McMahon, S., Henderson, T.D. II, Griffey, S.M. and Cheng, L.W. Ricin toxicokinetics and its sensitive detection in mouse sera or feces using immuno-PCR. *PLoS One* 5(9), 2010. e12858. doi: 10.1371/journal.pone.0012858. PMID: 20877567; PMCID: PMC2943921.

Kannan, K., Chapter 7, Toxicokinetics, in: *Casarett and Doull's Toxicology. The Basic Science of Poisons*, (pp. 401–430), Klaassen, C.D. (Ed.), 9th edition, McGraw Hill, New York, 2019.

Renwick, A. G., Chapter 4, Toxicokinetics, in: *General and Applied Toxicology*, Ballantyne, B., Marrs, T. and Syversen, T.M. (Eds.), 2nd edition, Macmillan, Basingstoke, 1999.

Slitt, A.L., Chapter 5, Absorption, distribution and excretion of toxicants, in: *Casarett and Doull's Toxicology: The Basic Science of Poisons*, (pp. 159–192), Klaassen, C.D. (Ed.), 9th edition, McGraw-Hill, New York, 2019.

Timbrell, J. A. *Principles of Biochemical Toxicology*, 4th edition, Informa Healthcare, New York, 2009.

Zbinden, G., Biopharmaceutical studies, a key to better toxicology, *Xenobiotica*, 18(1), 9, 1988.

Metabolism of Xenobiotic Compounds

Chapter Outline

This chapter discusses the principles of the metabolic fate of chemicals in biological systems and their importance to toxicity.

5.1	Objectives of Metabolism	66
5.2	Phase I Reactions	68
	5.2.1 Oxidation Reactions	68
	5.2.1.1 Cytochrome P450	69
	5.2.2 Types of Oxidation Reactions	70
	5.2.3 Reduction Reactions	71
	5.2.3.1 Hydrolysis	72
	5.2.3.2 Hydration	73
5.3	Phase II Reactions	74
	5.3.1 Sulfation	74
	5.3.2 Glucuronidation	74
	5.3.3 Glutathione Conjugation	75
	5.3.4 Acetylation	76
	5.3.5 Amino Acid Conjugation	77
	5.3.6 Methylation	77
5.4	Toxification versus Detoxification	78
5.5	Factors Affecting Toxic Responses	78
	5.5.1 Species	79
	5.5.2 Strain of Animal	79
	5.5.3 Gender Differences	80
	5.5.4 Genetic Factors and Human Variability in Response	80
	5.5.5 Environmental Factors	81

5.5.6 Pathological State		82
5.6 Summary and Learning Objectives		82
Review Questions		83
Short Answer Questions		84
Notes		84
Bibliography		84

5.1 Objectives of Metabolism

As discussed in the previous chapters, xenobiotic compounds absorbed into biological systems by passive diffusion are generally lipid soluble and consequently not ideally suited for elimination. For example, highly lipophilic substances, such as dichlorodiphenythreechloroethen (DDT) and polychlorinated biphenyls, are poorly eliminated through the water-soluble components of the kidneys and hence remain in the mammalian system for years, particularly the lipid compartments.

After a xenobiotic compound has been absorbed into a biological system, it undergoes metabolism (biotransformation). The metabolic fate of the compound has an important influence on its toxic potential, disposition in the body, and its elimination. The products of metabolism are usually more water-soluble than the original compound. In mammals, biotransformation is directed at increasing water solubility with subsequent elimination through the water-soluble compartment of the urinary system. Facilitating the removal of a compound means that its biological half-life is *reduced*, thus rendering its potential toxicity to a *minimum*. In conjunction with the process of elimination, metabolism also affects biological activity of a xenobiotic chemical. For example, administration of the short-acting anesthetic drug **succinyl-choline** results in skeletal muscle relaxation. Its duration of activity is short, only a few minutes, principally because metabolic enzymes rapidly cleave choline molecules to yield inactive succinic acid, which is readily eliminated in the urine (Figure 5.1).

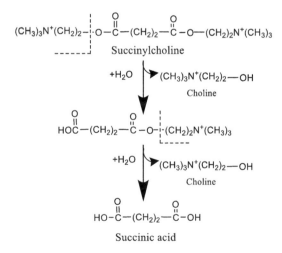

Figure 5.1 Enzymatic hydrolysis of the drug succinylcholine showing cleavage of acetyl groups (dashed lines) with the addition of water molecules.

Metabolism, therefore, is an important component of disposition since it is a major factor in the biological activity of the compound. Overall, the biochemical goal of metabolism is generally to *increase* polarity, which improves water solubility, thereby *enhancing* elimination. For example, the analgesic drug acetaminophen has a renal clearance value of 12 mL/min, whereas one of its major metabolites, the sulfate conjugate, is cleared at a faster rate of 170 mL/min.

Consequently, the objectives of metabolism promote:

1. transformation of the molecule into more polar metabolites;
2. increase in molecular weight and size of the chemical;
3. facilitation of elimination from the organism.

The consequences of these changes include:

a. *decrease* in the half-life of the compound;
b. *shortening* of exposure time;
c. *reduction* in accumulation;
d. *alteration* in extent and duration of biological activity.

Sometimes metabolism has the opposite effect by decreasing water solubility, thus reducing the ability for elimination. For example, addition of an acetyl group to the parent compound during metabolism (acetylation) *decreases* the solubility of sulfonamide antibiotics in urine, leading to crystallization of the drug in kidney tubules after high doses, the consequence of which risks necrosis of the tissue.

Metabolism is divided into two phases: (1) phase I and (2) phase II. Phase I involves alteration of the original xenobiotic molecule, whose purpose is to add a functional group to the parent molecule, the product of which is then conjugated in phase II. Figure 5.2 illustrates phase I metabolism of the organic solvent benzene, a highly lipophilic molecule not readily excreted from the systemic circulation except as a volatile compound in expired air. Phase I metabolism inserts a hydroxyl group which converts benzene into several metabolites, the major one of which is phenol. This allows for the phase II conjugation reaction to occur when the polar sulfate group is added. The final metabolite is a sulfate derivative, which is water soluble and readily eliminated in urine.

Most biotransformation reactions are divided into phase I and II reactions, although some xenobiotic molecules already possess functional groups suitable for phase II reactions (e.g. phenol).

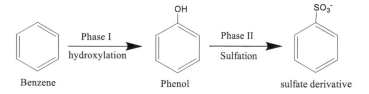

Figure 5.2 Metabolism of benzene. Phase I hydrolysis reaction adds a hydroxy group while phase II sulfation reaction inactivates the molecule to a water-soluble sulfate derivative.

Table 5.1 Features and Characteristics of Major Biotransformation Reactions

Features	Phase I Reactions	Phase II Reactions
Chemical modification	Oxidation, dealkylation, deamination, reduction, hydrolysis, dehalogenation	*Conjugation reactions:* glucuronidation, sulfation, acetylation; with glutathione
Enzymatically mediated	Hepatic microsomal, mitochondrial enzymes; cytochrome-P450 enzymes	Specific transfer enzymes; **microsomal**, cytosolic enzymes
Chemical modification of metabolite	Increased polarity; water soluble	Further increase in polarity and preparation for renal elimination
Toxicologic activity of metabolite	Variable (increase or decrease)	Mostly inactivation; some conversion to more toxic metabolites
Primary biotransformation organs	Liver; kidney, lung & skin	Primarily liver

Metabolism is usually catalyzed by enzymes usually found most abundantly in the mammalian liver – the organ possesses a protective physiological gateway. Many external compounds enter the body via the gastrointestinal (GI) tract, where they encounter the portal blood supply, which directs the complex toward the liver. However, it is important to note that enzymes are involved in the metabolism of xenobiotic compounds that are found in many tissues as well as the liver. They are also localized in one cell type of an organ and are not always specific for external compounds and have a major role in normal endogenous metabolism.

Enzymes involved in biotransformation are localized in the subcellular fractions of the cytoplasm – in the **endoplasmic reticulum**, cytosol, and a few in mitochondria. Features and characteristics of metabolic and biotransformation reactions are shown in Table 5.1.

5.2 Phase I Reactions

5.2.1 Oxidation Reactions

Most oxidation reactions are catalyzed by the cytochrome P450 (CYP_{450}) monooxygenase family, located in the smooth endoplasmic reticulum (SER) of the cell, and isolated in the microsomal fraction obtained by cell fractionation. The liver has the highest concentration of oxidizing enzymes although they are found in most tissues. The catalyzed reactions also require nicotinamide adenine dinucleotide phosphate hydrogen (reduced) (**NADPH**), molecular **oxygen**, and **magnesium**, and are represented as follows:

$$SH^- + O_2 + NADPH + H^+ \rightarrow S\text{-}OH + H_2O + NADP^+$$

where SH^- is the reduced substrate and S-OH is the oxidized product.

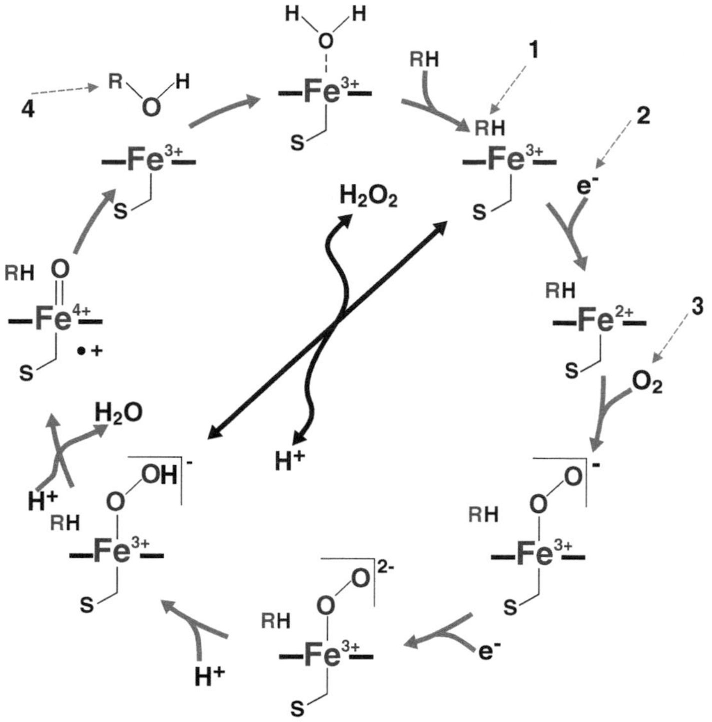

Figure 5.3 The cytochrome P450 catalytic cycle. The pathway illustrates the main site of the enzymatic reactions with the ferric (Fe^{+3}) heme iron in the center of the enzyme complex (not shown), coupled with a water molecule ($H2O$). The binding of reduced substrate (RH) displaces the water ligand. A further single electron reduction allows for a series of oxidation reactions, eventually forming the hydroxylated product (ROH). P450 enzyme is restored to its resting state. The double-headed arrow crossing the cycle between the substrate-bound ferric (Fe^{+3}) P450 and RH compound describes the reaction mechanism for related peroxygenase P450s (Fe^{+3}–O–O$^-$). (From: Belcher et al., 2014.)

Figure 5.3 illustrates the sequence of metabolic reactions involving four steps of the hydroxylation reaction:

1. coupling of the enzyme to the substrate (RH);
2. transfer of an electron;
3. addition of oxygen and molecular rearrangement; and,
4. loss of water and hydroxylation of the substrate (R-O-H).

5.2.1.1 Cytochrome P450

The CYP_{450} **monooxygenase** family of enzymes is a collection of **isoenzymes** (at least forty in humans) based on a heme protein, at the center of which is an iron atom. The system also requires NADPH CYP_{450} reductase, which donates electrons to the CYP_{450}. Although the enzyme is mainly located in the SER other organelles such as the nucleus are involved. There are at least twenty-seven gene families in the CYP_{450} gene superfamily. The enzyme protein is designated CYP and there are three main families involved with the metabolism of xenobiotics – CYP1, CYP2, and CYP3.[1] Many of the isozymes show genetic polymorphisms which influence the metabolism of drugs and other chemicals. The proportion of isoenzymes varies between different tissues in the same animal and among different species of animal.

CYP_{450} conducts about sixty different types of reactions, where the isozymes have broad and overlapping substrate specificity.

Although there is a large variety of substrate types for CYP_{450}, most are lipophilic. There is also a correlation between metabolism and lipophilicity of chemicals metabolized by the enzyme, with preference for more lipophilic substrates.

Cytochrome P450 expresses several polymorphisms which affect metabolism of drugs and chemicals and possess individual differences affecting their ability to metabolize drugs and chemicals.

5.2.2 Types of Oxidation Reactions

Aromatic and aliphatic hydroxylation, such as oxidation reactions of benzene (Figure 5.2) and vinyl chloride (Figure 5.4), respectively, involve addition of oxygen across a double bond. Hydroxylation of the aliphatic moiety in benzene occurs at one of four positions (Figure 5.5). Alicyclic and heterocyclic rings also undergo hydroxylation.

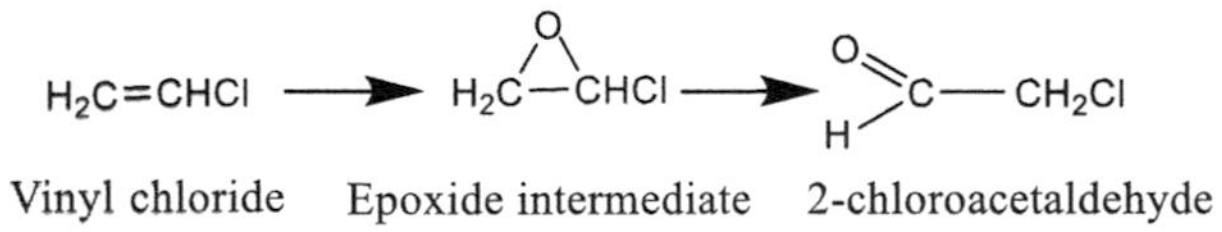

Vinyl chloride   Epoxide intermediate   2-chloroacetaldehyde

Figure 5.4 Oxidation of vinyl chloride showing epoxide intermediate.

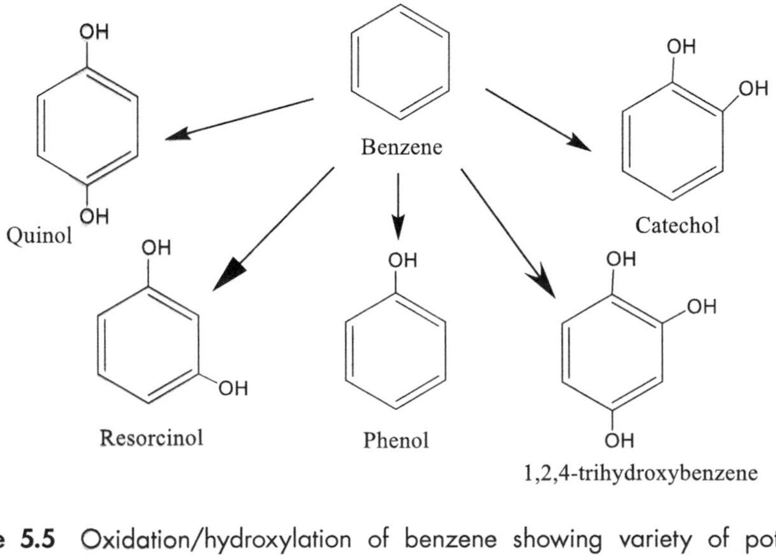

Figure 5.5 Oxidation/hydroxylation of benzene showing variety of potential derivatives.

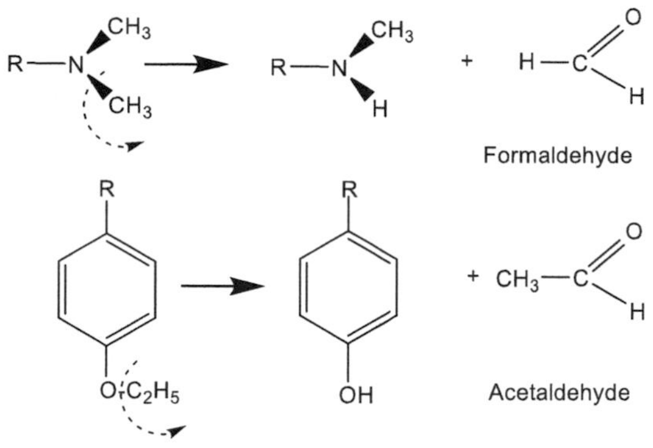

Figure 5.6 Dealkylation reaction. Dashed arrow represents enzymatic cleavage target.

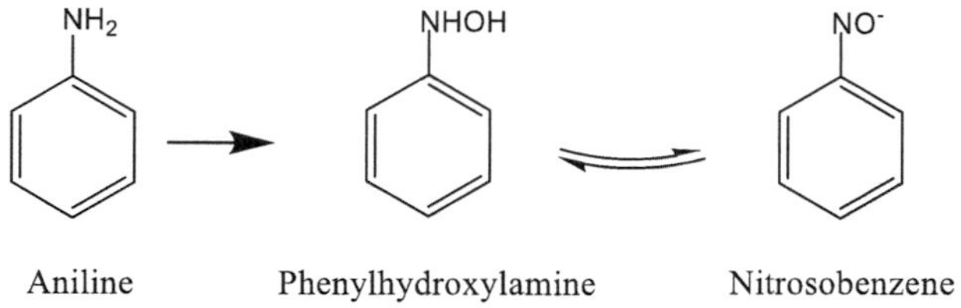

Aniline   Phenylhydroxylamine   Nitrosobenzene

Figure 5.7 N-hydroxylation of an aromatic amino group.

Alkyl groups attached to N, O, or S atoms are removed by dealkylation reactions which involve oxidation of the alkyl group followed by rearrangement and loss to form the respective aldehyde (Figure 5.6). Nitrogen and sulfur atoms in xenobiotics are oxidized by microsomal enzymes (Figure 5.7), while sulfur and halogen atoms are removed oxidatively (Figures 5.8 and 5.9).

Certain oxidation reactions are catalyzed by other enzymes such as alcohol dehydrogenase (Figure 5.10), xanthine oxidase, microsomal amine oxidase, monoamine, and diamine oxidases.

Peroxidases represent another important group of enzymes that catalyze oxidation reactions for xenobiotic chemicals. For example, benzene, a toxic solvent responsible for induction of aplastic anemia, is metabolized by peroxidases in the bone marrow. The antihypertensive vasodilator drug hydralazine is also metabolized by this system.

5.2.3 Reduction Reactions

Reduction reactions are catalyzed by microsomal or cytosolic reductases and GI bacteria[2] that possess reductases. The most common type of reaction is the reduction of nitro and azo groups present in the molecular structure of the food-coloring agent tartrazine (Figure 5.11). Less common reduction reactions include the reduction of aldehyde and keto groups, epoxides, and double bonds.

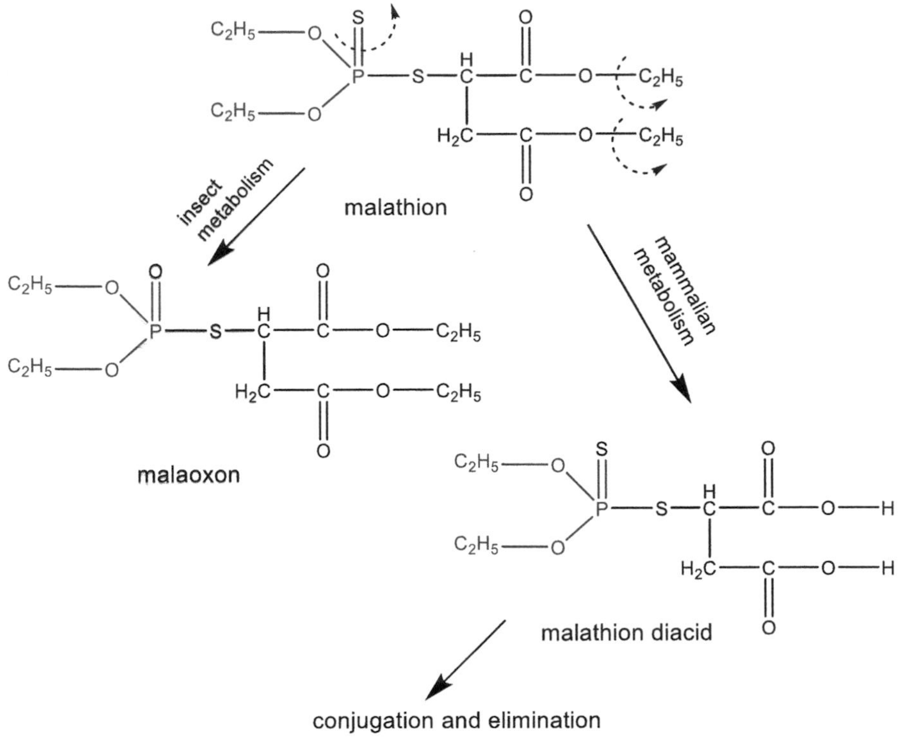

Figure 5.8 Metabolism of the insecticide, malathion. Dashed arrow represents enzymatic cleavage target.

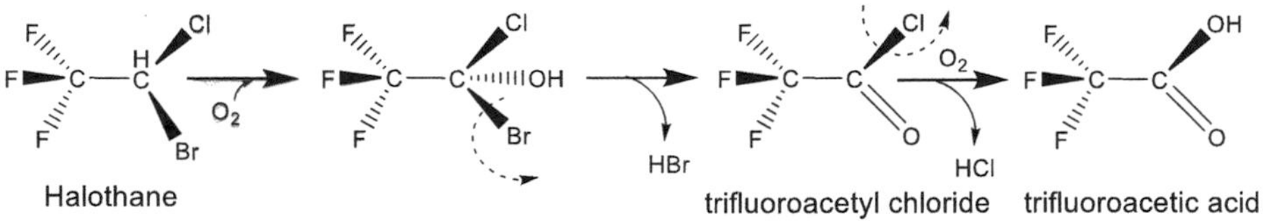

Figure 5.9 Metabolism of the anesthetic, halothane, showing the oxidative pathway. The penultimate product, trifluoroacetyl chloride, is a reactive intermediate which acylates liver proteins.

Reductive dehalogenation, catalyzed by the microsomal enzyme system, is an important route of metabolism for general anesthetics such as halothane (Figure 5.9).[3]

5.2.3.1 Hydrolysis

Esters and amides are hydrolyzed by esterases and amidases, respectively. Several of these enzymes are found in the cytosol of cells in a variety of tissues, as well as in the plasma component of blood, while microsomal esterases have also been identified.

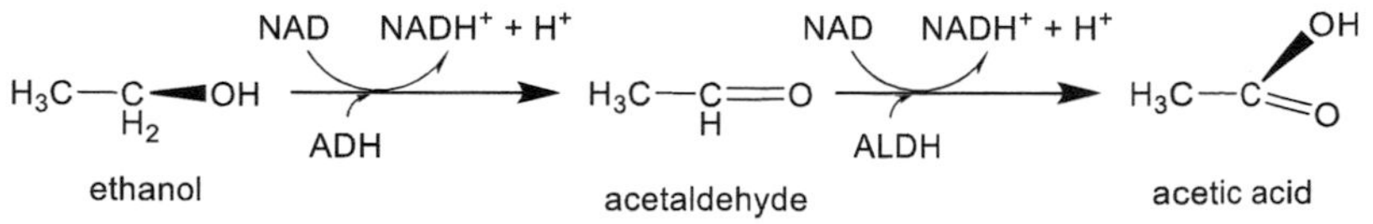

Figure 5.10 Oxidation of ethanol showing the typical oxidative progression from alcohol to aldehyde to acid.

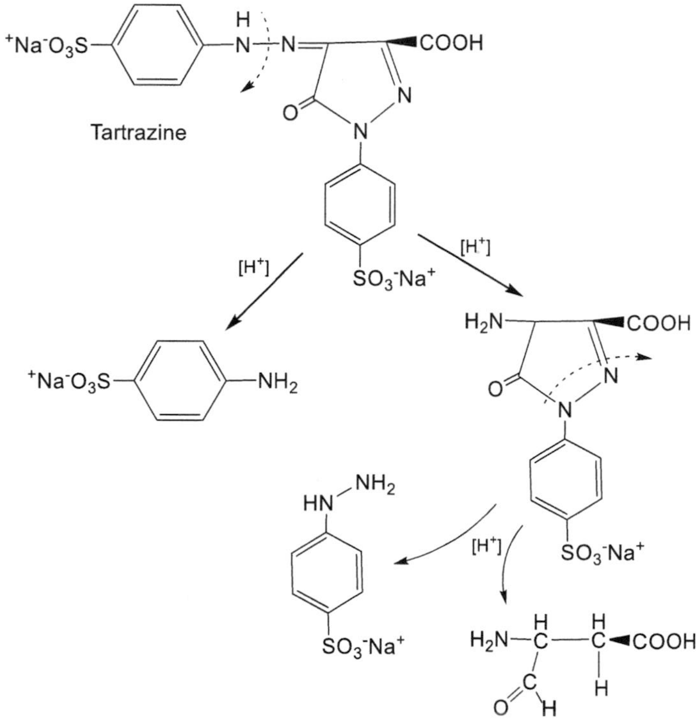

Figure 5.11 Metabolic reduction of the food-coloring agent tartrazine, showing reduction reactions and removal of side chains (dashed arrows).

Typical esterase and amidase reactions are shown in Figure 5.12. The shorter duration of action of procaine is due to its rapid hydrolysis in plasma by esterases. The amide bond in procainamide renders the molecule more resistant to amidases, thus accounting for its longer duration of action as an anti-arrhythmic drug.

5.2.3.2 Hydration

Epoxides are stable metabolic intermediates that undergo hydration catalyzed by the enzyme epoxide hydrolase, located in the microsomal fraction. The *detoxification* reaction yields dihydrodiol products that are less reactive than epoxides.

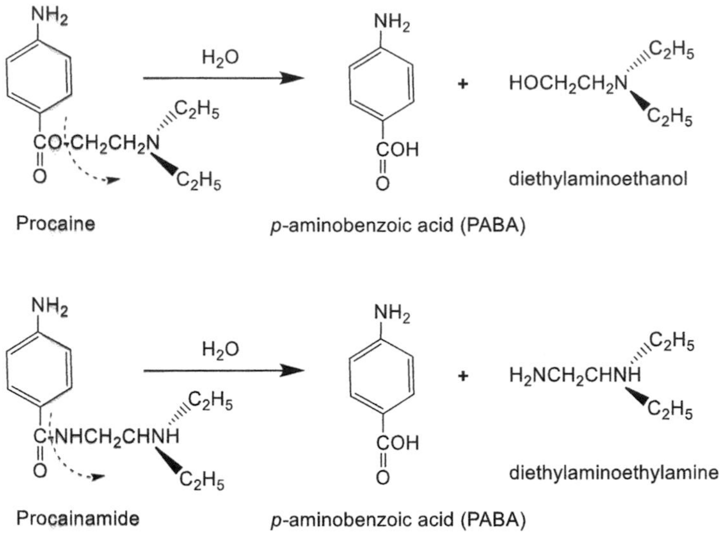

Figure 5.12 Hydrolysis of the anesthetic drug procaine (an ester) and the antiarrhythmic drug procainamide (an amide), showing removal of side chains at the ester and amide links, respectively (dashed arrows).

5.3 Phase II Reactions

Phase II reactions, also known as conjugation reactions, involve the addition of polar groups to xenobiotic molecules. The polar group is conjugated either to an existing molecule or to one added in from the previous phase I reaction, such as a hydroxyl group. The polar group renders the xenobiotic chemical *more* water soluble that is readily cleared from the systemic circulation and less likely to exert a toxic effect. Groups donated in phase II reactions are commonly complexed in intermediary metabolism. Conjugation reactions are considered below.

5.3.1 Sulfation

The addition of the sulfate moiety to a hydroxyl group is a major route of conjugation for xenobiotic compounds. This reaction is catalyzed by a cytosolic sulfotransferase enzyme and incorporates coenzyme phosphoadenosine phosphosulfate (PAPS). The resulting product is a polar and water-soluble ester. Both aromatic and aliphatic hydroxyl groups are conjugated with sulfate as N-hydroxy groups and amino groups, respectively (Figure 5.13).

5.3.2 Glucuronidation

Glucuronic acid is a polar and water-soluble carbohydrate molecule that is added to hydroxyl, carboxylic acid, amino groups, and thiols (Figure 5.14). This process

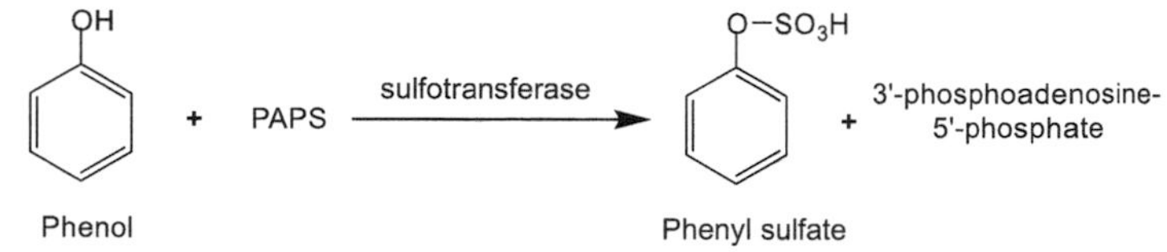

Figure 5.13 Conjugation reaction of phenol.

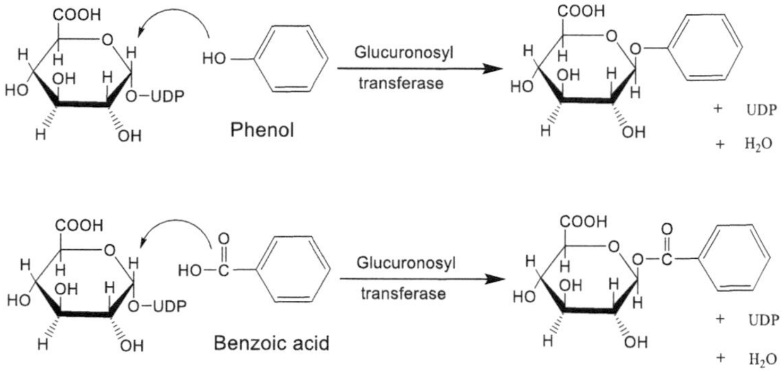

Figure 5.14 Conjugation of phenol and benzoic acid (a carboxylic acid) with UDP-glucuronic acid. UDP is released along with a water molecule.

is a major route of phase II metabolism and utilizes glucuronosyl transferases, microsomal enzymes, with uridine diphosphate (UDP) glucuronic acid as the cofactor. Other carbohydrates are also involved in conjugation, such as glucose, incorporated by insects to form glucosides. Ribose and xylose are also involved in conjugation reactions.

5.3.3 Glutathione Conjugation

Glutathione conjugation is an important route of phase II metabolism involved in the removal of reactive intermediates. **Glutathione (GSH)** is a tripeptide found in mammalian tissues, especially in the liver. It has a major *protective* role in the body as a reducing agent for reactive oxidizing intermediates (eg oxygen radicals), combining with the reactive center in the radical thus reducing or neutralizing toxicity. In general, the sulphydryl group of glutathione acts as a nucleophile and displaces atom or attacks an **electrophilic** site (Figure 5.15). Glutathione reacts in enzyme-catalyzed reactions with substrates that are electrophilic metabolites produced in phase I reactions. The reactions are catalyzed by glutathione transferases located in the cytosolic soluble fraction or, less frequently, in the microsomal fraction. The substrates include aromatic, heterocyclic, alicyclic and aliphatic epoxides, aromatic halogen and nitro compounds, and unsaturated aliphatic compounds. The resulting conjugates are either excreted into bile or metabolized further, via phase 3 reactions, to yield N-acetylcysteine conjugates (mercapturic acid; Figure 5.15).

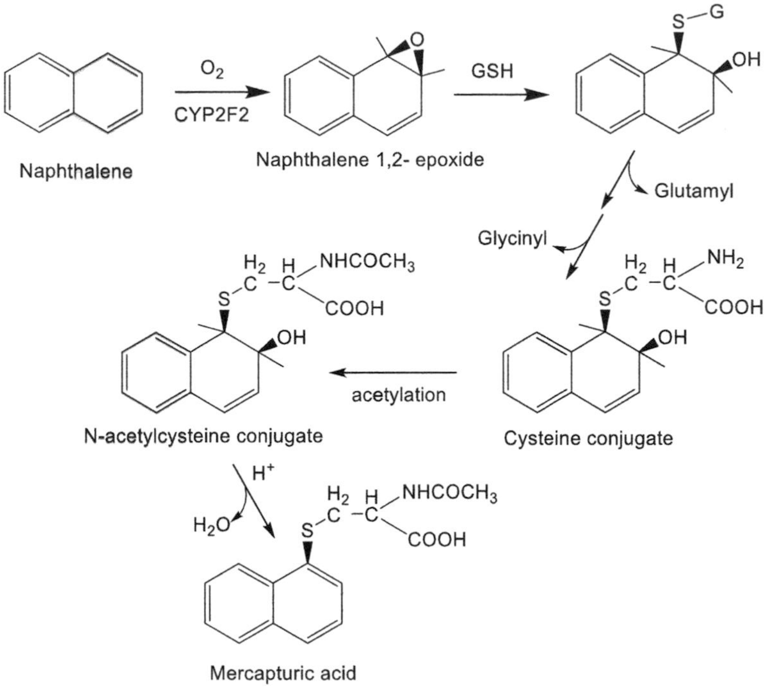

Figure 5.15 Phase II conjugation reactions with naphthalene, its epoxide derivative (primary metabolite), and glutathione, with subsequent formation of N-acetylcysteine conjugate (mercapturic acid). CYP2F2 is the major P450 enzyme for naphthalene.

5.3.4 Acetylation

Acetylation is unusual in that the product is *less water soluble* than the parent compound. Substrates for acetylation are aromatic amino compounds, sulfonamides (Figure 5.16), hydrazines, and hydrazides.

Acetylation reactions are catalyzed by acetyltransferase enzymes found in the cytosol of cells in the liver, gastric mucosa and in white blood cells. The enzymes utilize acetyl coenzyme A as cofactor. Among different mammalian species, including human and rabbit, the two isoenzymes (NAT1, NAT2) differ markedly in activity and substrate. In both species possession of one isoenzyme (NAT2) is genetically determined and yields two distinct phenotypes, 'rapid' and 'slow' acetylators. The predominance of either enzyme plays an important role in the toxicity of certain drugs such as the antihypertensive drug hydralazine, anti-tuberculosis drug isoniazid, and anti-arrhythmic drug procainamide, illustrating the importance of genetic factors in toxicology.

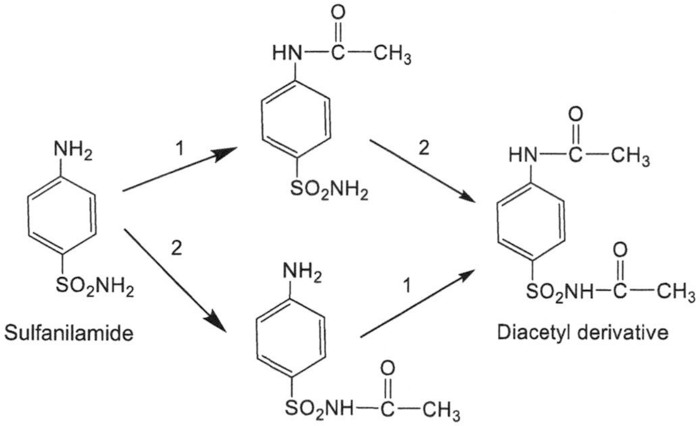

Figure 5.16 Acetylation of the antibiotic drug sulphanilamide at the amino (reaction 1) and at the sulphonamido (reaction 2) groups.

5.3.5 Amino Acid Conjugation

Xenobiotic organic acids undergo conjugation with amino acids (as well as with glucuronic acid). Any specific amino acid involved in the reaction depends on the species.[4] Glycine is the most common amino acid used. The carboxylic acid group first reacts with coenzyme A and then with the amino acid. Mitochondrial acylase enzymes catalyze the reaction.

5.3.6 Methylation

Hydroxyl, amino, and thiol groups in molecules are methylated by one of a series of methyltransferases. This occurs particularly with endogenous compounds but xenobiotics are also substrates. As with acetylation, this reaction tends to *decrease* rather than increase water solubility.

An important toxicological example is methylation of heavy metals such as mercury. Environmental microorganisms are responsible for many methylation reactions the importance of which changes the physicochemical characteristics of mercury from a water-soluble inorganic ion to a lipid-soluble organic compound. The lipid-soluble metabolite is more likely to bind within lipid stores of aquatic life, such as shellfish. When ingested, a corresponding *change* in its toxicity renders the mercuric ion preferentially toxic to the mammalian kidney, while organomercury is selectively toxic to the nervous system.

It is important to note that although a molecule is extraneous to a living organism, it still is a substrate for an enzyme involved in normal metabolic pathways, provided its chemical structure is appropriate, thus widening the scope of potential metabolic reactions. Xenobiotic compounds are metabolized by several different enzymes simultaneously in the same mammal, allowing for a variety of metabolic routes occurring simultaneously. The equilibrium between these routes often determines the toxicity of the compound.

5.4 Toxification versus Detoxification

Metabolism of xenobiotic compounds is also referred to as detoxification because the process generally converts compounds into more water-soluble, readily eliminated metabolites with *decreasing* toxicity. Occasionally a metabolite is produced which is *more* toxic than the parent compound. A well-documented example is the analgesic opioid drug meperidine where one of the two pathways of metabolism renders the parent compound neurotoxic (Figure 5.17). In the liver, the drug is hydrolyzed to meperidinic acid by carboxylesterases and demethylated to normeperidine by microsomal enzymes. Both metabolites are active, but chronic ingestion of the parent compound results in the production of the neurotoxic derivative, responsible for tremors, muscle twitching, and convulsions. The example illustrates the balance between the different pathways that alter eventual toxicity.

5.5 Factors Affecting Toxic Responses

As previously indicated, metabolism is a major factor in determining toxicity of a compound. Chemical or biological factors that affect disposition consequently determine toxicity. Biological factors include species, genetics, diet, age, gender, and pathological state. Chemical factors include physicochemical characteristics such as pK_a, lipophilicity, molecular size and shape, and chirality (type of isomer). All influence metabolism and toxicity of the compound. For example, isomers of the same molecule are often metabolized differently, displaying dissimilar

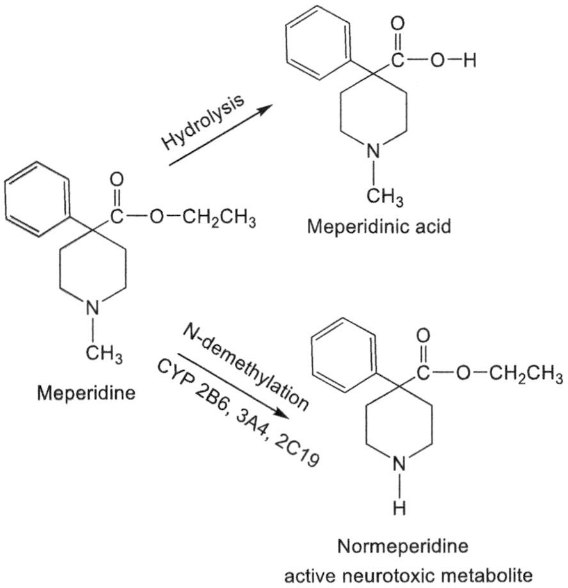

Figure 5.17 Metabolism of the opioid analgesic drug, meperidine. The parent drug is hydrolyzed to meperidinic acid by carboxyesterases and demethylated to normeperidine by microsomal enzymes, the latter of which is neurotoxic.

biological activity. In mammals, genetic differences affect metabolism and consequently toxicity. Diverse species possess a variety of metabolic capabilities and influence susceptibility to toxic effects. Dietary constituents also interact with metabolic pathways or rate of metabolism, regardless of toxicity of the compound. These factors and others are discussed in greater detail in subsequent chapters.

5.5.1 Species

Species often vary widely in their responses to drugs and chemicals which bear significance in the fields of veterinary medicine and environmental toxicology. For instance, drugs are tested in animals for eventual applications in humans, but since human response is not identical to those of rodents, significant issues arise when the drug undergoes **clinical trials**.

Similarly, it is important that species differences in animal response to veterinary products are understood, particularly in relation to treatment of farm animals versus household pets. For example, felines are mostly susceptible to the toxic effects of acetaminophen, because conjugation with glucuronic acid is deficient in cats. This species, therefore, relies on sulfate conjugation as the principle method for detoxification, which is easily saturated. In addition, CYP_{450}-mediated pathways produce toxic metabolites which become more significant, thus rendering cats susceptible to liver damage.

Environmentally large numbers of broadly diverse species react differently when exposed to pesticides. For example, insecticides, such as organophosphorus compounds and DDT, are more toxic to insects than to humans and other mammals because of their metabolic differences. The insecticide **malathion** is metabolized by *hydrolysis* in mammals but is *oxidized* in the insect to malaoxon which then binds to and inhibits the enzyme cholinesterase (Figure 5.8).

One problem associated with species differences in metabolism occurs during safety evaluation of drugs and chemicals. Regulatory testing of agents is mandatory in animals prior to human or veterinary applications but choosing the appropriate animal model is complex, especially when human metabolism of chemicals varies from commonly used experimental species. Also, as noted above, intraspecies variation to chemical response is as important as interspecies metabolic differences.

5.5.2 Strain of Animal

Just as different species vary in their metabolism and response to toxic compounds, different strains of the same species also show distinctions. For example, different strains of mice vary widely in their ability to metabolize barbiturates, resulting in a magnitude of pharmacological effects among the strains.

5.5.3 Gender Differences

Male and female genders differ in their reactions due to their respective metabolic and hormonal differences. In some species, males metabolize compounds *more rapidly* than females. Sex differences in *routes* of elimination also underlie differences in *susceptibility*. For example, dinitrotoluene-induced hepatic tumors occur predominantly in males due to the differences in the route of elimination. Biliary elimination of a glucuronide conjugate is favored in males while urinary elimination predominates in females. In addition, the glucuronide conjugate is packaged in the intestine by gut bacteria, the products of which are reabsorbed, causing the hepatic tumors. The difference in susceptibility to chloroform-induced kidney damage explains differences between male and female mice, which has a metabolic and hormonal basis. Male mice are more susceptible, but this difference is neutralized by sterilization and restored by androgens.[5]

5.5.4 Genetic Factors and Human Variability in Response

Genetic variation is particularly important in the mammalian population which accounts for many examples of toxic drug reactions due to genetic defects or differences in metabolism. For instance, the acetylator phenotype is the product of the development of mutant alleles where the metabolic acetylation reaction produces variations. This mutation results in rapid and slow acetylators among individuals where the latter have *less functional* acetyltransferase enzyme. This is an important factor in a number of adverse drug reactions including the hydralazine-induced lupus syndrome, procainamide-induced lupus syndrome, isoniazid-induced liver damage, and isoniazid-induced **peripheral neuropathy**.

The first genetic polymorphism of CYP_{450} identified affected CYP_{450} 2D6 which catalyzes the metabolism of important therapeutic drugs, such as the antidepressant paroxetine and the cardiac beta-blocker carvedilol. Two phenotypes result from this polymorphism – *poor* metabolizers and *extensive* metabolizers. As a result of mutations, poor metabolizers do not possess functional cytochrome CYP_{450} 2D6 metabolic capacity; accordingly, they have reduced metabolic activity which accounts for higher–than-expected blood levels of the compound. These mutations produce abnormal mRNA, and hence abnormal enzyme protein. Poor metabolizers succumb to increased toxicity from drugs such as penicillamine, which causes skin rashes, and phenformin, which is associated with lactic acidosis. The poor metabolizer phenotype occurs in approximately 5%–10% of the Caucasian population. A similar genetic polymorphism occurs with cytochrome CYP_{450} 2C, which is particularly common in the Japanese population.

Among other enzymes involved in drug metabolism that are also subject to genetic variation include alcohol dehydrogenase and esterases, which underlie toxic or exaggerated responses. For instance, increased sensitivity to ethanol (alcohol) results from reduced metabolism in individuals of North American Indian and Asian populations. The cause is a variant of alcohol dehydrogenase that oxidizes at a slower rate in susceptible individuals.

Similarly, polymorphisms in esterases interfere with the metabolism of the muscle relaxant drug succinylcholine which results in considerable variation in the duration of action of the drug. Thus, in affected individuals, muscle relaxation after administration of succinylcholine lasts a matter of minutes, whereas in a few individuals with a particular isoform of pseudocholinesterase, metabolism is reduced and life-threatening relaxation endures for over an hour.

Toxic responses to xenobiotic chemicals show large genetic disparities among patients. Just as genetically determined metabolic differences occur, genetic differences in receptors or in immunological parameters produce differences in toxicological and pharmacological responses to drugs and chemicals. In some cases, however, rare idiosyncratic reactions[6] account for toxic reactions (e.g. antihypertensive drug hydralazine). Interestingly much of the variability seen in humans is not encountered in inbred experimental animals and consequently rare, severe, life-threatening toxic reactions are not demonstrated in toxicity studies in animals. However, genetically modified animals with programmed genetic manipulations are commercially available to examine the experimental interactions of genetic variations on drug toxicity. Otherwise, these developments are only observed after post-clinical trial introduction of drugs into the larger population.

5.5.5 Environmental Factors

Chemicals in the diet, ambient air, habitable soil, and groundwater influence physiological responses, leading to toxicity. Unlike experimental animals, many humans also ingest medications while exposure to industrial, household, commercial, or occupational chemicals occurs. These clinical drugs interact with environmental pollutants and the reactions to the chemical. The intake of one drug affects the response to another. Repeated exposure of animals to chemicals increases *in vivo* activity of enzymes involved with the metabolism of xenobiotics. In some cases, these enzymes are responsible for metabolism of the same chemical, known as enzyme induction, and are attributed to increased amounts of the same or similar enzyme, possibly as a result of increased synthesis. There are several enzymes involved with xenobiotic metabolism which are induced, the most important of which is $CypP_{450}$. Phase II enzymes are also induced such as glucuronosyl transferase. Induction of these enzymes leads to either increased or decreased toxicity of a compound. Therefore, exposure to drugs or environmental chemicals has a significant effect on the toxicity of other substances, such as a co-administered drug or environmental chemical. For example, high doses of acetaminophen carry a significant risk for serious liver damage if the victim is also exposed to large amounts of alcohol or sedative/hypnotics (tranquilizers), both of which *induce* drug-metabolizing enzymes and thereby **increase** *in vivo* activity. Similarly, Western diets contain substances that influence enzymes of drug metabolism such as the microsomal enzyme inducer and aryl hydrocarbon receptor (AHR) agonist β-naphthoflavone found in green vegetables.[7] As with enzyme inhibitors, cigarette smoking and alcohol intake are also known to induce drug metabolism and pharmacological and toxicological responses.

Conversely, some drugs and chemicals act as enzyme inhibitors, similarly altering the metabolism of other chemicals, thus increasing their toxicity. Unlike enzyme inducers, inhibitors usually have an effect after a single exposure. Both enzyme inducers and inhibitors are natural constituents of the diet or are properties of therapeutic drugs, such as alcohol, tobacco, or prescription medications.[8]

Compounds that inhibit metabolic pathways by blocking specific enzymes also factor in toxic responses. In the case of workers exposed to the solvent dimethylformamide, it is suggested that they are more likely to suffer alcohol-induced facial redness (flushes) than those not exposed, due to *inhibition* of alcohol metabolism.

Although enzyme induction and inhibition are important regarding the disposition and toxicity of environmental chemicals, it is probably more often a significant problem with drugs. This is because concurrent multiple drug use is common, for extended periods and at higher concentrations than those of environmental chemicals.

5.5.6 Pathological State

The influence of disease states on metabolism and toxicity is well documented. Diseases of the liver affect metabolism albeit differently. Infectious disease states such as respiratory influenza also impact drug-metabolizing enzymes via production of interferon.

5.6 Summary and Learning Objectives

This chapter discusses metabolism or biotransformation of chemicals – enzyme-catalyzed conversion of molecules to products with altered physicochemical and biological properties. These reactions yield products that are more water-soluble, less lipid-soluble, and often of greater molecular weight than the original substrates. The consequences of metabolism, therefore, are increased elimination, shortened half-life, reduced accumulation, and exposure of the biological system to potentially toxic compounds. The metabolism of a chemical is determined by its structure, properties, and available enzymes with an affinity for the chemical. It is divided into two phases: (1) phase I predominantly oxidation but also reduction and hydrolysis and (2) phase II, conjugation. Phase I results in the generation of a functional group; phase II involves addition of an endogenous moiety to that functional group to increase water solubility. The most important family of enzymes involved in phase I oxidation reactions is the CYP_{450} system. The system is located in the SER, is comprised of 27 gene families, 3–4 of which are involved with chemical metabolism. Many isoforms exist and some demonstrate genetic polymorphisms. Other oxidative enzymes not within the cytochrome family include alcohol dehydrogenase, xanthine oxidase, microsomal amine oxidase, monoamine and diamine oxidases, and peroxidases. Reduction is commonly catalyzed by reductases (azo- and nitro-) in GI bacteria. Hydrolysis (ester and amide) is catalyzed by esterases. Hydration of epoxides, a detoxification reaction, is catalyzed by microsomal epoxide hydrolase.

Phase II reactions incorporate the addition of glucuronic acid, sulfate, glutathione, amino acids, and acetylation catalyzed by transferases. Glutathione conjugation is an important detoxification reaction.

Metabolism is affected by chemical, biological, and environmental factors. Chirality, size, shape, and lipophilicity are important physicochemical factors that dictate metabolic direction. Species and strain, genetic differences in humans, age, gender, pathology, and nutritional status are biological factors that also influence metabolism. Species differences are important for drug safety testing and pesticide design while genetic factors are accounted for in human responses. Pathologic conditions impact metabolism, while environmental factors include the influence of other drugs, food constituents, or environmental contaminants, such as inducers or inhibitors.

Review Questions

Choose the answer which is most appropriate.

1. Metabolism of a xenobiotic chemical leads to: (a) accumulation of the chemical in tissues; (b) increased elimination in urine; (c) decreased toxicity; (d) altered chemical structure; (e) increased toxicity.
2. Indicate which of the following statements is true and which is false. Cytochrome P450 is an enzyme which is: (a) found in lysosomes; (b) responsible for the conjugation of drugs; (c) a central part of the drug-metabolizing system; (d) one of the enzymes in the mitochondrial electron transport chain; (e) c and d are correct.
3. Phase II metabolism usually involves: (a) microsomal enzymes; (b) decreasing polarity of a chemical; (c) increasing toxicity of compounds; (d) addition of an endogenous moiety; (e) hydrolysis.
4. Indicate which of the following is true and which is false: Glutathione is a(n): (a) protein; (b) tripeptide; (c) enzyme involved in detoxification; (d) substance found in the kidneys; (e) vitamin.
5. Answer (a) if true and (b) if false. Cytochrome P450 mainly catalyzes phase I metabolism of chemicals.
6. Select (a) if 1, 2, and 3 are correct, (b) if 1 and 3 are correct, (c) if 2 and 4 are correct, (d) if only 4 is correct, or (e) if all four are correct. Which of the following are essential aspects of the microsomal enzyme system responsible for the metabolism of xenobiotic compounds? (1) magnesium ions; (2) addition of two electrons; (3) molecular oxygen; (4) the substrate is bound to an iron atom in the active site.
7. Answer (a) if true or (b) if false: The acetylator phenotype is: (a) not found in dogs; (b) found exclusively in Asian populations; (c) responsible for toxicity of amines; (d) an inherited trait affecting a particular metabolic reaction; (e) associated with the HLA genotype.

8. The phenomenon of enzyme induction encompasses: (a) an increase in synthesis of enzyme; (b) an increase in activity of enzyme; (c) increase in liver weight; (d) change in substrate specificity of enzyme; (e) increase in bile flow.

Short Answer Questions

9. Describe the following topics: (a) enzyme-mediated dealkylation; (b) alcohol dehydrogenase; (c) glucuronic acid conjugation; (d) phase I and phase II metabolism.
10. Describe the following topics concerning drug toxicity: (a) ethnic origin; (b) cytochrome P450 isozymes; (c) enzyme induction; (d) acetylator phenotype.

Notes

1. CYP4 is responsible for metabolism of fatty acids but is also involved in the metabolism of xenobiotics.
2. Normal flora or microbiome of the GI tract.
3. Interestingly, reductive dechlorination of carbon tetrachloride exacerbates its toxicity.
4. Species within a similar evolutionary group tend to utilize the same amino acid.
5. Testosterone influences microsomal enzyme-mediated metabolism of chloroform to give greater metabolism in males.
6. Of unknown origin.
7. β-Naphthoflavone is also a putative chemopreventive agent.
8. Alcohol is a potent enzyme inducer in relation to drug use and abuse. Naturally occurring inhibitors, such as the flavonoid found in grapefruit juice, is a potent inhibitor of $CYP_{450}3A4$.

Bibliography

Belcher, J., Mclean, K., Matthews, S., Woodward, L., Fisher, K., Rigby, S., Nelson, D., Potts, D., Baynham, M., Parker, D., Leys, D. and Munro, A., Structure and biochemical properties of the alkene producing cytochrome P450 OleTJE (CYP152L1) from the *Jeotgalicoccus* sp 8456 bacterium. *Journal of Biological Chemistry*, 289, 2014. Doi: 10.1074/jbc.M113.527325.

Kemper, R.A., Taub, M.E., Bogdanffy, M.S., Chapter 4. Metabolism: A determinant of toxicity, in: *Principles and Methods of Toxicology*, (pp. 141–214), Hayes, A.W. (Ed.), 6th edition, Taylor & Francis, Philadelphia, PA, 2014.

Olson, K., Anderson, I., Benowitz, N., Blanc, P., Clark, R., Kearney, T., Kim-Katz, S. and Wu, A., *Poisoning and Drug Overdose*, 7th edition, McGraw-Hill, Lange, New York, 2018.

Parkinson, A., Oglivie, B.W., Buckley, D.B., Kazmi, F. and Parkinson, O., Chapter 6, biotransformation of xenobiotics, in: *Casarett and Doull's Toxicology, The Basic Science of Poisons*, (pp. 193–400), Klaassen, C.D. (Ed.), 9th edition, McGraw-Hill, New York, 2019.

Ramírez, J., Innocenti, F., Schuetz, E.G., Flockhart, D.A., Relling, M.V., Santucci, R. and Ratain, M.J., CYP2b6, CYP3a4, and CYP2c19 are responsible for the *in vitro* N-demethylation of meperidine in human liver microsomes. *Drug Metabolism and Disposition*, 32, 930–936, 2004.

Timbrell, J.A., *Principles of Biochemical Toxicology*, 4th edition, Taylor & Francis Ltd., London, 2009.

Timbrell, J.A., Marrs, T.C., Chapter 4, Biotransformation of Xenobiotics, in: *General and Applied Toxicology*, Ballantyne, B., Marrs, T. and Syversen, T. (Eds.), 3rd edition, John Wiley & Sons, London, 89–126, 2009.

Target Organ Toxicity

Chapter Outline

6.1   Introduction   87
6.2   Liver Toxicity   88
6.3   Kidney Toxicity   89
6.4   Cardiac Toxicity   89
6.5   Toxicity of the Nervous System   91
6.6   Pulmonary Toxicity   92
6.7   Direct Toxic Action: Tissue Lesions   92
6.8   Summary and Learning Objectives   93
Review Questions   93
        Short Answer Question   94
Note   94
Bibliography   94

6.1 Introduction

The mammalian liver, kidney, heart, nervous system, and lungs are common target organs for toxic compounds and serve to illustrate both the reasons that organs are targeted and the mechanisms underlying different types of toxicologic pathology. The basic mechanisms underlying toxic responses are similar in all organs and are divided into primary, secondary, and tertiary. Primary events are those occurring at the molecular level such as covalent binding to crucial macromolecules or lipid peroxidation. These reactions cause enzyme inhibition or depletion (e.g. removal of thiols with glutathione) as an example. Secondary events from chemical exposure include damage to macromolecules (e.g. deoxyribonucleic acid [DNA]) or changes in structure or function of organelles (e.g. mitochondrion or endoplasmic reticulum). Tertiary events involve **blebbing**, necrosis, apoptosis, or steatosis.

DOI: 10.1201/9781003188575-6

6.2 Liver Toxicity

Biological explanations for the liver as a target for toxic substances include its: (1) anatomical position in the body in relation to its blood supply (Figure 6.1); (2) physiological structure; (3) role in intermediary and xenobiotic metabolism; and (4) biological function.

Most toxic substances are ingested orally. Following absorption from the gastrointestinal tract (GIT), the capillary circulation surrounding the duodenum and proximal small intestine quickly transports absorbed chemicals to the liver via the portal vein – known as the "first pass phenomenon". The liver receives 25% of the systemic circulation from the heart. Chemicals are then attracted into liver cells (hepatocytes) either actively or by passive diffusion, depending on the chemical structure.

Hepatocytes, which make up the majority of liver structure, process a variety of biochemical reactions essential for functioning of the whole organism, such as protein synthesis, removal of excess nitrogen (ammonia detoxification as urea), and lipid metabolism. Interference with such essential intermediary metabolic activity by exogenous chemicals results in hepatotoxicity. Consequently, chemicals that inhibit protein synthesis are toxic to the liver. Two chemicals that produce liver abnormalities by interfering with intermediary metabolism are galactosamine, which interferes with uridine nucleoside synthesis, and ethionine, which blocks the recycling of adenosine in the methionine cycle. Hepatotoxic chemicals

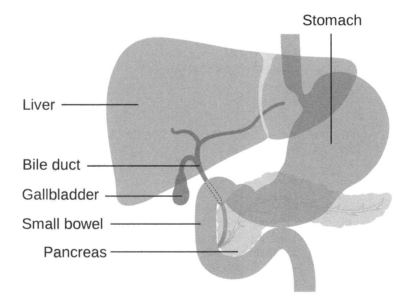

Figure 6.1 Diagram of the mammalian liver and its relation to the stomach and circulatory system. (Cancer research, UK., https://commons.wikimedia.org/wiki/File: Diagram_showing_the_ position_of_the_liver_and_the_gallbladder_CRUK_351. svg. Creative Commons© CC 3.0.)

also reduce lipid transport from the liver because of inhibition of protein synthesis. For example, interaction of the solvent carbon tetrachloride results in accumulation of fat in the liver (fatty liver or steatosis) via this mechanism.

Hepatocytes are active in metabolism of xenobiotic chemicals producing reactive intermediates in the process. Direct targeting of hepatocytes by chemicals such as the solvent carbon tetrachloride, for example, renders the liver as a primary focus of toxicity. The solvent is metabolized to a reactive **free radical** that damages the endoplasmic reticulum, and hence disrupts protein synthesis. Other examples discussed in subsequent chapters are acetaminophen and vinyl chloride.

The liver also has an excretory function, producing bile, which incorporates and transports waste products. Xenobiotics and their metabolites are excreted by this route, rendering the liver as a primary target organ. As an active process, chemical concentrations reached in the bile are high, which leads to direct impairment of the bile duct. Alternatively, high doses of a chemical normally excreted into the bile saturate the excretory processes leading to accumulation and high concentrations in the hepatocyte. For instance, the diuretic drug furosemide causes dose-dependent liver necrosis in animals because of accumulation in the organ. Although the liver has resourceful capacity to recover from chemical injury, continuous chronic or high-dose acute exposure cause irreversible destruction of its cells, reversible biochemical disturbances such as fatty liver (hydrazine), immune-mediated pathology (halothane), or development of cancer (vinyl chloride).

6.3 Kidney Toxicity

Another common target organ for toxic effects of chemicals is the kidneys. Like the liver, the kidney has a relatively high metabolic activity and blood flow and is an excretory organ. Compounds, such as the heavy metal mercury and the antibiotic drug gentamycin, cause kidney damage by concentrating within the organ. The industrial chemical hexachlorobutadiene undergoes metabolism in the kidney producing a reactive metabolite that damages mitochondria in proximal tubular cells.

6.4 Cardiac Toxicity

The important functions of the cardiovascular system include:

1. Maintenance of the cardiac pump;
2. Preservation of vascular integrity; and
3. Conservation of blood volume and composition, including water and electrolyte balance.

The extensive network of blood flow is initiated through the vasculature that extends between the heart and peripheral tissues. The vasculature is divided into a pulmonary circuit, which transports blood through the gas exchange surfaces of the lungs, and a systemic circuit, which carries blood throughout the rest of the body. To maintain the complete circuit continuously from the pulmonary to the systemic circulations, venous blood returns to the heart and must complete the pulmonary circuit to become oxygenated before reentering the systemic circuit.

Consequently, a toxic chemical enters and is maintained in the systemic circulation by the pumping action of the heart. Through this dynamic circulation propelled by the heart, compounds have access to target organs, including the heart. Most substances that interact with the cardiovascular system also have cardiac specificity. In fact, drugs that have been developed to improve cardiac function also have the potential for cardiac toxicity. For instance, digoxin is derived from the leaves of the common foxglove plant, *Digitalis purpurea*. The drug remains widely used today in the face of increasing rates of heart failure despite the emergence of newer medications. Its narrow therapeutic index and toxicity, however, have become more relevant as aging, comorbid diseases, and multiple drug ingestion increase patient population vulnerability.

Table 6.1 outlines some therapeutic drugs that cause significant cardiac toxicity.

Table 6.1 Features and Characteristics of Therapeutic Drug Classes with Significant Cardiac Toxicity

Classification	Compound Example	Indications[a]	Mechanism of Action	Signs & Symptoms of Toxicity
Digitalis glycosides	Digoxin	CHF	Positive inotropic[a] effect; decreases sympathetic NS activity	Bradycardia, prolongation of conduction, heart block
β-Adrenergic receptor antagonists (β-blocker)	Propranolol	Cardiac arrhythmias; hypertension	β1 receptor inhibition	Bradycardia, decreased cardiac contraction, hypotension
Anti-arrhythmic agents	Procain-amide	Cardiac arrhythmias	Decrease conduction velocity	Tachycardia, ventricular fibrillation
	Amiodarone	Cardiac arrhythmias	Prolong cardiac action potential	Bradycardia, hypotension Respiratory depression
Barbiturates	Secobarbital	Sedative/ hypnotics	Bind to GABA$_A$ receptors	CNS depression, coma

[a] Indications refers to pathology conditions for which the drug is approved for use; Inotropic is the force of contraction of the heart.

Abbreviations: β, beta; CHF, congestive heart failure; CNS, central nervous system; GABA$_A$, gamma-amino butyric acid, inhibitory neurotransmitter.

6.5 Toxicity of the Nervous System

The development of **psychoactive drugs** has been prompted by understanding the mechanisms of neurotoxicants that target the same receptors. Thus the study of neurophysiology explains many concepts of how neurotoxicants exert their pathologic effects. Figure 6.2 is a representative diagram of the neuron and some of its components. Examination of the components of the neuron makes it possible to envision the types of damage, a neurotoxic agent is capable of eliciting. Some pathologic effects include: neuronopathies, axonopathies, myelopathies, and interference with neurotransmission.

Table 6.2 classifies select important neurotoxic agents according to these major categories and their sites of action. The agents are chemically and

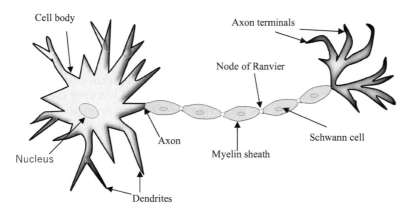

Figure 6.2 Schematic diagram of the neuron, the functional cell unit of the nervous system. (Barile, 2019.)

Table 6.2 Toxic Agents, Mechanisms, and Anatomical Sites of Neurotoxicity

Representative Toxic Agents	Mechanism of Neurotoxicity	Anatomical Sites of Toxic Action
Doxorubicin, methyl mercury, catecholamines, MPTP[a]	Neuropathy	Spinal ganglia, autonomic ganglia, visual cortex, cerebellum; midbrain, thalamic, hypothalamic centers
Carbon disulfide, acrylamide, chloroquine, lithium, organophosphates	Axonopathy	Central and peripheral NS axons, ascending and descending spinal cord axons
Hexachlorophene, lead	Myelopathy	Central and peripheral myelinated axons
Nicotine, cocaine, amphetamines	Interference with neurotransmission	Central cognitive and motor centers; adrenergic and cholinergic systems

[a] MPTP = 1-methyl-4-phenyl-1,2,3,6-tetrahydropyridine (causes Parkinson-like syndrome).

therapeutically unrelated representing a variety of classifications, such as the anticancer drug doxorubicin and the metal methylmercury. Their action uniformly affects any aspect of the central (CNS), autonomic and peripheral nervous systems (PNS), thus leading to a variety of complications and effects, including but not limited to:

- CNS and PNS effects – headache, depression, memory loss, cognition, behavioral consequences, spinal reflexes;
- motor effects – **ataxia** (muscular incoordination), muscular movement, paralysis, **paresthesias**, pain;
- autonomic nervous system (ANS) – effects on sympathetic and parasympathetic systems involving adrenergic and cholinergic neurons (motor, hormonal, and behavioral effects).

6.6 Pulmonary Toxicity

The pulmonary system is composed of at least 40 different cell types that are readily exposed to chemicals. The lungs have unique features that categorize them as a target for chemicals, including direct airborne exposure, high surface areas for absorption of volatile and particulate substances (e.g. asbestos), increased volume of blood flow, and significant metabolic activity. In addition, high oxygen concentrations and particle uptake mechanisms render the lungs more susceptible to primary chemical substance injury (e.g. herbicide paraquat).[1]

6.7 Direct Toxic Action: Tissue Lesions

Direct toxicity to tissues results in tissue damage often manifested as necrosis. **Necrosis** is an irreversible process during which the cell degenerates, the nucleus becomes fragmented and proteins denature. The cells swell, accumulate fluid, undergo cell lysis and contents leak out. The underlying mechanism involves derangement of biochemical pathways or the production of reactive intermediates which interact directly with cellular components such as enzymes or structural proteins. Highly reactive compounds also react with cell membranes and cause instant cell death by damaging the membrane sufficiently to allow rapid loss of contents and influx of external ions. Some toxic compounds interfere directly with vital cellular functions such as respiration, which results in rapid cell death. Toxicity occurs either acutely or chronically, causing cell death to occur more slowly (e.g. lead).

An alternative mode of cell death is apoptosis, i.e. programmed cell death. Understood to be part of biological tissue turnover and renewal, apoptosis is also stimulated by toxic chemicals. One apparent function of apoptosis is removal of damaged DNA which cannot be repaired, which triggers activation of the process. Severe damage to the cell compromises the apoptotic process developing into necrosis. Apoptosis involves production of specific proteins resulting from expression of regulatory genes (e.g. *fos*, *myc*, *max*, and *jun*). The process involves condensation of chromatin and cytoplasmic components, fragmentation of DNA, and inhibition of cell division. The cell contracts as a result, disconnects from neighboring cells, and is removed by phagocytosis. Consequently, there is no inflammatory response.

Dermal toxicity represents a version of direct tissue injury, commonly associated with industrial chemicals. Chemically-induced skin reactions are associated with direct toxicity leading to sensitization, irritation, and corrosion. After a single insult to the epidermis, the primary response is a local inflammatory reaction. Acute inflammation is the immediate response to a sensitizing or irritant chemical, and is characterized by dilation of subcutaneous blood vessels, increased blood flow, accumulation of fluid in the epidermal and dermal tissues, and invasion of white blood cells. The resulting symptoms are milder in a sensitization reaction but lead to redness, heat, pain, and swelling. Corrosive chemicals, such as liquid or solid sodium hydroxide, however, cause more extensive reactions of tissues.

6.8 Summary and Learning Objectives

Many organs are specifically targeted by toxic agents, such as the **liver**, **kidney**, **heart**, and **nervous systems**, primarily a result of metabolic role, anatomical position, structure, and function. Hepatocytes are metabolically active cells but are damaged by compounds that produce steatosis, necrosis, and damage to the biliary system. The kidney is a target due to its high metabolic activity and role in elimination of waste. Toxic effects in organs and tissues involve primary (e.g. lipid peroxidation), secondary (e.g. damage to specific proteins or DNA), and tertiary (e.g. necrosis) events.

Direct tissue damage and pathology result from *local corrosion* or *systemic effects* leading to liver necrosis, often due to direct interaction with macromolecules. Apoptosis is programmed cell death designed to protect the organs from chemical trauma and from aging.

Biochemical lesions are due to interference with a specific enzyme or pathways which lead to cell dysfunction and death of the organism. Some effects are reversible such as the interaction of carbon monoxide with hemoglobin. Pathological lesions such as steatosis and phospholipidosis are the result of biochemical lesions.

Pharmacological or physiological effects such as changes in blood pressure or vascular dilation are often due to neurotoxic agents with specific target actions. However, effects such as bronchoconstriction and production of excessive amounts of secretions may also occur with other chemicals that affect the ANS, such as organophosphate pesticides.

Review Questions

1. Choose the most appropriate answer for the question. Which of the following is *most important* in determining the extent of toxicity of a chemical: (a) chemical structure; (b) dose; (c) metabolism; (d) excretion; (e) metabolic detoxification.

2. Indicate which of the following is/are true. The liver is a target organ for toxic effects of chemicals because of its: (a) highly complex structure; (b) ability to metabolize chemicals; (c) blood supply; (d) excretory function; (e) low levels of glutathione.

3. Choose the most appropriate answer for the question. The most common toxic response of the liver following exposure to chemicals is: (a) cancer; (b) cholestasis; (c) blebbing; (d) necrosis of sinusoidal cells; (e) steatosis.

Short Answer Question

4. Describe the cardiac toxicity associated with the cardiac drug, digoxin.

Note

1. The blood–brain barrier (BBB) however is organized to exclude polar chemicals, most drugs and inorganic molecules.

Bibliography

Aldridge, W.N. Chapter 2. Stages in Induction of Toxicity, in: *Mechanisms and Concepts in Toxicology*, (pp. 10–15), Taylor & Francis, London, 1996.

Barile, F.A. Chapter 4. Classifications of toxins in humans, in: *Barile's Clinical Toxicology: Principles and Mechanisms*, (pp. 47–68), 3rd edition, Barile, F.A. (Ed.), CRC Press, Taylor & Francis, New York, 2019.

Campen, M.J., Chapter 18. Toxic responses of the heart and vascular system, in: *Casarett and Doull's Toxicology, The Basic Science of Poisons*, (pp. 909–952), Klaassen, C.D. (Ed.), 9th edition, McGraw-Hill, New York, 2019.

Gardner, D.E., Toxicology of the lung, 4th edition, in: *Target Organ Toxicology Series*, A.W. Hayes, J.A. Thomas, D.E. Gardner (series editors), CRC Press, Taylor and Francis, Boca Raton, FL, 2005.

Glaister, J.R., *Principles of Toxicological Pathology*, Taylor & Francis, London, 1986.

Harry, G.J., and Tilson, H.A., Neurotoxicology, 3rd edition, in: *Target Organ Toxicology Series*, A.W. Hayes, J.A. Thomas, D.E. Gardner (series editors), CRC Press, Taylor and Francis, Boca Raton, FL, 2016.

Plaa, G.L., and Hewitt, W.R., Toxicology of the liver, 2nd edition, in: *Target Organ Toxicology Series*, A.W. Hayes, J.A. Thomas, D.E. Gardner (series editors), Routledge/CRC Press, Taylor and Francis, Boca Raton, FL, 1998.

Timbrell, J.A., Biomarkers in Toxicology. *Toxicology* 129, 1–12, 1998.

Timbrell, J.A., *Principles of Biochemical Toxicology*, 4th edition, Taylor & Francis Ltd, London, 2009.

Turton, J.A. and Hooson, J. (Eds.), *Target Organ Pathology*, Taylor & Francis, London, 1998.

Chapter 7

Carcinogenic and Mutagenic Compounds

Chapter Outline

This chapter discusses potential, suspected, and known teratogenic and mutagenic drugs and chemicals to which humans and animals are exposed.

7.1	Introduction	95
7.2	Mechanisms of Chemical Carcinogenesis and Mutagenesis	96
7.3	DNA Repair Mechanisms	98
7.4	Multistage Carcinogenesis	98
7.5	Chemical Carcinogens	99
7.6	Cancer Chemopreventive Agents	100
7.7	Summary and Learning Objectives	101
	Review Questions	101
	Notes	102
	Bibliography	102
	Review Articles	103
	Suggested Readings	105

7.1 Introduction

Cancer is an arrangement of diseases where uncontrolled proliferation of cells expresses varying degrees of faithfulness to their precursor cells of origin. This cell proliferation occurs in almost all tissues throughout a lifespan and is influenced by a variety of circumstances. Mutations in deoxyribonucleic acid (DNA), caused by the influence of suspect or known chemicals, have the potential to lead to cancer development by disrupting its normal regulation. Thus, the carcinogenic process is often a response to a mutation occurring within the genetic material of normal cells, resulting in uncontrolled cell division and transformation to the immortal phenotype. Consequently, the initiation of a cancer is due to an abnormal and uncontrolled progression of cells.

Carcinogenesis represents the unwarranted appearance or increased incidence of abnormal cell proliferation. A **carcinogen** is any chemical or viral agent that increases the frequency or distribution of new tumors, results in their appearance within a low-risk group, or results in the introduction of new pathological growths otherwise absent in normal populations or experimental controls.

Most chemical carcinogens require metabolic activation before demonstrating carcinogenic potential. As with most toxic phenomena, a minimum dosage is necessary to elicit a carcinogenic event. Mutagenesis refers to the ability of a virus or chemical agent to induce changes in the genetic sequence of mammalian or bacterial cells, thus altering the phenotypic expression of cell characteristics. Genotoxicity is the ability of an agent to induce heritable changes in genes that normally exercise homeostatic control in somatic cells. Genotoxic substances induce genotoxicity by either binding directly to DNA or by indirectly altering the DNA sequence resulting in irreversible damage. It is also important to note, however, that genotoxic substances are not necessarily carcinogenic.

The causes of most human cancers remain unidentified; however, considerable evidence suggests that besides chemical agents, environmental and lifestyle factors are important contributors. For example, tobacco smoking is responsible for approximately 30% of all cancer deaths in developed countries.

Thus, understanding the molecular and cellular processes underlying chemical carcinogenesis and mutagenesis is of critical importance for carcinogenic development.

7.2 Mechanisms of Chemical Carcinogenesis and Mutagenesis

The induction of a neoplasm[1] is a multistage process that occurs over a long period of time, the stages of which include initiation, promotion, and progression (Figure 7.1). Carcinogenic agents initiate cancer progression through one of two pathways:

1. parent chemicals cause cancers directly, such as heavy metals;
2. some chemicals require metabolic activation to reactive intermediates to affect the carcinogenic process (*procarcinogens*); e.g. organic chemicals, such as benzo(a)pyrene, are first converted to an electrophilic intermediate which then covalently binds to cellular macromolecules. Figure 7.2 illustrates the metabolic activation of benzo(a)pyrene. The multistage process is discussed in further detail below.

Cytochrome P450 phase I and phase II enzymes are involved in the metabolism of carcinogens and usually result in the formation of reactive metabolites. Phase II enzyme-catalyzed reactions often lead to detoxification and elimination, which

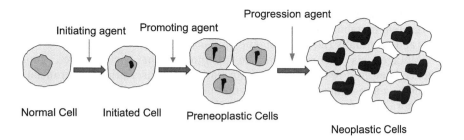

Figure 7.1 Multistage process for chemical carcinogenesis illustrating the initiation, promotion, and progression processes.

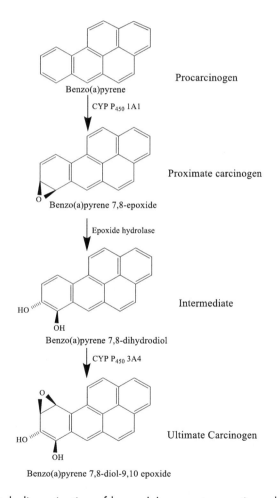

Figure 7.2 Metabolic activation of benzo(a)pyrene to reactive substrates.

usually protect against chemical carcinogenesis. The constant assault of cells with reactive metabolites over time leads to interaction with cellular macromolecules and eventually the carcinogenic process.

Mutagenesis occurs when the mammalian or bacterial cell genetic sequence is altered resulting in transformation of transcription and translation. This induces a modification of the phenotypic expression of cell characteristics, which more often results in permanent pathologic changes rather than beneficial adjustments. In general, carcinogens are separated into genotoxic and nongenotoxic classifications. Thus, a genotoxic carcinogen interacts with DNA directly, leading to mutations. The production of mutations is due primarily to chemical or physical alterations in the structure of DNA that result in inaccurate replication of that gene. In contrast, nongenotoxic (epigenetic) carcinogens do not directly affect DNA in the induction of cancer.[2]

7.3 DNA Repair Mechanisms

Interaction of carcinogens with DNA results in the formation of various DNA adducts, which prompts the cellular machinery to repair the structural alteration. It is estimated that more than one hundred genes are dedicated to DNA repair, the purpose of which is to correct the structural damage induced by carcinogens, thus preventing mutagenesis. Alternatively, the persistence of DNA-carcinogen adducts is indicative of the insufficiency of DNA repair.

7.4 Multistage Carcinogenesis

The process of carcinogenesis is divided into three experimentally defined stages: *tumor initiation, tumor promotion,* and *tumor progression.* This multistage development of carcinogenesis requires the conversion of benign hyperplastic[3] cells to the malignant state, involving invasion and metastasis as manifestations of further genetic changes.

Tumor initiation by a chemical involves irreversible genetic alterations. The formation of a carcinogen-DNA adduct is central to the theory of chemical carcinogenesis and is a prerequisite for tumor initiation. The formation of DNA adducts causes either *activation* of a proto-oncogene or *inactivation* of a tumor-suppressor gene. One important characteristic of this stage is its irreversibility, such that the genotype/phenotype of the initiated cell is conferred during the process. Chemicals capable of initiating cells are referred to as initiating agents.

Tumor promotion comprises the selective clonal expansion of initiated cells through a mechanism of gene activation. Tumor promoters are generally non-mutagenic, are not solely carcinogenic, and often are able to mediate their biological effects without metabolic activation. In addition, they do not directly interact with DNA. Interestingly, tumor promotion is reversible, although the continued presence of the promoting agent maintains the state of the promoted cell population (pre-neoplastic lesion). Examples of typical tumor promoters include tetradecanoyl phorbol acetate (TPA), phenobarbital, and 2,3,7,8-tetrachlorodibenzo-ρ-dioxin (TCDD).

Tumor progression comprises the expression of the malignant phenotype and the tendency of malignant cells to acquire more aggressive characteristics over time. Further genetic changes occur, including the activation of proto-oncogenes and the functional loss of tumor-suppressor genes. It is important to note that it is the accumulation of these mutations, and not the order or the stage of tumorigenesis in which they occur, that appears to be the determining factor.

7.5 Chemical Carcinogens

Chemical carcinogens are classified according to their chemical characteristics, such as:

1. **Organic chemicals**: Benzo(a)pyrene, aflatoxin B1, and benzene;
2. **Inorganic chemicals:** Arsenic, cadmium, chromium, and nickel; and
3. **Hormonal substances:** Estrogens, anabolic, and androgenic steroids.

Furthermore, chemical carcinogens are classified as genotoxic or non-genotoxic (epigenetic) carcinogens, based on reactivity with DNA, or as animal or human carcinogens, depending on evidence of carcinogenicity in animals and humans. The International Association for Research on Cancer (IARC) evaluates and categorizes human carcinogens accordingly:

Group 1 – these agents have sufficient epidemiological evidence of carcinogenicity in humans; as such they are labeled as known human carcinogens; e.g. arsenic, aflatoxin B1, benzene, estrogens, vi1nyl chloride, nickel, and chromium;

Group 2A – these substances possess sufficient evidence of carcinogenicity in animals, but have limited evidence of carcinogenicity in humans, therefore labeled as probably carcinogenic to humans; e.g. benz(a) anthracence, polychlorinated biphenols, and styrene oxide;

Group 2B – possess either limited evidence of carcinogenicity in humans, or have sufficient evidence of carcinogenicity in animals and inadequate evidence of carcinogenicity in humans; labeled as possibly carcinogenic to humans; e.g. styrene, urethane;

Group 3 – this group is not classifiable as to carcinogenicity;

Group 4 – these chemicals possess inadequate evidence of carcinogenicity in both animals and humans, and thus are probably not carcinogenic to humans.

Not all carcinogenic chemicals are equally successful in inducing neoplasia, i.e. they exhibit different carcinogenic potencies. The carcinogenic potential of a chemical is defined as the slope of the dose-response curve for induction of neoplasms. This definition, however, is not sufficient for estimating carcinogenic potential based on data from chronic carcinogenesis bioassays. Historically, several methods have been developed to measure the carcinogenic potential, particularly the tumorigenesis dose rate 50 (TD_{50}). This value has been popular for the estimation of the carcinogenic potential of several chemicals. The TD_{50} is calculated as the dose rate (mg/kg body weight/day) of carcinogen, which when administered chronically for a standard period, induces neoplasms in half of the test animals. The value is adjusted for spontaneous neoplasms and is an important component of carcinogenic risk assessment.

Approximating carcinogenic risk based on uncomplicated laboratory data requires major assumptions to extrapolate carcinogenic information from bioassays and **epidemiology** to humans. The actual levels of human exposure to a particular potential carcinogenic chemical are generally much lower than those used in laboratory animal experiments. Therefore, applying the carcinogenic data obtained in animals treated with high doses of a test substance to the carcinogenic potential in humans whose exposure to that agent is considerably lower poses a significant hurdle in extrapolation statistics.

Of the various environmental hazardous compounds, cigarette smoke enjoys the highest causal relationship with cancer risk in humans. Tobacco smoking plays a major role in the etiology of lung, oral cavity, and esophageal cancers, as well as a variety of chronic degenerative diseases. Although cigarette smoke is a mixture of about 4,000 chemicals, including more than 60 known human carcinogens, 4-methylnitrosamino-1-(3-pyridyl)-1-butanone (nicotine-derived nitrosamine ketone, NNK) is the most carcinogenic tobacco-specific nitrosamine. NNK induces lung tumors in mice, rats, and hamsters, and the International Agency for Research on Cancer has designated NNK and NNN (N-nitrosonornicotine) as known human carcinogens. NNK is metabolically activated by CYP P-450 enzymes in the lung and generates O6-methylguanine in DNA. The reaction generates G:C to A:T mutations, with the subsequent activation of K-Ras proto-oncogene and development of tumor initiation.

Radiation also contributes to the causative physical factors that induce human cancers. Radiation promotes double-strand breaks (DSBs) in DNA that lead to chromosome aberrations and cell death and generate a variety of oxidative DNA damage. Because of its genotoxicity potential, radiation at high doses evidently results in the appearance of various tumors in humans. Even at low doses, residential exposure to radioactive radon and its decay products, for instance, accounts for about 10%–20% of all lung cancer deaths worldwide.

7.6 Cancer Chemopreventive Agents

Several potential targets for cancer chemoprevention have recently been identified. Chemopreventive agents most often cited include:

1. selective estrogen receptor modulators, such as tamoxifen and raloxifene;
2. anti-inflammatory agents, including aspirin and celecoxib;

3. antioxidants and phase 2 enzyme-inducers, such as vitamin C, vitamin E, omega-3 fatty acids, isothiocyanates, and dithiolethiones; and
4. agents that selectively modulate cellular receptors and signal transduction, such as retinoids and vitamin D analogs.

The mechanisms underlying the protective effects against a particular carcinogen operate according to the following:

1. mechanisms leading to *alteration of toxicokinetics* of carcinogens; and,
2. mechanisms resulting in the *inhibition of the multistages* of carcinogenesis.

Chemopreventive agents alter carcinogen toxicokinetics by either inhibiting the absorption of carcinogens or increasing their detoxification. This is actuated primarily by inducing phase 2 and antioxidative enzymes. Alternatively, chemopreventive drugs inhibit the three stages of carcinogenesis, i.e. initiation, promotion, and progression, by modulating a number of cellular mechanisms, and pathways, such as (1) stimulation of DNA repair, (2) inhibition of cell proliferation, (3) stimulation of immune system, and (4) inhibition of neovascularization.

7.7 Summary and Learning Objectives

The causes of most human cancers remain unidentified; however, considerable evidence suggests that besides chemical agents, environmental and lifestyle factors are important contributors. For example, tobacco smoking appears to be responsible for approximately 30% of all cancer deaths in developed countries. Thus, understanding the processes underlying chemical carcinogenesis and mutagenesis is of critical importance for cancer development.

Chemical mutagenesis involves changes in the genetic sequence of mammalian cells with subsequent alteration of the phenotypic expression of cell characteristics. A *genotoxic* chemical induces heritable changes in genes that normally exercise homeostatic control in mammalian cells. Genotoxic substances induce genotoxicity by either binding directly to DNA or by indirectly altering the DNA sequence resulting in irreversible damage. Genotoxic substances are not necessarily carcinogenic.

Review Questions

1. Match the following terms on the left with its description in the right column:

Aneuploidization	addition or alteration of the number of base pairs
Clastogenesis	loss or acquisition of a complete chromosome
Mutagenesis	loss, addition, or rearrangement of parts of chromosomes

2. Describe the multistage process of carcinogenesis. Indicate the stages and chemicals involved for each stage.

Notes

1. Refers to an abnormal "new growth" of cells or tissues.
2. The National Toxicology Program (NTP) report on chemical carcinogenicity estimates that 40% of chemicals classified as carcinogens are non-genotoxic (epigenetic) carcinogens, with the liver as the most common target organ (NTP, 2009).
3. An increased growth in the number of abnormal cells.

Bibliography

Au, W.W., Usefulness of biomarkers in population studies: From exposure to susceptibility and to prediction of cancer, *International Journal of Hygiene and Environmental Health*, 210, 239, 2007. Doi: 10.1016/j.ijheh.2006.11.001.

da Costa, A.N. and Herceg, Z. Detection of cancer-specific epigenomic changes in biofluids: Powerful tools in biomarker discovery and application. *Molecular Onolology*, 6, 704, 2012. Doi: 10.1016/j.molonc.2012.07.005.

Jacobson-Kram, D. and Contrera, J.F., Genetic toxicity assessment: Employing the best science for human safety evaluation. Part I: Early screening for potential human mutagens, *Toxicological Sciences*, 96, 16, 2007. Doi: 10.1093/toxsci/kfl191.

Kirkland, D.J, Aardema, M., Banduhn, N., Carmichael, P., Fautz, R., Meunier, J-R. and Pfuhler, S., *In vitro* approaches to develop weight of evidence (WoE) and mode of action (MoA) discussions with positive *in vitro* genotoxicity results, *Mutagenesis*, 22, 161, 2007. DOI: 10.1093/mutage/gem006

Klaunig, J.E., Acrylamide carcinogenicity, *Journal Agricultural Food Chemistry*, 56, 5984, 2008. Doi: 10.1021/jf8004492.

Little, M.P., Heidenreich, W.F., Moolgavkar, S.H., Schöllnberger, H. and Thomas, D.C., Systems biological and mechanistic modelling of radiation-induced cancer, *Radiation and Environmental Biophysics*, 47, 39, 2008. Doi: 10.1007/s00411-007-0150-z.

Lorge, E., Lorge, E., Gervais, V., Becourt-Lhote, N., Maisonneuve, C., Delongeas, J-L. and Claude, N., Genetic toxicity assessment: Employing the best science for human safety evaluation part IV: A strategy in genotoxicity testing in drug development: Some examples, *Toxicological Sciences*, 98, 39, 2007. Doi: 10.1093/toxsci/kfm056.

Marks, F., Fürstenberger, G. and Müller-Decker, K., Tumor promotion as a target of cancer prevention, *Recent Results Cancer Research*, 174, 37, 2007. Doi: 10.1007/978-3-540-37696-5_3

National Toxicology Program (NTP), Department of Health and Human Services, Report on Carcinogens (RoC), http://ntp.niehs.nih.gov, 2009. Last accessed November 2022.

Nishigori, C., Hattori, Y. and Toyokuni, S., Role of reactive oxygen species in skin carcinogenesis, *Antioxidants Redox Signaling*, 6, 561, 2004. Doi: 10.1089/152308604773934314.

Nomura, T., Transgenerational effects from exposure to environmental toxic substances, *Mutation Research*, 659, 185, 2008. Doi: 10.1016/j.mrrev.2008.03.004.

O'Brien, J., Renwick, A.G., Constable, A., Dybing, E., Müller, D.J.G., Schlatter, J., Slob, D., Tueting, W., van Benthem, J., Williams, G.M. and Wolfreys, A., Approaches to the risk assessment of genotoxic carcinogens in food: A critical appraisal, *Food Chemical Toxicology*, 44, 1613, 2006. Doi: 10.1016/j.fct.2006.07.004.

Romani, M., Pistillo, M.P. and Banelli, B., Environmental Epigenetics: Crossroad between Public Health, Lifestyle, and Cancer Prevention. *Biomedical Research International*, 587983, 2015. Doi: 10.1155/2015/587983.

Siddiqui, I.A., Afaq, F., Adhami, V.M. and Mukhtar, H., Prevention of prostate cancer through custom tailoring of chemopreventive regimen, *Chemical Biological Interactions*, 171, 122, 2008. Doi: 10.1016/j.cbi.2007.03.001.

Trosko, J.E., Dietary modulation of the multistage, multi-mechanisms of human carcinogenesis: Effects on initiated stem cells and cell-cell communication, *Nutrition Cancer*, 54, 102, 2006. Doi: 10.1207/s15327914nc5401_12

Valavanidis, A., Fiotakis, K. and Vlachogianni, T., Airborne particulate matter and human health: Toxicological assessment and importance of size and composition of particles for oxidative damage and carcinogenic mechanisms, *Journal Environmental Sciences and Health: C. Environmental Carcinogens Ecotoxicology Reviews*, 26, 339, 2008. Doi: 10.1080/10590500802494538.

Wu, K.M., Ghantous, H. and Birnkrant, D.B., Current regulatory toxicology perspectives on the development of herbal medicines to prescription drug products in the United States, *Food Chemical Toxicology*, 46, 2606, 2008. Doi: 10.1016/j.fct.2008.05.029.

Review Articles

Bode, A.M. and Dong, Z., Molecular and cellular targets, *Molecular Carcinogenesis*, 45, 422, 2006. Doi: 10.1002/mc.20222.

Carnero, A., Blanco-Aparicio, C., Kondoh, H., Lleonart, M. E., Martinez-Leal, J. F., Mondello, C., Scovassi, A. I., Bisson, W. H., Amedei, A., Roy, R., Woodrick, J., Colacci, A., Vaccari, M., Raju, J., Al-Mulla, F., Al-Temaimi, R., Salem, H. K., Memeo, L., Forte, S., Singh, N., Hamid, R.A., Ryan, E.P., Brown, D.G., Wise, J.P. Sr., Wise, S.S. and Yasaei, H. Disruptive chemicals, senescence and immortality, *Carcinogenesis*, 36, S19, 2015. Doi: 10.1093/carcin/bgv029.

Christofori, G., New signals from the invasive front, *Nature*, 441, 444, 2006. Doi: 10.1038/nature04872.

Claxton, L.D. and Woodall, G.M. Jr., A review of the mutagenicity and rodent carcinogenicity of ambient air, *Mutation Research*, 636, 36, 2007. Doi: 10.1016/j. mrrev.2007.01.001.

Ghanayem, B.I. and Hoffler, U., Investigation of xenobiotics metabolism, genotoxicity, and carcinogenicity using Cyp2e1(-/-) mice, *Currents Drug Metabolism*, 8, 728, 2007. Doi: 10.2174/138920007782109760.

Goodson, W.H. III, Lowe, L., Carpenter, D.O., Gilbertson, M., Manaf Ali, A., Lopez de Cerain Salsamendi, A., Lasfar, A., Carnero, A., Azqueta, A., Amedei, A. and Charles, A.K., Assessing the carcinogenic potential of low-dose exposures to chemical mixtures in the environment: The challenge ahead. *Carcinogenesis*, 36, S254, 2015. Doi: 10.1093/carcin/bgv039.

Gonzalez, F.J. and Kimura, S., Study of P450 function using gene knockout and transgenic mice, *Archives Biochemistry Biophysics*, 409, 153, 2003. Doi: 10.1016/s0003-9861(02)00364-8.

Guengerich, F.P., Forging the links between metabolism and carcinogenesis, *Mutation Research*, 488, 195, 2001. Doi: 10.1016/s1383-5742(01)00059-x.

Hengstler, J.G., Bogdanffy, M.S., Bolt, H.M. and Oesch, F., Challenging dogma: Thresholds for genotoxic chemicals? The case of vinyl acetate, *Annual Reviews Pharmacology Toxicology*, 43, 485, 2003. Doi: 10.1146/annurev. pharmtox.43.100901.140219.

Kuper, H., Boffetta, P. and Adami, H.O., Tobacco use and cancer causation: Association by tumor type, *Journal Internal Medicine*, 252, 206, 2002. Doi: 10.1046/j.1365-2796.2002.01022.x.

Laconi, E., Doratiotto, S. and Vineis, P., The microenvironments of multistage carcinogenesis, *Seminars Cancer Biology*, 18, 322, 2008. Doi: 10.1016/j. semcancer.2008.03.019.

Mohan, C.G., Gandhi, T., Garg, D. and Shinde, R., Computer-assisted methods in chemical toxicity prediction, *Miniature Reviews Medicinal Chemistry*, 7, 499, 2007. Doi: 10.2174/138955707780619554.

Preston, R.J., Quantitation of molecular endpoints for the dose-response component of cancer risk assessment, *Toxicological Pathology*, 30, 112, 2002. Doi: 10.1080/01926230252824798

Preston, R.J. and Williams, G.M., DNA-reactive carcinogens: Mode of action and human cancer hazard, *Critical Reviews Toxicology*, 35, 673, 2005. Doi: 10.1080/10408440591007278.

Richardson, S.D., Plewa, M.J., Wagner, E.D., Schoeny, R. and Demarini, D.M., Occurrence, genotoxicity, and carcinogenicity of regulated and emerging disinfection by-products in drinking water: A review and roadmap for research, *Mutation Research*, 636, 178, 2007. Doi: 10.1016/j.mrrev.2007.09.001.

Saha, S.K., Lee, S.B., Won, J., Choi, H.Y., Kim, K., Yang, G-M., Dayem, A.A. and Cho, S-G., Correlation between oxidative stress, nutrition, and cancer initiation, *International Journal Molecular Sciences*, 18, 1544, 2017. Doi: 10.3390/ijms18071544.

Shaughnessy, D.T., McAllister, K., Worth, L., Haugen, A.C., Meyer, J.N., Domann, F.E., Van Houten, B., Mostoslavsky, R., Bultman, S.J., Baccarelli, A.A., Begley, T.J., Sobol, R.W., Hirschey, M.D., Ideker, T., Santos, J.H., Copeland,

W.C., Tice, R.R., Balshaw, D.M. and Tyson, F.L., Mitochondria, energetics, epigenetics, and cellular responses to stress, *Environmental Health Perspectives*, 122, 1271, 2014. Doi: 10.1289/ehp.1408418.

Sporn, M.B. and Suh, N., Chemoprevention: An essential approach to controlling cancer, *Nature Reviews: Cancer*, 2, 537, 2002. Doi: 10.1038/nrc844

Suggested Readings

Atienzar, F.A. and Jha, A.N., The random amplified polymorphic DNA (RAPD) assay and related techniques applied to genotoxicity and carcinogenesis studies: A critical review, *Mutation Research*, 613, 76, 2006. Doi: 10.1016/j.mrrev.2006.06.001.

Gately, S. and Li, W.W., Multiple roles of COX-2 in tumor angiogenesis: A target for antiangiogenic therapy, *Seminars in Oncology*, 31, 2, 2004. Doi: 10.1016/j.ijheh.2006.11.001.

Klaunig, J.E., Wang, Z., Chapter 8. Chemical carcinogenesis, in: *Casarett & Doull's Toxicology: The Basic Science of Poisons*, (pp. 433–496), Klaassen, C.D., (Ed.), 9th edition, McGraw-Hill Companies, Inc., New York, 2019.

Trosko, J.E., Chang, C.C., Upham, B.L. and Tai, M.H., Ignored hallmarks of carcinogenesis: Stem cells and cell-cell communication, *Annals N.Y. Academy of Sciences*, 1028, 192, 2004. Doi: 10.1196/annals.1322.023.

Chapter 8

Drugs as Toxic Substances

There are no safe drugs, only safe ways of using them. Doctors put drugs of which they know little, into our bodies of which they know less, to cure diseases of which they know nothing at all.

Voltaire

Chapter Outline

This chapter illustrates types of drug toxicity associated with historically specific drug examples:

8.1	Types of Drug Toxicity	108
8.2	Acetaminophen (Paracetamol in UK, EU)	108
8.3	Aspirin (Acetylsalicylic Acid, Acetylsalicylate, ASA)	110
8.4	Hydralazine	113
8.5	Halothane	115
8.6	Debrisoquine	116
8.7	Thalidomide	117
8.8	Drug Interactions	118
8.9	Altered Responsiveness: Glucose-6-Phosphate Dehydrogenase Deficiency	119
8.10	Summary and Learning Objectives	120
	Review Questions	121
	Short Answer Question	121
	Notes	121
	Bibliography	122
	Suggested Readings	122

DOI: 10.1201/9781003188575-8

8.1 Types of Drug Toxicity

Drugs are chemical substances *designed* to have pharmacological activity for public health benefits. However, it is common knowledge that adverse or toxic effects occur with acute, chronic, or improper administration. Consequently, because of their major contributions to human and animal health, there is a risk/benefit association with these therapeutic agents.

An historical medical tragedy first made public dramatically demonstrated the risks associated with drug treatment caused by the sedative **thalidomide**. Consequential events that resulted from improper administration during pregnancy proved to be a major watershed for awareness of drug toxicity and the need for better legislation in testing for the safety of pharmaceuticals. Events surrounding thalidomide that illustrate the problem of teratogenesis are discussed below.

There are several different types of drug toxicity: adverse drug reaction (ADR, i.e. side effects) described as regular undesirable occurrences during proper therapeutic usage; acute toxicity due to overdosage; idiosyncratic reactions which occur rarely during regular therapeutic usage; toxic effects resulting from drug interactions, physiological reactions of desired drugs in the presence of other drugs or substances administered concurrently; and unintentional habituation or abuse of drugs leading to chronic toxicity. Drug overdoses are studied within the boundaries of clinical toxicology as with accidental ingestion of hazardous substances, whereas drug abuse including use for illegal purposes is within the domain of forensic toxicology.

Basic mechanisms underlying these types of toxicity are also summarized accordingly:

1. direct, predictable toxic effects due to altered or inhibited metabolism;
2. toxic effects occurring after repeated therapeutic doses with a metabolic. pharmacological, or immunological basis;
3. direct, unpredictable toxic effects occurring after single therapeutic doses, due to idiosyncratic metabolism or a pharmacodynamic response;
4. toxicity occurring with other drugs or substances co-administered with the desired compound, interfering with the disposition or pharmacological response of the initial drug.

Examples of drug toxicity are considered below.

8.2 Acetaminophen (Paracetamol in UK, EU)

One of the most commonly used drugs involved in overdose events in the US and the UK is acetaminophen, estimated at 12.5% of all chemical substance poisonings per year. These include intentional, suicidal, and accidental poisoning. Since the medication is available over-the-counter[1], self-administration of drug without professional guidance is interpreted as harmless. In addition, patients are not aware that the compound is also a common ingredient of numerous cough and cold preparations, all of which are available OTC. Thus, repeated ingestion of

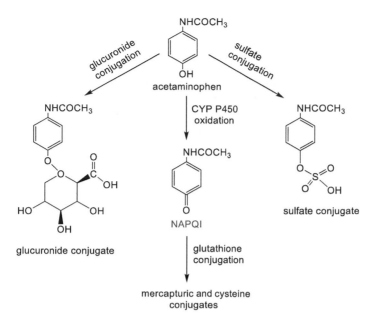

Figure 8.1 Structure and metabolism of the analgesic drug acetaminophen.

acetaminophen tablets, both as acute overdose and upon chronic administration, has led to serious consequences in many cases.

Acetaminophen is a useful and popular analgesic if ingested at recommended therapeutic doses.[2] The consequence of an acute overdose or chronic ingestion is liver damage. Understanding the mechanism underlying acetaminophen toxicity has led to development of treatment with an antidote, a method available to prevent fatal outcomes.

Acetaminophen is metabolized mainly by conjugation with sulfate and glucuronic acid. Only a minor proportion is metabolized by oxidation, catalyzed by microsomal mono-oxygenases (Figure 8.1). The latter reaction produces N-acetyl-p-benzoquinone imine (NAPQI), a toxic metabolite, which is normally detoxified by interaction with glutathione (GSH). However, experimental evidence reveals that after an overdose several changes take place in this metabolic scheme. Pathways of conjugation are saturated and cofactors, especially sulfate, are depleted. As a result, *more* acetaminophen is metabolized by the oxidative pathway yielding the toxic metabolite. Sufficient NAPQI is produced in the liver to deplete all GSH available. Therefore, the toxic metabolite reacts with liver proteins instead of GSH resulting in direct tissue damage and hepatic necrosis.

These findings suggest that a reactive metabolite of paracetamol is responsible for hepatotoxicity and covalent binding rather than the parent drug. More recent immunohistochemical studies using anti-paracetamol antibodies have shown that covalent binding of a paracetamol metabolite occurs in damaged centrilobular regions of the human liver after overdoses. There is, thus, a marked dose threshold for toxicity which occurs when hepatic GSH is depleted by at least 80% of control levels.

Several cellular target proteins for the reactive metabolite of paracetamol have distinguished cytosolic proteins from those in the endoplasmic reticulum and mitochondria. The reactive metabolite starts a cascade of events, such as increases in cytosolic Ca^{++} inhibition of various enzymes and loss of adenosine triphosphate (ATP), as well as reduction in the ability to replenish GSH, culminating in damage to critical proteins and hepatotoxicity.

Another factor of importance in relation to susceptibility to toxicity is individual variation in metabolism, possibly because of drug interactions. For example, excessive alcohol intake prior to acetaminophen overdose increases liver damage through induction of the isoenzyme of cytochrome P450 involved in metabolic activation of acetaminophen. Elucidation of this mechanism has led to development of an antidote to regenerate GSH or replace it with an alternative. Currently, the antidote, N-acetylcysteine (NAC), is administered orally or intravenously (i.v.), most effective in preventing liver damage when administered within 10–12 hours of overdose.

Further study has demonstrated that NAC: promotes the synthesis of GSH; relieves the saturation of sulfate conjugation which occurs during paracetamol overdose; is involved in the reduction of NAPQI; and, prevents further formation of oxidized protein thiols.

8.3 Aspirin (Acetylsalicylic Acid, Acetylsalicylate, ASA)

Acetylsalicylic acid, commonly known as aspirin, is widely used as a minor analgesic, alone or along with other salicylate derivatives. The drug, however, is still an important cause of human poisoning resulting both from overdoses and inappropriate therapeutic use, responsible for a significant number of deaths each year throughout the world. In children, most deaths are from therapeutic overdose, toxic effects of which are biochemical and physiological, with no clear target organ. Interestingly, aspirin poisoning illustrates how chemicals cause toxicity or lethality without damaging tissues or organs specifically.

When used repeatedly, aspirin at therapeutic doses accumulates in patients and eventually reaches toxic concentrations, explained by saturable metabolic reactions. Most of the circulating acetylsalicylic acid (ASA) is hydrolyzed by esterases to salicylic acid (Figure 8.2), followed by conjugation with glucuronic acid or glycine. However, conjugation steps are saturable and therefore elimination is reduced (GSH) as dose increases or accumulates. Figure 8.3 is a schematic diagram of the mechanism of aspirin toxicity and how it contributes to the production of metabolic acidosis.

The primary result of high serum concentrations of salicylic acid is interference with acid-base balance. The normal physiological ratio of bicarbonate ions to carbonic acid (HCO_3^-/H_2CO_3) is 20/1.[3] As salicylic acid levels rise, pH decreases, triggering a stimulation of the medullary respiratory center, resulting in an increase in ventilatory rate (hyperventilation). With a rise in respirations per minute (RPMs), the victim expels more CO_2. This increases the bicarbonate:carbonic acid ratio due to the decreasing concentrations of CO_2 and precipitates a temporary increase in blood pH (respiratory alkalosis). Accordingly, a temporary but significant response from the kidney is triggered. The renal cells of the tubules

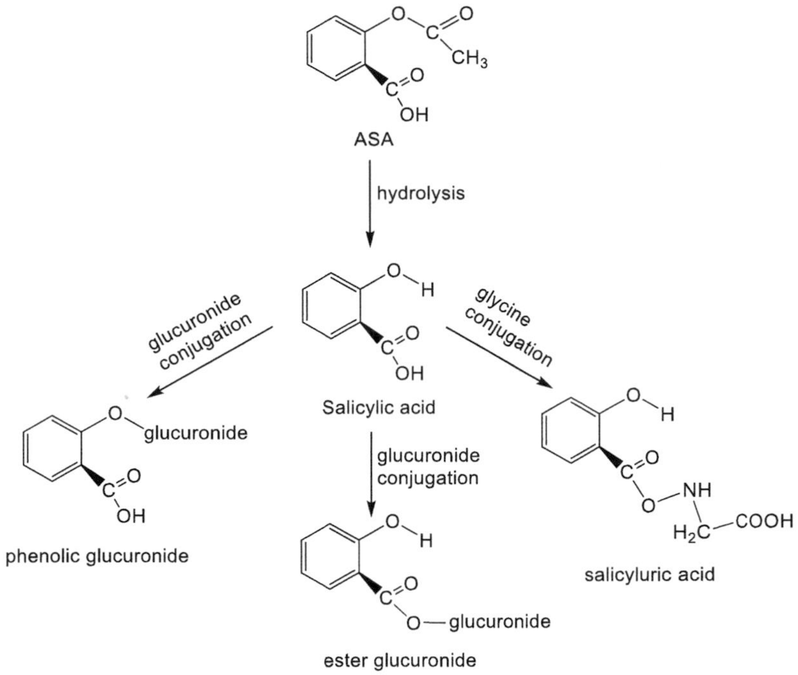

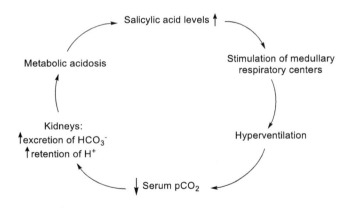

Figure 8.2 Metabolism of aspirin. Hydrolysis yields salicylic acid, the major metabolite, followed by glucuronide and glycine conjugation.

Figure 8.3 Diagram of mechanism of aspirin toxicity.

compensate for the rise in pH by *retaining* H^+ and *eliminating* HCO_3^-, initiating a decrease in serum pH and *compensatory* metabolic acidosis.

   In addition, salicylate intoxication interferes with the function of the electron transport chain in mitochondria, leading to uncoupling of ATP production.

Subsequent decrease in production of ATP, increased utilization of oxygen and increased production of carbon dioxide enhances metabolic acidosis.

In children, and after overdoses in adults, fall in pH is extensive and the patient enters metabolic acidosis.[4] The result is a shift in distribution of salicylate, the main metabolite of aspirin. Acid elimination into urine triggers further complicates the kidney's compensatory mechanism. As the flow of acidic filtrate passes through kidneys, organs are activated to reabsorb filtrate, resulting in decrease excretion. Distribution of acidic molecules into tissues, particularly brain, increases as a greater proportion of salicylate is in nonionized form, which stimulates the effect of salicylate on mitochondrial respiration in critical organs. Overall, the patient suffers from lack of ATP in the brain and heart and body temperature rises since energy is not incorporated into production of ATP but dissipates as heat. Elimination of bicarbonate occurring in response to rise in blood pH also results in loss of sodium with plasma water and rise in temperature stimulates sweating.

Consequently, the patient becomes dehydrated. As urine pH decreases, salicylate and its metabolites are not readily excreted, the drug is not eliminated, and the condition deteriorates. Salicylate also has other effects such as inhibition of parts of Krebs' cycle and increased glycolysis (to produce missing ATP) which compounds acidosis. The biochemical sequence resulting in aspirin toxicity is complicated by the low levels of ATP production and subsequent acidosis.

Unlike acetaminophen, there is no specific antidote for therapeutic intervention of aspirin toxicity. In addition, serum salicylate levels are not dependable for guiding treatment. However, a drop in serum concentration of 10% every 3–4 hours is a good indicator of recovery.

Treatment is supportive and involves the ABCs[5] of emergency guidelines, essentially reducing acidosis by increasing blood pH, supplying glucose as a source of energy, and stimulating elimination of salicylate. These are achieved by infusing bicarbonate solution containing glucose (7.5% D_5W).[6] Bicarbonate increases the pH of blood, causing salicylate to dissociate and diffuse out of tissues, drawing the ion from brain. It also increases the pH of urine which facilitates elimination of salicylate through the kidneys and from the systemic circulation.

As the pH of renal filtrate becomes more alkaline, salicylates in ultrafiltrate produced by kidney are more highly ionized. Consequently, less is reabsorbed back into systemic circulation. Understanding the dynamics of ionization and the pK_a of salicylic acid, it is possible to calculate the shift in urine pH from 6 to 8, with a concomitant 100-fold increase in ionization of acid, outlined in the following calculation:

Using the Henderson–Hasselbalch equation:

$$pH = pKa + Log\left[\frac{[\text{ionized salicylate}]^-}{[\text{nonionized acid}]}\right]$$

When filtrate pH = 6 and pK_a of salicylic acid = 3, the ratio of ionized to nonionized salicylic acid is:

$$6 = 3 + \text{Log} \frac{[\text{ionized}]}{[\text{nonionized acid}]}$$

$$\text{Then Log} \frac{[\text{ionized}]}{[\text{nonionized acid}]} = 6 - 3$$

anti-log $3 = 1,000$.

Therefore, at pH 6, there are 1,000 times more ionized species than nonionized, favoring elimination into urine. At pH 8 the same calculation yields 100,000, demonstrating that salicylic acid is more highly ionized in urine at pH 8 than at pH 6, enhancing elimination.

Similarly, in blood at physiologic pH 7.4, the ratio of ionized to nonionized salicylic acid is about 25,000 whereas at pH 6.8 it is 6,300. Therefore when a patient is suffering from the consequences of metabolic acidosis, there is more nonionized salicylic acid able to diffuse into tissues than at normal blood pH.

8.4 Hydralazine

The antihypertensive drug hydralazine represents another example of clinical drug toxicity which follows *normal therapeutic dosage* leading to adverse effects in a significant number of patients. This is of particular interest because it illustrates the importance of the combination of several **factors** in development of and susceptibility to an ADR.

Hydralazine causes the syndrome lupus erythematosus which has some similar immunological origins to other autoimmune diseases such as rheumatoid arthritis. When the drug was first introduced in the 1950s, relatively high doses were used; incidence of adverse effects was high, occurring in over 10% of patients. As use of drug declined and lower doses were incorporated as part of antihypertensive combination therapy, the incidence of adverse effects was reduced. Several factors have since revealed predisposition of patients to this adverse event including: dose, acetylator phenotype, human leukocyte antigen (HLA) phenotype, gender, and duration of treatment. Toxicity manifests features characteristic of an allergic type III immune reaction.

Dose: As mentioned above, a high occurrence of toxicity is frequent when doses of 800 mg daily or greater were used compared with 200 mg daily, which was shown later to be as effective for lowering high blood pressure. It has since been determined that the *risk of toxicity* is *dose related,* since no cases were reported at 50 mg daily.[7]

Acetylator phenotype: Hydralazine is metabolized by the acetylation route, a phase II metabolic transformation for xenobiotic compounds with an amine, sulfonamide, or hydrazine group. The acetylation reaction is subject to *genetic influence control* in the general population but subdivides into individual phenotypes according to rapid or slow acetylators. With hydralazine, adverse effects occur almost exclusively in slow acetylators. As the drug undergoes acetylation, differences in metabolism are responsible for development of the syndrome. The parent drug found in slow acetylators initiates an immunological reaction. Figure 8.4

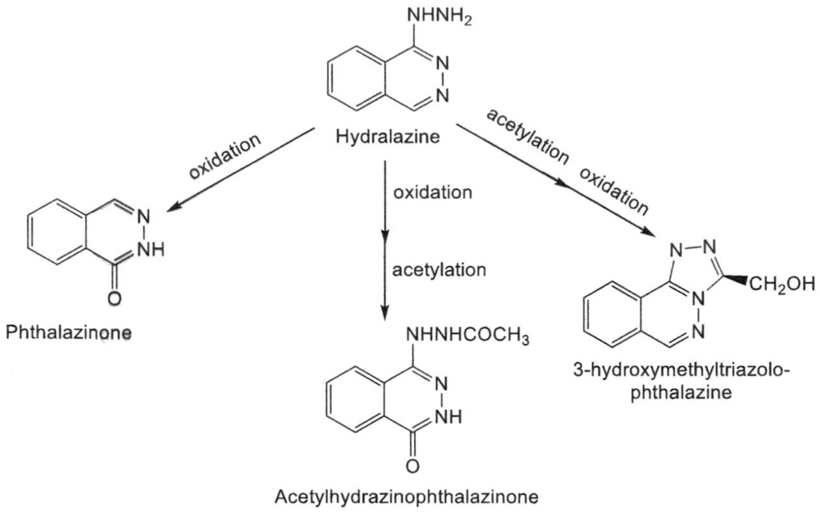

Figure 8.4 Metabolism of the antihypertensive drug hydralazine.

demonstrates that other pathways of metabolism are also important in slow acetylators, such as the oxidative pathway catalyzed by mono-oxygenases. However, peroxidase enzymes, such as in leucocytes, activate hydralazine to yield similar damaging metabolites (phthalazine and phthalazinone).

Human leukocyte antigen phenotype: Patients with **HLA type** DR4, present in white blood cells or in tissue, are more susceptible to the toxic syndrome development from hydralazine metabolism than those individuals who do not express the phenotype. That is, the incidence of HLA DR4 occurs in 60% of patients with hydralazine-induced lupus compared to 27% DR4 occurrence in the general population. A causal relationship of HLA type development of the syndrome is unknown, although biomarkers are identified with genetic predisposition for the disease.

Gender: Adverse effects associated with hydralazine metabolism occur *more commonly in women* than in men (about 2:1).[8] Currently no explanation has been proposed for this gender difference since gender differences in acetylator phenotype or HLA type distribution between males and females do not account for metabolic variances.

Duration of treatment: On average, the development of the syndrome occurs typically 18 months after treatment initiation

These factors highlight hydralazine-induced lupus syndrome as a particularly interesting example of how adverse drug reactions develop. Recognition of predisposing factors allows for estimation of risk occurrence and, consequently, avoidance; presence of HLA phenotype DR4, slow acetylation, higher doses, and females are at higher risk for syndrome development. Screening of prospective patients and use of other effective antihypertensive drugs have contributed to lowering adverse events associated with this and other drugs.

8.5 Halothane

A rare, idiosyncratic reaction is associated with the anesthetic halothane. This ADR causes liver damage from 1:10,000 to 1:100,000 patients. This severe and rare hepatic damage involves centrilobular hepatic necrosis. Patients present with fever, rash, and arthralgias; about 25% develop serum tissue anti-microsomal autoantibodies.

Mild liver dysfunction is more commonly encountered (about 20% of patients receiving the drug) which involves a separate mechanism. Liver dysfunction is thought to be due to a direct toxic action of a reductive free radical halothane metabolite, which binds covalently to liver protein, leading to lipid peroxidation. Figure 8.5 illustrates the metabolite involved in direct toxicity.

Like hydralazine, halothane hepatotoxicity involves predisposing factors including:

1. multiple exposures, which sensitize patients to future exposures;
2. gender predisposition where females are more commonly affected than males (1.8:1);
3. obesity, 68% of patients affected were clinically obese;
4. history of allergies, previous history of allergy is noted in one-third of patients.

Halothane appears to sensitize the liver via an immunological mechanism. Antibodies bind to *altered* hepatocyte cell membranes stimulating CD4/CD8 lymphocyte attachment to the antibodies. The cell-mediated response triggers

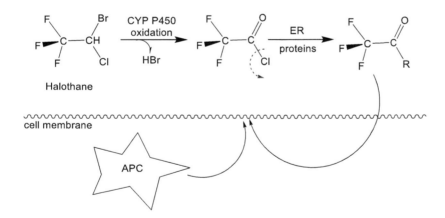

Figure 8.5 Metabolism of the anesthetic drug halothane with cytochrome P450 yielding the trifluoroacetyl (CF3COCl) reactive metabolite, which binds covalently to proteins in the endoplasmic reticulum (ER). The metabolite-protein conjugate (——R) is transported to the cell surface where it elicits antigenic responses from antigen-presenting cells (APC) in susceptible patients.

hepatocellular cytolysis *destroying* liver cells of the patient, resulting in hepatitis (Figure 8.5). Reactive metabolites involved in the immunological reaction include trifluoroacetyl chloride, which acetylates cellular proteins. The acetylation reaction produces antigenic enzymes of cytochrome P450, in endoplasmic reticulum triggering the immunological response.

8.6 Debrisoquine

Although not frequently used due to the advent of newer, less damaging, and more effective drugs, debrisoquine is an antihypertensive drug that produces marked inter-individual variation primarily due to genetic predisposition.

Within normal recommended therapeutic dose ranges, debrisoquin causes an *exaggerated* pharmacological effect represented by an *excessive* fall in blood pressure in genetically predisposed individuals. The genetic marker, expressed as poor metabolizers of debrisoquine, is distributed in 5%–10% of the Caucasian population of the EU and North America. Poor metabolic capacity is due to a *defect* in the monooxygenase system which catalyzes hydroxylation of debrisoquine at the number 4 position of the molecule in the major metabolic reaction (Figure 8.6), resulting in almost complete absence of cytochrome P450 isozyme activity.

The oxidation reactions are *major* routes for removal of the drug from the body; thus, patients with genetic predispositions have *higher* plasma levels of unchanged drug after normal therapeutic doses. Since debrisoquine is responsible for the hypotensive effect, the result is an excessive fall in blood pressure (Figure 8.7). This often unrecognized but predictable metabolic consequence occurs in a small proportion of susceptible patients.

Similarly, toxicity of **succinylcholine**, a short-acting neuromuscular blocker, occurs in genetically susceptible individuals. The reaction occurs from reduced metabolism in certain individuals due to an enzyme variant. Succinylcholine,

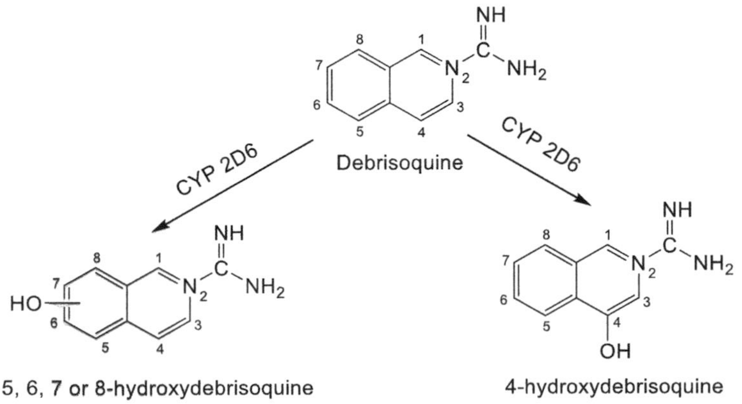

Figure 8.6 Metabolism of the antihypertensive drug debrisoquine showing the major hydroxylation reaction at the 4-position. CYP 2D6 is the primary cytochrome P450 oxidizing enzyme. Numbers indicate structural positions.

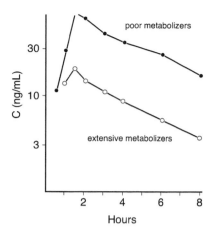

Figure 8.7 Plasma concentration (C) vs. time (hours) of debrisoquine after single oral dose (10 mg) in human subjects expressing extensive (O) and poor (•) metabolizer phenotypes. (Data from: Sloan et al., 1983.)

used as a muscle relaxant in abdominal surgery or operations involving lower extremities, is rapidly removed by metabolic hydrolysis, accounting for its short duration of action. Individuals with a *defect* in the cholinesterase enzyme responsible for hydrolysis, however, decrease the rate of metabolism and consequently relaxation of muscle is *excessive* and *prolonged*. The subsequent danger is uncontrollable respiratory inhibition.

8.7 Thalidomide

Thalidomide is historically known for causing limb deformities in children born to women who had used the sedative during pregnancy. The drug is well established as a known human teratogen. The thalidomide disaster is particularly important as it was the *watershed* for drug safety evaluation since it was a *major* example of unrecognized drug-induced toxicity. The sedative was used for treatment of morning sickness, which appeared as relatively non-toxic. However, it eventually became apparent that its use during pregnancy was associated with phocomelia, a rare and characteristic limb deformity in which arms and legs of the infant were foreshortened. Further investigation revealed that the deformities were associated with widespread prescriptions of thalidomide on days 24–29 of pregnancy.[9] Malformations were initially not reproducible in most animal toxicity studies and had not been detected in limited toxicity studies conducted by the company manufacturing the drug. Although poorly understood, the mechanism underlying the effect is associated with the formation of an *unstable* molecule, producing several polar metabolites that are derivatives of glutamine and glutamic acid. Interestingly one of the isomers of thalidomide, S-enantiomer, is more embryotoxic than the D- or L- isomer, thus illustrating the importance of chirality as a chemical factor affecting toxicity.

Thalidomide is an *unstable* molecule, producing several **polar metabolites** initially thought to be involved in the toxicity; however, the mechanism is now understood to involve the parent drug.

The molecule exists in two isomeric forms, R and S, which are mirror images. Only the S form is teratogenic, and the R form is responsible for the sedative action. Unfortunately, the liver converts the R form into the teratogenic S form precluding the therapeutic use of the drug. It appears that the three-dimensional shape of the molecule of thalidomide is crucial for its teratogenic conversion. Only the S form of the thalidomide molecule fits into a particular section of DNA in the nucleus of the cell, which then interferes with the production of growth factors, which are involved with the production of new blood vessels. Crucial in the development of an embryo, formation of limbs must be supplied with blood. Other growth factors are also recruited for the development of limb buds, accounting for the toxic specificity of thalidomide to the embryo.

Thalidomide is an exceptionally *potent* teratogen, but because it had low maternal toxicity in humans and in experimental animals, it was approved for use as a sedative during pregnancy. It was detected to cause deformities after post-clinical and marketing epidemiological data revealed the problem, when local physicians reported exceedingly unusual effects coinciding with use of the drug.

8.8 Drug Interactions

Drug interactions are a major cause of hospital emergency visits, particularly with growth in polypharmacy and multiple drug prescribing. Although physicians and pharmacists are aware of well-documented drug interactions, new and unexpected occurrences appear. Interactions are due to a variety of mechanisms, such as interference in metabolism of one drug by another, interference in the normal disposition of the drugs as a result of their simultaneous presence or alteration of pharmacological response in the presence of both or many compounds.

Many drugs interfere with normal metabolic processes by inducing or inhibiting enzymes involved in the reactions. Barbiturates, such as phenobarbital, which induce mono-oxygenase enzymes and *alter* the *rate* or *route* of metabolism of pharmacologically active compounds, *influence* their toxicity. Acetaminophen overdoses are *more severe* if administered in the presence of other enzyme-inducing drugs; metabolism via the toxic pathway catalyzed by microsomal mono-oxygenases is enhanced. Enzyme induction also *decreases* pharmacological or toxicological effects of a compound. For instance, concomitant use of rifampicin, an antibiotic drug used in the treatment of tuberculosis, and is also a microsomal enzyme inducer, increases metabolism of contraceptive steroids, thus reducing the birth-control efficacy of the latter. Whether toxicity of a particular drug is altered depends on the interacting drugs and their mechanisms.

Interference in disposition of interacting drugs is common, particularly involving *displacement* of compounds from binding sites, typically from binding to plasma proteins. A notorious example is displacement of the anticoagulant warfarin from plasma protein binding sites by anti-inflammatory and moderate analgesic compounds such as aspirin. About 97% of warfarin binds to circulating plasma proteins, allowing approximately 3% of the circulating drug to react at target sites. Even a 3% displacement from the protein in the presence of aspirin, doubles the therapeutic plasma level of warfarin, leading to excessive anticoagulant activity and hemorrhage.

8.9 Altered Responsiveness: Glucose-6-Phosphate Dehydrogenase Deficiency

Occasionally drug toxicity occurs in select individuals due to unique sensitivity, i.e. idiosyncratic reactions. Acute, drug-induced **hemolytic anemia** is triggered by a *deficiency* in glucose-6-phosphate (G-6-P) dehydrogenase, a critical enzyme in glycolysis. This enzyme has a major role in intermediary metabolism in the pentose phosphate pathway and is important in maintaining normal nicotinamide adenine dinucleotide phosphate (NADPH) concentrations in red blood cells. NADPH is necessary for balancing the level of reduced and oxidized **glutathione (GSSG)** in red cells, which protects oxidation reactions of drug metabolites:

$$GSSG + NADPH + H^+ \rightarrow 2GSH + NADP^+$$

$NADP^+$ then combines with G6P

$$Glucose\text{-}6\text{-}phosphate + NADP^+ \xrightarrow{G6PD}$$

to yield

$$6\text{-}phosphogluconate + NADPH + H^+$$

regenerating NADPH

Patients who carry this genetic defect suffer from acute hemolytic anemia when they ingest primaquine, an antimalarial antibiotic, or are exposed to aniline derivatives, such as amino-containing compounds. Fava beans contain aniline products that precipitate hemolytic anemia in vulnerable individuals, hence the term *favism*.

Deficiency in G-6-phosphate dehydrogenase activity is the result of variants in enzyme function rather than complete absence. Enzyme variants are intrinsic to red blood cells which are also responsive *in vitro*. *In vitro* challenge with a suitable drug causes hemolysis of the red blood cells. Also, GSH levels in red cells are *lower* in predisposed patients[10] than in individuals without the genetic defect. The defect is carried on the X chromosome, although sex-linked inheritance is not guaranteed. Overall, 5%–10% of African American males have the deficiency and develop acute hemolytic anemia if challenged with primaquine. The highest incidence (53%) is found in male Sephardic Jews from Kurdistan.

8.10 Summary and Learning Objectives

Drugs are chemicals with biological activity with common toxicological effects. Toxicity following *overdoses* (e.g. acetaminophen, aspirin) or with *therapeutic doses* (e.g. debrisoquine, hydralazine, halothane) represents common pathological consequences of drug administration. Such toxic events are not always *predictable as exaggerated pharmacological, physiological,* or *biochemical responses*. In fact, the *unpredictable* nature of chemical activity is often idiosyncratic and unrelated to its pharmacology.

Drug toxicity is affected by genetic factors that alter susceptibility or is influenced by environmental or public health issues such as multidrug use and alcohol intake. Adverse reactions also result from interactions between two or more drugs or with other chemicals.

Acetaminophen causes *liver necrosis* following overdoses as a result of metabolic activation, depletion of GSH, and interaction of reactive metabolites with cellular proteins. Toxicity is increased by enzyme induction due to alcohol use or abuse or in the presence of barbiturates.

Aspirin poisoning is manifested by means of physiological and biochemical disturbances (metabolic acidosis, uncoupling of ATP production, rise in temperature, and **hypoglycemia**), which follow accidental, suicidal, or therapeutic overdose, the latter resulting from saturation of elimination.

Hydralazine causes an *immunologically-induced* toxic reaction following long-term therapy particularly in susceptible individuals (females, slow acetylator phenotypes, high dose, HLA type DR4). The resulting events are manifested as lupus erythematosus-like syndrome with joint pain, skin rashes, and antinuclear antibodies.

Halothane also causes an *immunologically-related* toxic event but is much more severe than hydralazine. The autoimmune response presents as destruction of the liver with a high fatality rate. As with hydralazine predisposing factors are evident (female gender, multiple exposures, obesity, history of allergies). Toxic events involve metabolic activation of halothane, subsequent interaction of metabolites with liver cell proteins, and combination of antibodies with lymphocytes targeting and destroying liver cells.

Toxicity of debrisoquine involves reactive overdose as a result of *genetic deficiency* in metabolism. Pharmacologically, the active parent drug is not metabolized in a proportion of the population (approximately 6%–8% of Caucasians) leading to predictable, exaggerated loss of blood pressure.

Thalidomide caused birth defects (phocomelia) when prescribed during pregnancy for treatment of morning sickness. Although relatively non-toxic to the mother, it presented as a potent teratogen in the developing fetus when exposed during critical days of the first trimester.

Combinations of drugs lead to unexpected toxic effects because of the pharmacological interactions when prescribed and ingested simultaneously. These **drug interactions** are presented as interference with metabolism of one drug in the presence of another (synergistic or inhibition); displacement from plasma protein binding sites, or alteration of pharmacological response.

Toxic events are also manifested as a result of altered responsiveness as with G-6-P dehydrogenase deficient individuals who develop hemolytic anemia upon exposure to primaquine and sulfonamides. Susceptible individuals lack protective GSH in red blood cells, rendering them prone to pathologic consequences.

Review Questions

Choose the answer which is most appropriate.

1. Acetaminophen is an analgesic drug that causes liver damage following overdoses. This is the result of: (a) depletion of body stores of sulfate, (b) inhibition of cytochrome P450, (c) production of a glutathione conjugate, (d) metabolic activation by microsomal enzymes, (e) biliary excretion and metabolism by gastrointestinal bacteria.
2. Which of the following are shown as predisposing factors in the toxicity of hydralazine: (a) genetic polymorphism of metabolism, (b) gender, (c) dose, (d) alcohol intake, (e) glucose-6-phosphate dehydrogenase.
3. Indicate which statements are true and which are false. Thalidomide is a drug that: (a) only causes malformations in rats, (b) results in morning sickness in women, (c) is responsible for the development of phocomelia in newborns when administered during pregnancy, (d) is only toxic in the R-isomer configuration.
4. Indicate which statements are true and which are false. The anesthetic drug halothane: (a) induces cytochrome P450 enzymes, (b) destroys lymphocytes, (c) causes liver damage more commonly in females, (d) produces allergic reactions.
5. Select: (a) if 1, 2 and 3 are correct, (b) if 1 and 3 are correct, (c) if 2 and 4 are correct, (d) if only 4 is correct, (e) if all four choices are correct.
   Adverse effects of drugs in humans is caused by: (1) exaggerated pharmacological effects following overdoses, (2) idiosyncratic effects following normal doses, (3) toxicity unrelated to pharmacological effect following inappropriate doses, (4) interactions with dietary constituents.

Short Answer Question

6. What is the mechanistic role of plasma and urinary pH in aspirin poisoning?

Notes

1. OTC or without the need for a physician's prescription.
2. 325–500 mg every 4 fours not to exceed 4,000 mg/day for 10 continuous days of administration.

3. This ratio is physiologically maintained at a pH 7.4. Besides the lungs, adjustments of serum pH are accomplished by the kidney through reabsorption of filtered bicarbonate and/or hydrogen ions.
4. Note that in pathologic conditions, such as with aspirin overdose, biologic compensation that usually adjusts blood pH in routine physiologic activity is no longer normal.
5. Maintain Airway clearance, support Breathing, ensure Cardiac integrity.
6. 7.5% sodium bicarbonate in water containing 5% dextrose.
7. 5.4% incidence occurred after 100 mg daily which increased to 10.4% with 200 mg daily.
8. Incidence of 19.4% of women taking 200 mg daily compared to 4.9% of men when measured 3 years after starting therapy.
9. First trimester of gestation.
10. And demonstrate a bimodal distribution.

Bibliography

Barile, F.A., Chapter 18. Acetaminophen, salicylates, and non-steroidal anti-inflammatory drugs (NSAIDs), in: *Barile's Clinical Toxicology: Principles and Mechanisms*, (pp. 271–286), 3rd edition, CRC Press, Boca Raton, FL, 2019.

Reid, L. Chapter 135. *Toxicological considerations of pharmaceutical products in General and Applied Toxicology* (pp. 323–3250) Ballantyne, B., Marrs, T. and Syversen, T.L.M.(Eds), 3rd edition, John Wiley and Sons, Hoboken, NJ. 2009

Sloan, T.P., Lancaster, R., Shah, R.R., Idle, J.R. and Smith, R.L., Genetically determined oxidation capacity and the disposition of debrisoquine. *British Journal Clinical Pharmacology* 15, 443–450, 1983. Doi: 10.1111/j.1365-2125.1983. tb01528.x.

Utrecht, J. Idiosyncratic drug reactions: Current understanding. *Annual Reviews Pharmacology1.Toxicology*, 47, 513–539, 2007.

Suggested Readings

Aronson, J.K., (ed.) *Meyler's Side Effects of Drugs: The International Encyclopedia of Adverse Drug Reactions and Interactions*, 16th edition, Elsevier, Netherlands, 2015.

Stockley, I.H., *Drug Interactions*, Pharmaceutical Press, Wallingford, 1996.

Talbot, J. and Aronson, J.K., *Stephens' Detection and Evaluation of Adverse Drug Reactions: Principles and Practice*, 6th edition, Wiley-Blackwell, New York, 2011.

Timbrell, J. A., *Principles of Biochemical Toxicology*, 4th edition, Taylor & Francis Ltd., London, 2009.

Chapter 9

Industrial Toxicology

Chapter Outline

This chapter describes hazards of exposure to industrial chemicals, including occupational and commercial examples.

9.1 Occupational and Commercial Use of Industrial Chemicals   123
9.2 Means of Exposure   124
9.3 Toxic Effects   124
9.4 Examples of Hazardous Industrial Chemicals   126
9.5 Regulatory Legislation   130
9.6 Summary and Learning Objectives   131
Review Questions   132
    Short Answer Question   132
Notes   132
Bibliography   133

9.1 Occupational and Commercial Use of Industrial Chemicals

Pathologies from chemical exposure have been known since the dawn of the industrial revolution of the 18th and 19th centuries. The exposures to chemicals range from use of household products, occupational diseases, as well as illicit incorporation into society. Notoriety of chemical hazards increased with continuous benefits that surrounded the agents, while some of these are still known by their original, colloquial names. Diseases resulting from occupational exposure

DOI: 10.1201/9781003188575-9

posed serious consequences socially, economically, and medically. Today, many occupations still carry risk of diseases or groups thereof. For instance, coal mining has always been a hazardous occupation that portends the risk of **silicosis** to miners, while asbestos workers with prolonged interaction with the fibers develop **asbestosis** and **mesothelioma**, and workers in paper and printing mills are prone to dermal diseases. Consequently, the occupational environment is a major factor in determining health, especially since health hazards from chemical exposure were not well recognized. Although the working environment has improved immeasurably over the last century, some occupations are still approached with caution, notwithstanding legislation and regulations to improve conditions.

Thousands of chemical substances used in commercial and occupational industries are available in the marketplace and range from heavy metals and inorganic compounds to complex organic chemicals. Occupational and commercial workers therefore must be protected from the risks of exposure. Regulatory mandates require that exposure to these chemicals is minimized. This is often accomplished by handling chemicals in closed systems so that operators do not come into contact with them. In developing countries, however, some of which have rapidly industrialized, exposure levels are higher and industrial diseases are more common than in Western society. In fact, the lack of legislative agendas permits discarding of chemicals in environmentally sensitive areas, where communities thrive. Consequently, exposure to toxic substances in the workplace and in the residential areas is still hazardous. Furthermore, even in well-regulated industrial environments, intentional or accidental exposure is still a major concern.

9.2 Means of Exposure

Just as with environmental exposure, occupational handling of commercial chemicals occurs via three major routes: oral ingestion, inhalation, and dermal absorption, with inhalation and dermal occupying the most common routes. Gases, vapors, aerosols, volatile solvents and liquids, as well as dust, fibers, dirt, soot, and smoke, pose risks of contact with the skin and lungs.[1] Resulting toxicity is manifest as local reactions or, if absorbed, systemic toxicity.

9.3 Toxic Effects

Toxic effects of industrial chemicals are either acute or chronic. Acute inhalation of sufficient quantities of solvents causes asphyxiation, unconsciousness, coma, and death. Inhalation of irritant substances, such as methyl isocyanate, results in immediate bronchoconstriction and pulmonary edema, both of which are locally mediated rather than systemic effects. However, such acute effects are usually accidental and are less common than chronic industrial diseases.

Outcomes of inhalation of industrial gases, metal fumes, or organic solvents include acute or chronic irritation or corrosion of the respiratory tract. Chronic chemical or particulate exposure is associated with debilitating respiratory diseases and pulmonary cancer. The acute phase is manifest as pulmonary irritation or allergic responses. Absorption of substances via the lungs is efficient and rapid and leads to systemic effects, such as narcosis from solvents, or kidney damage from metal salts, such as with mercuric chloride or uranium dioxide.

Exposure of skin to occupational chemicals causes local irritation, where **contact dermatitis** is acute or progresses as a chronic skin disease. Some compounds are absorbed through the skin producing systemic reactions. Exposure to the insecticide parathion was shown to produce fatal poisoning following skin absorption.[2]

The respiratory and dermal systems are most commonly affected by industrial chemicals. In fact, the most prevalent occupational disease is dermatitis, accounting for more worker absentee days than all other industrial diseases together. Dermatitis has many causes including exposure to organic and inorganic chemicals. Furthermore, chemical agents act as sensitizers or irritants, where the symptoms result from induction of inflammation. The number of primary irritants is large and includes many different types of chemical substances such as acids, alkalis, metals, solvents, and solid organic and inorganic chemicals. The mechanism of toxicity varies from inflammation (redness, swelling, pain, and heat production) to corrosion and denaturing of dermal layers.

Skin sensitizers act via immunological mechanisms to cause contact dermatitis. As the chemical filters through the epidermis, its reaction with keratin proteins produces an antigenic response. Since small molecular weight chemicals usually do not act as antigens, their combination with resident proteins produces a hapten.[3] The hapten-antigen then initiates the production of humoral and cellular immunity.[4] Continuous exposure to the substance stimulates stronger allergic reactions. Table 9.1 lists a few of the large number of sensitizers available. Nickel and its salts are well-known causes of contact dermatitis (*nickel itch*), resulting from occupational exposure as well as from contact with nickel-containing jewelry.

Sensitization also follows inhalation exposure leading to systemic effects such as asthma. Toluene diisocyanate is a pulmonary sensitizer widely used as an industrial solvent and chemical initiator. Dermal contact with chlorinated

Table 9.1 Types of Skin Sensitizers

Commercial Applications	Chemical Class
Dye intermediaries	Aniline compounds
Dyes	p-Phenylenediamine
Photographic developers	Hydroquinone
Antioxidants	o- and p-Toluidine
Insecticides	Organophosphorus compounds
Resins	Urethane
Coal tar derivatives	Anthracene
Explosives	Picric acid
Metals	Nickel, chromium, and mercury

hydrocarbons is associated with occupational acne, due to denaturing of skin pores, dermal congestion, and increased production of keratin.

9.4 Examples of Hazardous Industrial Chemicals

Vinyl chloride: Vinyl chloride (vinyl chloride monomer, VCM) is an initiating gaseous substrate in the manufacture of the ubiquitous plastic polyvinyl chloride (PVC). Since the introduction of PVC in the 1950s as a versatile compound useful in the plumbing industry, occupational exposure to vinyl chloride soared. However, early safety standards in factories and working localities were not rigorous as they are today and not always observed. In some cases, workers were required to enter reaction vessels periodically to clean them, despite the presence of substantial amounts of vinyl chloride in the containers. The gas is inhaled but is also readily absorbed through the skin, with sufficient amounts to overcome some workers by solvent narcosis. The chronic toxic effect was not immediately apparent; the most severe lesion, development of hemangiosarcoma, a liver tumor, was rare and only observed in epidemiological studies of workers in the industry. Malignant hemangiosarcomas were generally confined to workers exposed to high concentrations of vinyl chloride, cases of which were later reproduced and identified in experimental animals. As with many historical episodes of toxic chemicals, hygiene and safety standards were promulgated and applied to occupational handling of vinyl chloride only in hindsight and with the benefit of retrospective studies.

Chronic exposure to vinyl chloride results in 'vinyl chloride disease' which comprises **Raynaud's phenomenon**, skin changes, alterations of bones of the hands, liver damage, and in some cases development of hemangiosarcoma. Bone deviations are due to ischemic damage following degeneration and **occlusion** of small blood vessels and capillaries. The liver becomes fibrotic. Recently, vinyl chloride syndrome has been identified with an immunological origin, as immune complexes are deposited in vascular epithelium and complement activation is featured.

Toxic effects of vinyl chloride result in part from *metabolic activation*, as it is metabolized by cytochrome P450 to the reactive intermediates, chloroethylene oxide or chloroacetaldehyde, which *alkylate* DNA. Metabolism is *saturable* as the incidence of liver tumors produced in experimental animals reaches a maximum. Tumor incidence, therefore, correlates with the amount of vinyl chloride metabolized rather than the dose. Reactive intermediates also interact with other macromolecules, causing tissue damage either directly or via an immunological reaction.

Historically, the vinyl chloride episode emphasizes the importance of stringent safety standards in industrial complexes. In addition, human epidemiologic and laboratory experimental evidence are important in risk assessment, as well as highlighting the type of toxic effects. Consequently, major Western countries have promulgated legislation that deals specifically with occupational conditions involving industrial chemicals. For example, UK regulations dictate that all chemicals produced in quantities of greater than 1 ton must undergo toxicity testing while strict occupational hygiene limits, such as Maximum Exposure Limits (MEL) or Threshold Limit Values (TLV) for industrial chemicals are enforced.

Cadmium: Cadmium is a valuable metal widely incorporated in industrial alloys, metal plating, batteries, and in pigments used in inks, paints, plastic, rubber, and enamel. It is also found naturally and is present in food, although poorly absorbed from the gastrointestinal lining (5%–8%). However, up to 40% of an inhaled dose is absorbed, especially as a component of cigarette smoke.

The major hazard encountered with cadmium as an industrial metal is from inhalation of cadmium metal or cadmium oxide. The metal has many toxic effects, primarily kidney damage, as a result of chronic exposure, and testicular damage following acute exposure; the latter occurrence is not a common feature in humans after occupational exposure. It is also a suspected carcinogen in experimental animals causing tumors in the testes as well as at the site of exposure.

Renal damage is a delayed effect even after repeated single doses, due to accumulation of cadmium in the renal glomerulus. The metal complexes metallothionein, a low molecular weight protein involved with systemic transport of metals. Due to its chemical similarity to zinc, upon exposure, 80%–90% of cadmium binds to metallothionein. The cadmium–metallothionein complex is transported to the kidney, filtered through the glomerulus, and reabsorbed by proximal convoluted tubular (PCT) cells, where the complex is degraded by proteases. Subsequent release of cadmium from the complex results in cellular disruption or recombines with available metallothionein.

Testicular pathology occurs within a few hours of a single exposure to cadmium and results in necrosis, degeneration, and complete loss of spermatozoa. The mechanism involves an effect on testicular vasculature. Cadmium reduces blood flow through the testes producing ischemic necrosis from oxygen and nutrient deprivation, thus indirectly affecting a critical physiologic parameter.

Half-life of cadmium in total body compartments is between 7 and 30 years and is excreted through the kidneys, particularly accelerated after renal damage.

Following acute inhalation exposure, lung irritation occurs along with diarrhea and malaise, while chronic inhalation results in emphysema occurring before kidney damage is observed. The metal also triggers disorders of calcium metabolism and subsequent loss of calcium from the body leading to **osteomalacia**. In 1979, a public health situation was highlighted in Japan when development of osteomalacia increased dramatically in women eating rice contaminated with cadmium.[5]

Aromatic amines (AA): Widely used in the rubber and dye industry AA are responsible for a variety of toxic effects. 2-Naphthylamine, formerly used in manufacturing of rubber products, is a known human carcinogen, highly associated with the production of bladder cancer. The earliest recorded cases of bladder cancer due to AA were reported in Germany in 1895 among aniline dye workers. It was eventually withdrawn from industrial use in 1949.

There are a number of different AA used in industry (Figure 9.1), some of which are known carcinogens in humans or animals. The toxic mechanism of bladder cancer initiation by 2-naphthylamine has been extensively studied and involves metabolic activation. The aromatic amine undergoes hydroxylation at the nitrogen atom followed by conjugation of the resulting hydroxyl group with

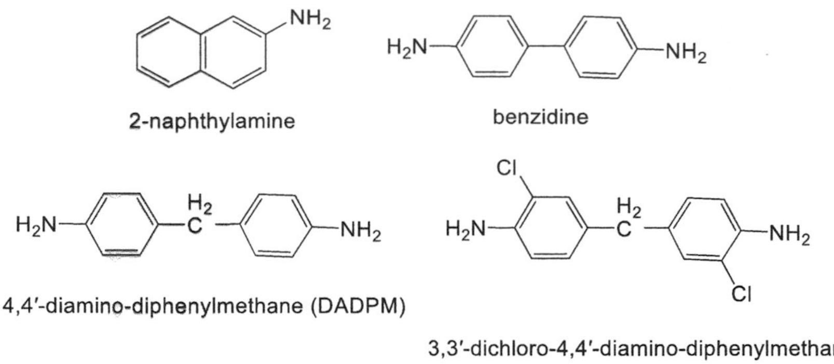

2-naphthylamine

benzidine

4,4′-diamino-diphenylmethane (DADPM)

3,3′-dichloro-4,4′-diamino-diphenylmethane*

Figure 9.1 Representative structures of carcinogenic aromatic amines. *Chemically also labeled as: 4,4′-methylene-bis-O-(2-chloroaniline), MBOCA.

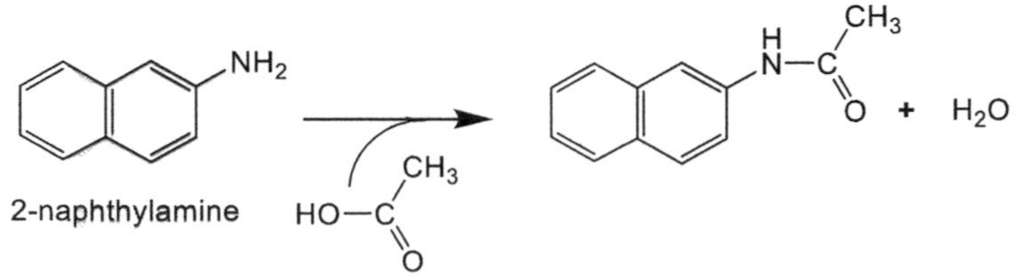

2-naphthylamine

Figure 9.2 Acetylation of 2-naphthylamine.

glucuronic acid. When the conjugate is excreted into urine, however, it is cleaved under acidic urinary conditions to yield a reactive metabolite, which reacts with cellular macromolecules.

Recently the acetylator phenotype is also associated with bladder cancer induced by AA. Acetylation is one route of detoxication for these compounds (Figure 9.2); consequently slow acetylators are more susceptible to extended exposure due to accumulation of AA.

Other commercially available *in vivo* carcinogenic AA includes *o*-tolidine, 4-aminobiphenyl, and diaminodiphenylmethane (DADPM). DADPM was responsible for Epping jaundice, an outbreak of liver inflammation in the UK. Case reports indicate that a solution of the chemical was spilt onto the floor of a lorry which subsequently carried sacks of flour. The substance contaminated the flour and produced jaundice in communities of people who ate the bread made from the ingredients. The chemical damages the bile duct resulting in production of liver tumors in rodents rather than bladder tumors. The target organ for the AA, however, is species-dependent; rodents develop liver tumors whereas bladder tumors occur more often in dogs.

Screening procedures, such as **cytological** examination of urine, are recommended for workers in occupational settings where exposure to AA is a risk. Aniline, the simplest aromatic amine, causes **methemoglobinemia** with **cyanosis** following acute exposure. Chronic exposure produces anemia with mild cyanosis.

Asbestos: Industrial diseases associated with exposure to asbestos demonstrate that even chemically inert substances have potential for serious toxicity. Asbestos includes a group of fibrous mineral silicates with divergent chemical compositions. Its wide use in industry relies on the mineral's ability to withstand heat and to provide insulation as a component of heat barriers. Chrysotile (white asbestos) is most commonly used and is relatively inert biologically. Crocidolite (blue asbestos) remains as a common contaminant of white asbestos, and is associated with production of mesothelioma and bronchial carcinoma.

Exposure to asbestos results in about 2,000–3,000 deaths/year in the UK and 10,000 per year in the US (1983–2021). There have been more than 400 known deaths from mesothelioma alone in the UK, solely associated with exposure to asbestos.

Extensive exposure to asbestos is widespread via inhalation——in factories manufacturing asbestos products, during its use as an insulating material, and in commercial housing developments where it was incorporated into structures for their fire-retardant properties. More recently, workers have been exposed to airborne asbestos released during demolition of buildings where it is present. In the automobile industry, asbestos was also incorporated into the manufacturing of brake linings. The mineral is also a contaminant of food and water, where its presence in production of water filters accounts for its appearance in drinking water. Although the toxicological importance of this route of exposure is currently uncertain, gastrointestinal tumors have been ascribed to asbestos after inhalation exposure.

The following pathologic conditions are associated with exposure to asbestos via inhalation:

1. Asbestosis, or interstitial fibrosis of the lung;
2. Benign pleural disease;
3. Bronchial carcinoma;
4. Malignant mesothelioma.

Asbestosis is a dose-related disease which requires continuous prolonged exposure. Particles of asbestos are detected in fibrotic areas of the lung and in sputum; alveolar spaces are infiltrated with **collagen**. Asbestos fibers are coated with iron-containing proteins. The disease develops over an extended but variable period of time with the development of progressive dyspnea.[6] Measurement of lung function capacity of exposed workers is indicated for monitoring effects of asbestos exposure.

Although the compound is chemically inert, the fibers are cytotoxic and hemolyze red blood cells. The length of the fiber is an important factor in toxicity—fibers *longer* than 10–20 μm cause fibrosis while shorter ones do not. This is due to *inability* of **macrophages** to completely *phagocytose* long fibers, leaving the macrophage cell membrane to leak enzymes. The outflow of enzymes and other cellular constituents is involved in the development of **fibrosis**. Although the lungs have a normal capacity to remove hazardous airborne exogenous particles, long asbestos fibers are not adequately dispensed. Immunologically, asbestos fibers distort the macrophage cell surface after ingestion, due to alteration of C3 receptors (and complement activation) and immunoglobulin G antibodies.

The use of crocidolite is prohibited in the UK and US; amosite (brown asbestos) is not encouraged, and general use of asbestos for insulation is banned. The control limit for crocidolite and amosite in the environment is 0.2 and 0.5 fibers/mL for other forms of asbestos.

Bronchial carcinoma results from prolonged exposure to asbestos and occurs in approximately 50% of workers who develop asbestosis. Development of disease correlates with dose and duration of exposure, as well as the type of exposure. The use of asbestos products, such as in textiles, where asbestos of a particular particle size is generated, is important in the development of the disease.

Mesothelioma is an uncommon form of cancer that affects the chest lining. It is associated with exposure to asbestos, especially but not exclusively, crocidolite. Crocidolite from the North-West Cape Province in South Africa is more *potent* than that from the Transvaal. Prolonged exposure to high levels of asbestos is not necessary for the development of mesothelioma nor is it limited to occupational exposure. Although the latent period is typically 30 years after exposure, once established, the disease progresses rapidly and is usually fatal within months. Tumors eventually spread to the lung and encase it.

The mechanisms underlying asbestos-induced cancer are currently unknown but do not seem to involve genotoxic mechanisms. Animal studies as well as human data have shown that asbestos fibers alone will cause cancer of the mesothelium. Unlike other types of chemical carcinogens, asbestos is not metabolized or activated *in vivo* but remains in tissue permanently. The fibers however are capable of migrating from the airways to the pleural cavity. Consequently, exposure to high levels for short periods of time is sufficient to eventually initiate mesothelioma.

The size of fibers is a critical factor; $0.3\,\mu m$ in diameter and $5\,\mu m$ in length are *most active*. In addition, the extent of exposure and concentration of fibers in inhaled air is also grave. There is a synergistic effect between smoking and asbestos in the induction of pulmonary carcinogenesis.

9.5 Regulatory Legislation

In the UK, US, and most other Western industrialized nations, legislation sets limits on the levels of toxic substances in the workplace. Exposure levels are based on results of human epidemiological data and on animal toxicity studies. Monitoring of the occupational environment for compliance is an essential component of enforcement. Experimental evidence of toxic effects usually includes determination of a dose-response relationship and no-effect levels *in vivo*. Screening for *in vitro* irritation and sensitization is also conducted.

Maximum exposure limit (UK) or TLV (US) is defined as the maximum level of exposure for a compound. MEL and TLV are calculated on the basis of exposure over a normal working day usually from knowledge of the toxicity of the compound (**no-observed-adverse-effect level [NOAEL]**) with a margin of safety included in the estimate. Regulatory agencies, such as the Health and

Safety Executive (UK) and National Institute for Occupational Safety and Health (NIOSH) (US), set the occupational exposure limits. The last 20 years has shown dramatic decreases in the rates of occurrence of industrial diseases, principally as a result of adherence and enforcement of regulations. Some diseases, however, such as cancer, require longer development times, allowing for appearance and progression of pathologies many years after initial, critical exposures.

Long latency periods also signal the difficulty associated with detection of industrial diseases, since sufficient rarity and increased frequency of the disease must occur within a population for epidemiological detection. In the US and the UK, however, recently enacted legislation requires that all new chemical substances not already covered by existing regulations undergo toxicity testing. In addition, legal requirements allow identification of hazards so that control measures, such as suitable labeling, can be affected. Despite this, however, new occupational diseases continue to appear when exposure occurs many years prior.

9.6 Summary and Learning Objectives

Many chemicals used in industry are reactive molecules and likely to interact with biological systems that cause damage.

Exposure is most common via skin and lungs. *Toxic effects* on skin, such as irritation, sensitization, and contact dermatitis, such as with nickel, are the most common occupational diseases with a probable immune basis. Similarly, allergic lung disease such as asthma results from exposure to industrial chemicals and extremely reactive irritant chemicals (e.g. toluene diisocyanate), responsible for pulmonary sensitization, edema, bronchoconstriction, coma, and death. Some industrial chemicals initiate cancer which develops many years after exposure.

High levels of exposure to vinyl chloride have occurred in manufacturing plants and resulted in rare liver cancer developing some years later. Vinyl chloride also caused liver damage and cancer as determined by interactive reactive metabolites produced when cytochrome P450 reacts with protein and DNA.

Cadmium is widely used in industry in various forms; however, its toxicity, following acute or chronic inhalation of cadmium fumes, includes renal damage, brittle bones (*Itai-Itai* disease), and lung irritation and emphysema. In rodents, testicular damage and tumors occur. Cadmium is bound to metallothionein but release of free cadmium from this complex in the kidney underlies the nephrotoxicity.

A variety of AA are employed in the industry such as the production of rubber. A number of these are suspect or known carcinogens such as 2-naphthylamine. Metabolic activation by cytochrome P450, conjugation of the hydroxylated product, and release of the reactive metabolite in urine allow interaction with bladder cell DNA. The resulting carcinogenic response is detoxified by acetylation, making the slow acetylator status a factor. Consequently, slow acetylators are more at risk from 2-naphthylamine-induced bladder cancer.

In contrast, asbestos is a relatively inert substance but causes lung cancer (mesothelioma, bronchial carcinoma) and asbestosis, a chronic lung disease. The fibers lodge in the lungs are ingested by phagocytic cells, which leak cell contents and damage surrounding tissue. Fiber size is a crucial factor. Exposure to such chemicals and minerals is now regulated by legislation and exposure levels (TLV and MEL) have since been established.

Review Questions

1. Indicate which statements is(are) true and which is(are) false. Skin sensitization is an important occupational disease and can be caused by: (a) vinyl chloride, (b) cadmium, (c) nickel, (d) asbestos.
2. Which of the following industrial chemicals are known human carcinogens? (a) cadmium, (b) vinyl chloride, (c) 2-naphthylamine, (d) asbestos.
3. Which of the following information is necessary to calculate the TLV for an industrial chemical? (a) latency period, (b) half-life, (c) NOAEL, (d) daily exposure level.
4. Toxicity of asbestos is affected by which of the following factors? (a) fiber size, (b) physical form, (c) route of exposure, (d) dose, (e) exposure period.
5. Which of the following pathologies is (are) triggered by both cadmium and vinyl chloride exposure? (a) testicular damage, (b) kidney damage, (c) **ischemia**.

Short Answer Question

6. Discuss the importance of acetylation and glucuronic acid conjugation in 2-naphthylamine carcinogenicity.

Notes

1. Particulate matter or PM (a.k.a. particle pollution) is a mixture of solid particles and liquid droplets found in ambient air. The topic is of high research interest in environmental toxicology.
2. Parathion has since been replaced in the U.S. by the less toxic malathion as an industrial insecticide, particularly for prevention of mosquito-borne diseases.
3. A chemical or drug which by itself cannot initiate an immunological response, but when combined with a larger stationary or circulating protein, produces an antigen with immunological capability.
4. B-cell (antibody-producing cell) and T-cell responses, respectively.
5. Later labeled as Itai-Itai ('Ouch-Ouch!') disease.
6. Difficulty breathing.

Bibliography

Dekant, W., Vamvakas, S., Occupational health and safety, in: Ullmann's Industrial Toxicology, (pp. 299–360), 2nd edition, Volume 1, Wiley-VCH, John Wiley & Sons, New York, **2005**.

Harbison, R.D., Bourgeois, M.M. and Johnson, G.T., *Hamilton and Hardy's Industrial Toxicology*, 6th edition, John & Wiley, New York, 2015.

Lewinsohn, H.C., Chapter 104. Occupation, Toxic Exposures and Health Effects, in: *General and Applied Toxicology*, (pp. 2583–2602), Ballantyne, B., Marrs, T. and Syversen, T.L.M. (Eds.), 2nd edition, Macmillan & Co., Basingstoke, 2009.

Newfang, D.A., G.T. Johnson, and R.D. Harbison, Chapter 2. Controls of Occupational Diseases, in: *Hamilton and Hardy's Industrial Toxicology*, (pp. 13–18), Harbison, R.D., Bourgeois, M.M. and Johnson, G.T., (Eds.), 6th edition, Wiley, New York, 2015.

Thorne, P.S., Chapter 34. Ecotoxicology, in: *Casarett and Doull's Toxicology, The Basic Science of Poisons*, (pp. 1551–1572), Klaassen, C.D. (Ed.), 9th edition, McGraw-Hill, New York, 2019.

Chapter 10

Food Additives and Contaminants

Chapter Outline

This chapter discusses toxicology of food additives and contaminants using specific examples.

10.1	Introduction	135
10.2	Tartrazine	138
10.3	Saccharin	139
10.4	Food Contaminants	140
	10.4.1 Botulinum Toxin	141
	10.4.2 Aflatoxin	141
	10.4.3 Ginger Jake	142
	10.4.4 The Toxic Oil (Spanish Oil) Syndrome	142
10.5	Summary and Learning Objectives	143
	Review Questions	144
	Short Answer Question	145
	Notes	145
	Bibliography	146
	Suggested Readings	146

10.1 Introduction

Besides the natural components of food that are consumed daily, human diets contain many different chemical substances – natural, intentionally added, and continuously present. Food additives are substances intentionally added to food products and are not a recent innovation. For instance, use of salt as a preservative and spices to enhance the taste of foodstuffs has been common practice for

DOI: 10.1201/9781003188575-10

Table 10.1 Classification of Food Additives and Representative Examples

Classification	Representative Examples
Coloring agents	Tartrazine
Antioxidants	Butylated hydroxytoluene
Stabilizers	Vegetable gums
Anti-caking agents	Magnesium carbonate
Flavors	Cinnamaldehyde
Preservatives	Sodium nitrate, EDTA
Emulsifiers	Polyoxyethylene sorbitan fatty esters
Acids/Alkalis	Citric acid
Buffers	Carbonates
Bleaches	Benzoyl peroxide
Propellants	Nitrous oxide
Sweeteners	Sorbitol, saccharin
Flavor enhancers	Monosodium glutamate (MSG)

centuries. However, treatment with additives has only reached the current level of industrialization relatively recently, on the order of 2,500 food additives currently in use. Incorporation of food additives on a wide scale has been questioned and monitored by toxicologists and nutritionists, especially as the long-term effects of substances are often not known. The public has questioned the value of food additives, which has prompted manufacturers to re-evaluate the growth, supply, and production of food products.

Table 10.1 classifies food additives according to their use, particularly as coloring agents and preservatives incorporated into food products, and as additive ingredients whose function is less obvious. In the EU, allowable food additives are provided with the E number, which also appears on the packaging of food.

According to the Joint FAO/WHO Expert Committee on Food Additives (Food and Agriculture Organization of the United Nations/World Health Organization; JECFA), the international body responsible for evaluating safety, food additives are substances added to food to maintain or improve its safety, freshness, taste, texture, or appearance. Food additives are checked for potential harmful effects on human health before they are approved (www.who.int/news-room/fact-sheets/detail/food-additives).

Historically, many food additives in current use have been incorporated into production for centuries. For example, preservatives[1] have maintained an important public health function in reducing the risk of microbiological contamination affecting food.[2] Preservatives reduce biological and chemical degradation and render the product with a longer shelf life, i.e. chemical preservatives slow decomposition of natural ingredients of foodstuff caused by molds, air, yeast, bacteria, and fungi.

A variety of other food additives, such as dyes (for color enhancement) and non-sugar sweeteners, are of less obvious benefit to consumers but have important functions for taste and appearance of consumables, for the producer as well as the consumer. They are added when food is prepared, packaged, transported, or stored, and they eventually become a component of the food. Thus, enhancing attractiveness of food is a good justification for their use, but consumers have questioned incorporation of these chemicals into food, and have demanded 'additive-free' consumables or the use of 'natural' additives. However, the misunderstanding that natural substances are always intrinsically safe is misleading since natural products can be at *least as toxic* as synthetic chemicals. 'Natural' or 'organic' food additives must be assessed independently, with the same rigorous testing requirements as with synthetic additives.

As outlined in Table 10.1, food additives comprise a wide range of chemical types from simple inorganic compounds such as preservatives, to complex organic molecules used as coloring and flavoring agents.[3]

As noted above, the independent, international expert scientific group, JECFA, is responsible for the worldwide risk assessment of human health from food additives. Only additives that have been evaluated according to the JECFA safety assessment and are found not to present an appreciable health risk to consumers, are then presented to national authorities for consumption, whether the additives are organic, natural, or synthetically derived. Toxicological tests usually include acute, short-term, and long-term studies that determine how the food additive is absorbed, distributed, and eliminated, and possible harmful effects of the additive or its by-products at certain exposure levels of experimental animals at several concentrations, usually several times greater than that expected to be consumed by humans. Post-experimental follow-up observations are also monitored in humans.

However, experimental testing in animals is confronted with complications of questionable predictive power since data from *in vivo* testing may not accurately reflect behavioral or immunological effects as in humans. In addition, differences in toxicokinetics, such as absorption, distribution, metabolism, and elimination are also of suspect applicability. Another confounding factor is that the administration of relatively large amounts of a chemical substance to experimental animals leads to accumulation from saturation of metabolic or excretory pathways. These kinds of issues encountered with a variety of previously investigated additives render interpretation of toxicological data from experimental animals difficult. Although quantities of food additives consumed by humans are in micrograms, and blood levels are measured in nanograms, consumption occurs over a *lifetime* and is considered *chronic* exposure (notwithstanding sporadic rather than continuous exposure). *In vitro* alternatives to animal testing, many with significant predictive power, have supplanted many of the required *in vivo* testing protocols previously mandated by legislative authorities.

Most of the concerns associated with food additives are related to allergic reactions. The incidence of intolerance to food additives in the population at large is uncertain, most data referring to patients who develop symptoms such as urticaria or asthma. Up to half of these reactions are associated with responses to food ingredients but the data varies widely. Additional factors that influence allergic reactions to food additives involve cross-reactivity between the original chemical and naturally occurring food contaminants, such as between salicy-lates and tartrazine. Interactions between synthetic sweeteners, cyclamate and saccharin (Figure 10.1), both of which suffered from what was interpreted as adverse animal toxicity data eventually forced a ban on the substitute in the US. Interestingly, the US[4] and the EU[5] have since changed their interpretation of the data on the sweetener.

10.2 Tartrazine

The food color tartrazine, also known as E102 in the EU and FD&C Yellow #5 in the US, is well documented for its intolerance studies, particularly in pharma-ceutical preparations. This widely used orange dye is incorporated in consumer juices (orange juice) and carbonated beverages, as well as in a variety of other foodstuffs and pharmaceutical preparations (Figure 10.1).

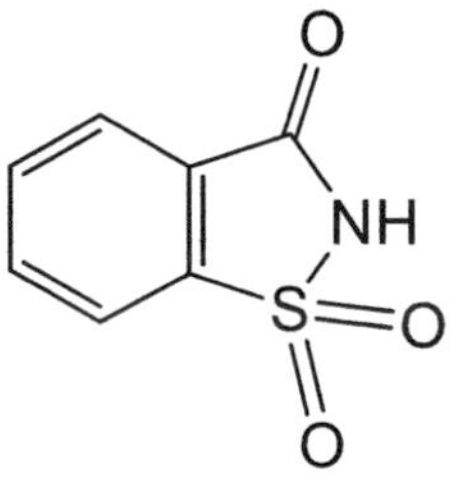

Saccharin
2-benzothiazole-1,1,3-trione

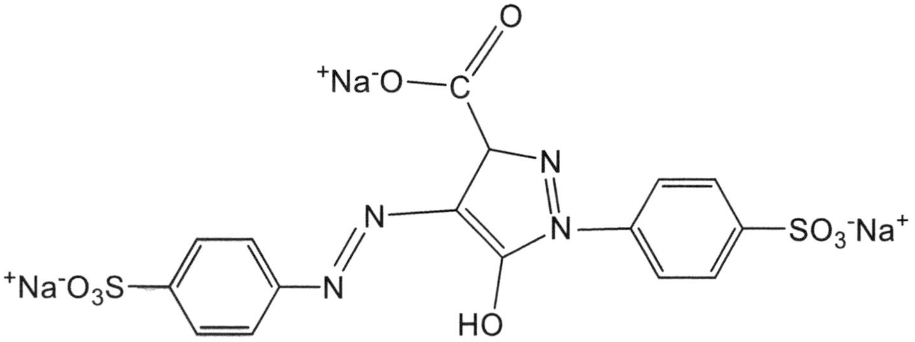

Tartrazine
trisodium carboxylate derivative

Figure 10.1 Structures of saccharine and tartrazine.

Toxic effects ascribed to tartrazine include induction of hyperkinetic behavior (energetic purposeless activity in children), and urticaria (skin rashes). **Hyperkinetic** behavior is difficult to diagnose and distinguish from ADHD[6] which has other unrelated causes. Causation associated with this syndrome and food additives is inconclusive since some studies have shown an improvement in behavior after switching to diets free from artificial colors and flavors.[7] Other data challenges the improvement claimed by altering the diet.

Tartrazine-induced urticaria is more widely accepted as an adverse effect and has been demonstrated in several studies. The mechanism involves a typical inflammatory reaction with the release of **histamine** from dermal and pulmonary mast cells resulting in the appearance of red wheals on skin. Itching, swelling, and redness are common symptoms. Other food coloring agents and food additives cross-react to produce urticaria, such as with the dyes erythrosine and sunset yellow. Asthma is also a symptom of tartrazine hypersensitivity. However, Ardern (2001) argued that there is no evidence that tartrazine makes asthma worse or avoiding it makes asthma patients any better.

Tartrazine sensitivity is often related to aspirin intolerance. Between 10% and 40% of aspirin-sensitive patients respond to tartrazine with reactions ranging from severe asthma to urticaria and mild rhinitis. The mechanism underlying tartrazine sensitivity and its relation to aspirin intolerance is unknown but does not involve **reaginic** antibodies or the prostaglandin synthesis system, as previously suspected. A range of antigenic substances in the diet that are absorbed from the gastrointestinal (GI) tract do not produce immune responses because most individuals develop immunological tolerance via a regulatory system that prevents adverse reactions to food constituents. However, 10% of the western population is predisposed to allergic diseases and does not become immunologically tolerant, hence develop adverse reactions to dietary constituents.

Tartrazine is metabolized by the normal GI[8] flora resulting in elevation of the aminopyrazolone and sulfanilic acid metabolites.

Although the food coloring agent is most implicated in reports of adverse reactions, other food dyes also trigger adverse effects including the 'natural' food color **annatto**. Sadowska et al. (2021) describe the relationship between annatto and production of urticaria.

10.3 Saccharin

This artificial sweetener, first used in the 19th century, has been extensively studied. Banned in 1981, saccharin has long been considered carcinogenic because it produced bladder tumors in rats. However, it is now approved for use in the US as a non-nutritive sweetener with more than 100 countries worldwide legitimately allowing saccharin as a food-sweetening additive. As a food additive, saccharin has low acute toxicity, with an LD_{50}[9] between 5 and 17.7 g/kg in experimental animals. It is not metabolized and volunteers taking large amounts for several months suffered no ill effects. Increased consumption of saccharin and a report showing another sweetener to be carcinogenic prompted further studies to be carried out. In one, saccharin and cyclamate were studied as mixtures with doses up to 2,500 mg/kg. Bladder tumors were observed and, as a result, cyclamate was banned. Still, further studies were carried out but proved inconclusive. Finally, in a comprehensive study Canadian authorities showed that saccharin could produce bladder tumors in rats and saccharin availability was suspended by Canadian and US regulators in 1977. The **Delaney Clause** of the Food, Drug and Cosmetic Act (U.S. Department of Health and Human Services, 1958) prohibits the use of any food additive which has been shown to produce cancer in laboratory animals. The public outcry against this amendment was significant since saccharin was the only general-purpose artificial sweetener approved and available for diabetics, as well as for other members of the public wishing to reduce their sugar intake. The result was a moratorium on the ban pending further evidence.

Epidemiologic studies showed no increased incidence of bladder tumors with saccharin but others have indicated a slight increase in bladder tumor risk (National Cancer Institute [NCI], 2022). Pharmacokinetic studies have since demonstrated that plasma clearance of saccharin is *saturated* at the higher exposure level, resulting in higher tissue concentrations than would be predicted from a linear extrapolation of data from lower dose studies (NCI, 2022). Consequently, such high-level exposures in animals are inappropriate with regard to normal human exposure.

The absence of detectable metabolism of saccharin after chronic low-level dietary exposure and negative mutagenicity data were summarized to indicate that saccharin was not a classical electrophilic carcinogen. Therefore, any carcinogenicity was probably due to the unmetabolized parent compound acting by an epigenetic mechanism. As a result, the National Toxicology Program (NTP), U.S. National Institutes of Health (NIH) concluded that saccharin should be removed from the list of potential carcinogens, nor was it necessary to bear the warning label.

The toxicological case for saccharin illustrates the wider social aspects as well as the scientific considerations involved with toxicology. Continuous monitoring of toxicological data has provided evidence for evaluating and updating judgments for human risk assessment.

10.4 Food Contaminants

Other synthetic and naturally occurring chemicals are also classified as food contaminants, particularly toxic bacterial or fungal by-products, toxic degradation products from food constituents,[10] or ingredients inadvertently added to food. Significant interest has resulted in understanding how toxic and carcinogenic compounds are produced as a result of high-heat cooking, including the chemical production of mutagenic compounds Trp1 and Trp2, and carcinogenic nitroso derivatives resulting from heating dietary amines in food.

Two examples of naturally occurring but toxic food contaminants are botulinum toxin and aflatoxin.

10.4.1 Botulinum Toxin

Botulism is the infectious disease caused by botulinum toxin from the bacterium *Clostridium botulinum*. This anaerobic bacterial organism contaminates poorly packaged, canned, or bottled food (see Chapter 13, Natural Products, for a complete discussion).

10.4.2 Aflatoxin

Aflatoxins are a group of related mycotoxins produced by the fungi (mold) *Aspergillus flavus* and *Aspergillus parasiticus*, which are abundant in warm and humid regions of the world. The mold grows typically on crops such as maize (corn), peanuts, cottonseed, and tree nuts in hot, humid climates, such as Sub-Saharan West Africa and Southeast Asia. The bacterium secretes four separately toxic compounds, B_1, B_2, G_1, and G_2.

Poisoning from the organism (aflatoxicosis) is a global problem, with chronic exposure occurring primarily in developing countries. Outbreaks of acute liver failure (jaundice, lethargy, nausea, death) have been observed in human populations since the 1960s. Epidemiological evidence has associated intake of aflatoxin B1 and liver cancer in humans.

Contaminated crops are difficult to sell to countries that have strict criteria on levels of mycotoxins. Accordingly, the tainted crops are then exported to or sold within poorer third-world nations. In addition, the syndrome is a major concern in the production of domestic and livestock pet food.

Animals fed on meals derived from contaminated feed, such as peanuts or corn, have developed tumors. The syndrome was identified when turkeys died en masse when fed moldy peanuts and pathology showed they suffered liver damage. Traces of aflatoxin have been detected in peanut butter, especially that made from peanuts not treated with chemicals to prevent mold growth, which were subsequently sold in international health and pet food shops labeled as 'natural'.

Aflatoxin B_1 is a potent liver carcinogen and hepatotoxin; 1 ppb[11] (in contrast to ppm) in the diet is sufficient to cause liver tumors, as evidenced by the higher incidence of liver cancer on the African continent. The mechanism of toxicity of aflatoxin B_1 involves metabolism to a chemically **reactive intermediate** (an epoxide) which binds covalently to protein and interacts with nucleic acids. This chemically reactive intermediate is responsible for both liver necrosis and liver tumors (Figure 10.2).

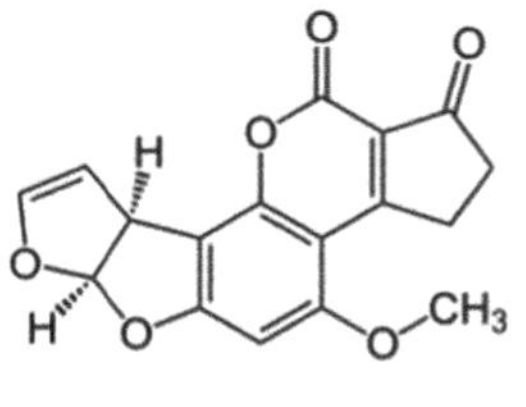

Figure 10.2 Structure of aflatoxin B1.

10.4.3 Ginger Jake

> Then he would eat of some craved food until he was sick; or he would drink Jake or whiskey until he was shaken paralytic with red wet eyes.
>
> *The Grapes of Wrath, John Steinbeck*

Tri-orthocresyl phosphate (TOCP) is a solvent used in industry in the preparation of lacquers and varnishes and was extensively used in the leather industry. It is odorless and tasteless. TOCP has been involved in a number of poisoning cases, including a notorious case in the 1930s. The poisoning was a result of the conditions during the US Prohibition where alternative ways of obtaining alcohol were prominent. One source was an alcoholic extract of Jamaica Ginger, an official US Pharmacopoeia preparation sold for the cure of common ailments. It could be sold despite the alcohol content as the large amount of ginger it contained was very irritating and unpalatable. However, adulterated versions were soon produced containing less ginger. At 35 cents per bottle, usually mixed with Coca–Cola®, it was fit to drink and contained more alcohol than a legal drink before Prohibition. Consequently, as a newly derived source of alcohol, it was particularly inviting within the poorer southern US States. However, batches of the illegal preparation were adulterated with poisonous TOCP, probably incorporated by 'bootleggers' as a solvent. The first reports appeared in 1930 and described the sudden onset of cramps and sore calf muscles followed quickly by paralysis in both legs. Its effect on the peroneal nerve caused foot drop.[12] Victims were mainly poor farmers and workers who were also unemployed during the Depression (1929). As many as 50,000 poisoning cases were documented, many of whom suffered permanent paralysis.[13]

The paralysis caused by the TOCP-contaminated popular drink, known as *Ginger Jake* or *Jake* was labeled Jake Leg. Phrases in music *blues* songs from that period refer to the episode:

> Jake liquor, Jake liquor, what in the world you tryin' to do?
> Everybody in the city messed up on account of you.
> I drank so much Jake it settled all in my knee.
> I reached for my loving baby but she turned her back on me.
>
> Blues Song, I shman Bracey, 1930

10.4.4 The Toxic Oil (Spanish Oil) Syndrome

Non-natural substances also contaminate food and a recent, tragic example was the contamination of cooking oil in Spain.

An unusual outbreak of pulmonary disease was reported around Madrid in May 1981 (Figure 10.3). The syndrome involved the formation of acute but severe pulmonary infiltrates, incapacitating myalgias, **exanthema**,[14] and peripheral eosinophilia.[15] Overall, more than 20,000 cases of the syndrome and 351 fatalities were reported. A toxic substance was suspected after which a causal relationship was established between the disease and the use of poorly manufactured, reduced-quality cooking oil (*rapeseed oil*). Action by the Spanish government to replace the oil with pure olive oil decreased the numbers of reported cases. The statistical correlation established between the consumption of the toxic oil, especially in the fraudulent market, and the development of the syndrome, helped to identify the causes, prevention, and treatment (Gelpí *et al.*, 2002).

The disease appeared after a latent period of at least 1–2 weeks and an apparent dose-response relationship was noted. However, the association between the intake of oil and the syndrome was circumstantial as the effects were not reproduced in experimental animals and the precise causative agent was not identified. The syndrome had an acute phase with mainly pulmonary interstitial edema, and a chronic neuromuscular phase with muscular atrophy, skin lesions, and weight loss. **Vasculitis** was also observed which affected peripheral blood vessels.

Spanish law required denaturation of imported rapeseed oil with the addition of aniline, so as to render it unusable for cooking. However, the oil was fraudulently refined and the resulting product was sold as suitable for human consumption. This practice was previously employed without production of the toxic effects, settling on the conclusion that the batch of oil responsible for the syndrome may have been altered differently. It was also mixed with other oils in some cases. Identification of the toxic constituents to date has been inconclusive. Epidemiologic studies and chemical analysis data suggest an autoimmune mechanism for TOS, such as high levels of soluble interleukin-2 receptor. In addition, the disease is strongly associated with the consumption of oils containing fatty acid esters of 3-(N-phenylamino)-1,2-propanediol (PAP). However, the causal relationship remains to be identified; it is unknown whether PAP esters are either simple markers of toxicity of the oils or have the capacity to induce the disease. In either case, the problem of obtaining samples of oil reliably associated with the syndrome and the absence of an animal model significantly hampered the research.

10.5 Summary and Learning Objectives

Food contains many unrelated substances: normal constituents, naturally occurring contaminants, and synthetic additives. Food additives are purposely used to color, preserve or flavor food products. Although many are tested for toxicity, humans are continuously exposed throughout a lifetime. Laboratory testing of additives in animals, such as high doses of the sweetener saccharin, however, lead to the development of pathological changes (bladder tumors) which were difficult to interpret in humans. Toxicokinetics of high-dose substances are confounded by elimination kinetics when pathways become saturated. Based on the toxicological understanding at the time, the sweetener was banned for commercial use.

Contaminants also appear from inappropriate treatment of foodstuffs such as in the case of Ginger Jake when tri-o-cresyl phosphate was used as a solvent for

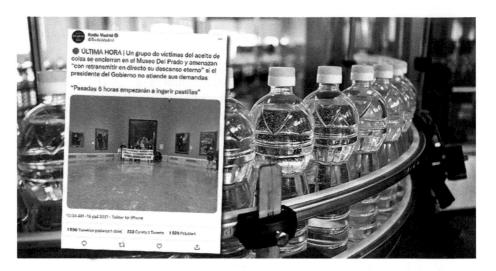

Figure 10.3 Headline alluding to the Spanish oil cases. (From: newsbeezer. com https://newsbeezer.com/polandeng/the-toxic-oil-syndrome-killed-hundreds-of-people-in-spain-they-thought-it-was-oil/.)

ginger in a pharmaceutical preparation bought for its alcohol content as a cheap drink during Prohibition. The organophosphate caused peripheral neuropathy resulting in paralysis and foot drop (*Jake leg*) in many victims. In the toxic oil (*Spanish oil*) syndrome (TOS), contaminated rapeseed oil was sold for cooking, leading to many deaths and victims of an unusual syndrome which included muscular atrophy, weight loss, and pulmonary edema. Products of mold, such as *Aspergillus flavus,* which grows on crops, include the aflatoxins. Aflatoxin B_1 causes liver cancer when its metabolite interacts with DNA. Other toxic agents are produced by bacterial contamination of food, as noted with *Salmonella* or *Clostridium botulinum* infections.

Review Questions

1. Match the food additives on the left (A–E) with the appropriate category on the right (a–e).

A. Erythrosine	a. flavor enhancer
B. Monosodium glutamate	b. antioxidant
C. Cinnamaldehyde	c. coloring agent
D. Butylated hydroxytoluene	d. bleach
E. Benzoyl peroxide	e. flavoring agent

2. Indicate which of the following statements is true and which is false? Tartrazine: (a) is a flavoring agent; (b) causes urticaria; (c) is reduced by gastrointestinal (GI) bacteria; (d) is known as F102; (e) is a derivative of aspirin.

3. Indicate which of the following statements is true and which is false? The sweetener saccharin: (a) causes bladder tumors in rats at high doses; (b) was discovered by Delaney et al.; (c) is banned for use as a sweetener worldwide; (d) has low acute toxicity; (e) shows saturation pharmacokinetics.

4. Indicate which of the following statements is(are) true and which is(are) false? The TOS: (a) was caused using adulterated sunflower oil for cooking; (b) was caused by TOCP used in cooking; (c) is a type of muscular dystrophy; (d) causes pulmonary edema.

Short Answer Question

5. Name three naturally occurring toxicants and briefly explain their appearance in food.

Notes

1. Preservatives include salt in dried meats or fish, sugar in marmalades, or sulfates in wine.
2. For instance, food poisoning from *Salmonella* contamination or botulinum toxin provokes serious bacterial pathological consequences for the unsuspecting consumer.
3. Historically food additives later discovered to possess significant toxicity, were inadvertently used; butter yellow (4-dimethylaminoazobenzene), a color dye for dairy products, proved to be carcinogenic capable of initiating liver tumors in experimental animals.
4. The U.S. National Toxicology Program (NTP) and The International Agency for Research on Cancer (IARC) support the U.S. Environmental Protection Agency's (EPA) conclusion that saccharin is safe "at human levels of consumption" because, after assessing many saccharin-sweetened human foods, no association between saccharin and cancer could be established (Touyz, 2011).
5. The WHO and the E.U. Scientific Committee for Food concluded that saccharin is safe at human levels of consumption. Consequently, saccharin has been removed from the list of substances hazardous to humans (WHO, 2022).
6. Attention deficit hyperactivity disorder.
7. Feingold diet; favorable conclusions by Miller and Nicklin (1984) were countered by Lin and Ho (1994).
8. Gastrointestinal.
9. Lethal dose 50%.
10. Pyrolysis products resulting from cooking.

11. Parts per billion.
12. Loss of control of dorsal extensor muscles of the foot and toes resulting in difficulty lifting the front part of the foot (*dragging*).
13. A series of cases occurred in Cincinnati (1932) where 2,500 people were affected. The episode did not receive much attention until 21 individuals and 6 corporations were indicted (1967).
14. Skin rash accompanying a disease or fever, which also includes allergic contact dermatitis.
15. A higher-than-normal level of eosinophils, a white blood cell of granulocyte classification.

Bibliography

Ardern, K. Cochrane airways group, tartrazine exclusion for allergic asthma, *Cochrane Database Systematic Reviews,* 2001(4), CD000460, 2001, Doi: 10.1002/14651858.CD000460.

Gelpí, E., de la Paz, M.P., Terracini, B., Abaitua, I., de la Cámara, A.G., Kilbourne, E.M., Lahoz, C., Nemery, B., Philen, R.M., Soldevilla, L. and Tarkowski, S., WHO/CISAT scientific committee for the toxic oil syndrome, *Environmental Health Perspectives,* 110, 457–464, 2002. http://ehpnet1.niehs.nih.gov/docs/2002/110p457-464gelpi/abstract.html.

National Academy of Sciences (U.S. NAS), *Saccharin: Technical Assessment of Risks and Benefits*, Report No. 1, Committee for a Study on Saccharin and Food Safety Policy, Washington, DC, 1978. https://nap.nationalacademies.org/catalog/20013/saccharin-technical-assessment-of-risks-and-benefits.

National Cancer Institute (NCI), U.S. National Institutes of Health (NIH). https://pubchem.ncbi.nlm.nih.gov/compound/saccharin. Last accessed April 2022.

Sadowska, B., Sztormowska, M. and Chełmińska, M., Annatto hypersensitivity after oral ingestion confirmed by placebo-controlled oral challenge, *Annals Allergy, Asthma, Immunology*, 127, 403–516, 2021. Doi: 10.1016/j.anai.2021.07.019.

World Health Organisation, *Toxic Oil Syndrome, Report on a WHO Meeting, Madrid 1983*, WHO, Copenhagen, 1984. https://www.euro.who.int/__data/assets/pdf_file/0005/98447/E84423.pdf, last accessed Nov. 2022.

World Health Organisation, *Assessing Chemical Risks*, https://www.who.int/activities/assessing-chemical-risks-in-food. Last accessed, April 2022.

Suggested Readings

Hanssen, M. and Marsden, J., *E for Additives*, Thorsons, Wellingborough, 1987.

Miller, K. and Nicklin, S., Adverse reactions to food additives and colors, in: *Developments in Food Colors*, vol. 2, Walford, J. (Ed.), Elsevier Applied Science, Amsterdam, 1984.

Rechcigl, M., *Handbook of Naturally Occurring Food Toxicants*, CRC Press, Boca Raton, FL, 1983.

Touyz, L.Z.G., Saccharin deemed "not hazardous" in United States and abroad, *Current Oncology*, 18(5), 213–214, 2011. Doi: 10.3747/co.v18i5.836.

Chapter 11

Pesticides and Herbicides

Chapter Outline

This chapter discusses toxicology of pesticides and herbicides using specific examples.

11.1	Introduction and Types of Pesticides and Herbicides	147
11.2	Dichloro-diphenyltrichloroethane	149
11.3	Organophosphorus Compounds	153
11.4	Paraquat	156
11.5	Fluoroacetate	158
11.6	Summary and Learning Objectives	159
	Review Questions	160
	Short Answer Questions	160
	Notes	160
	Bibliography	160
	Suggested Readings	162

11.1 Introduction and Types of Pesticides and Herbicides

Pesticides are substances designed for selective toxicity to a variety of organisms. Although their toxicity is selective, they are also toxic to other species. As well as being of interest in terms of their mode of action they are of concern to toxicologists for two reasons: (1) the substances are potentially toxic to humans either in acute poisonings or after chronic exposure, and (2) the compounds have toxic effects on unintentional target organisms in the environment.

Human poisonings from accidental exposure to pesticides have occurred since they were first used (Table 11.1). Occasionally, human poisonings occurred, sometimes fatally. Many of these cases were due to accidental contamination of food or inappropriate use. For example, organic mercury fungicides used to treat seed grain for animal feed resulted in several mass poisonings of humans.

DOI: 10.1201/9781003188575-11

Table 11.1 Human Poisonings from Accidental Exposure to Pesticides

Pesticide Involved	Year	Material Contaminated	No. Affected	No. of Deaths	Locations
Endrin	1967	Flour	159	0	Wales
Endrin	1967	Flour	691	24	Qatar
Parathion	1967	Flour	600	88	Colombia
Parathion	1968	Sugar	300	17	Tijuana
Hexachlorobenzene	1955–1959	Seed grain	>3,000	3%–11%	Anatolia
Methylmercury	1971	Seed grain	321	35	Iraq
Malathion	1976	For malaria	2,800	5	Pakistan
Pentachlorophenol	1967	Nursery linens	20	2	Missouri, U.S.A.

Source: Report of the Secretary's Commission on Pesticides and Their Relationships to Environmental Health. Washington D.C. U.S. Governmental Printing Office, 1969.

Occupational poisoning has also occurred in agricultural workers through accidental contamination or untimely use. Careless use of pesticides, such as spraying without adequate protection, also leads to exposure of the operator.

Chronic toxicity due to pesticides present in the environment is more difficult to identify although with development of improved analytical techniques; the detection of residues has become easier. Such techniques have shown the ability to universally measure exposure and detectable levels of pesticides. However, chemicals are an important part of society, especially for agricultural economics and food production. Although their use is curtailed in some instances, it is unlikely to be completely halted when risk/benefit considerations are presented.

Pesticides are divided into several groups, including insecticides, fungicides, herbicides, and rodenticides, depending on the target organism. Although the chemicals in each category are designed for specific target species, there is considerable overlap in the biological targets. For instance, selective toxicity of a pesticide is demonstrated with the anticoagulant warfarin, typically applied as a rodenticide. The chemical is effective since rodents *lack* a vomit reflex which renders them incapable of vomiting after ingesting the poison.

Other pesticides depend on diverse mammalian biochemical differences. For example, malathion is *hydrolyzed* in mammals to yield the dicarboxylic acid metabolite, which is readily excreted following further conjugation (Figure 11.1). In insects, however, the preferred metabolic route is *oxidation* to yield malaoxon, whose toxic action is through the inhibition of cholinesterase. Although pesticides are perceived as equally hazardous to humans, they vary in their toxicity to mammals, other non-target wildlife, and their effects on the environment.

Table 11.2 lists examples of the major pesticide types emphasizing the range of chemical classifications. As noted in Figure 11.1, selective toxicity to humans and mammals follows different mechanisms depending on the distinct metabolic pathways.

Table 11.2 Classification of a Variety of Pesticides

Pesticide Classifications	Types
Insecticides	Organophosphorus compounds; carbamate and organochlorines; natural products
Herbicides	Chlorophenoxy compounds; triazines, bipyridyls, substituted ureas, aromatic amides
Fungicides	Alkyl mercury compounds; chlorinated hydrocarbons, dialkyldithiocarbamates, organotin
Rodenticides	Anticoagulants, red squill, phosphorous, metals, α-naphthylthiourea

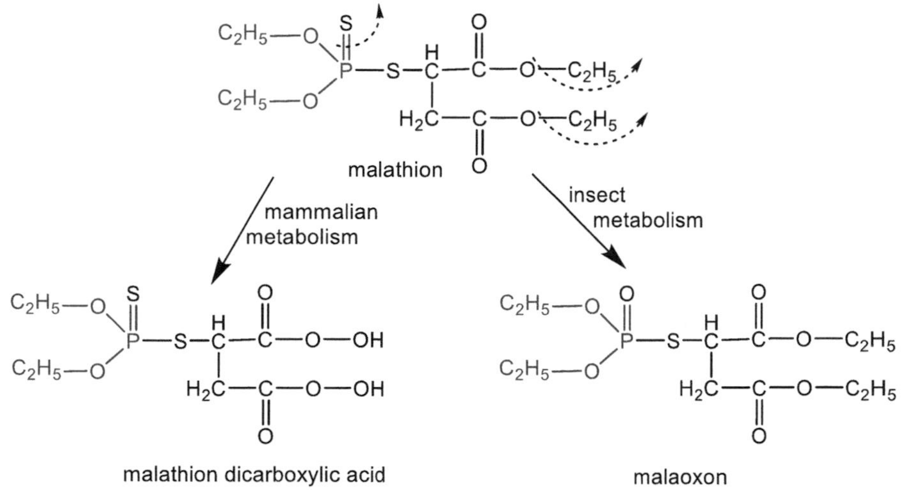

Figure 11.1 Comparative metabolism of malathion in mammals and in insects.

The following discussion represents characteristics of some toxicologically important examples of pesticides.

11.2 Dichloro-diphenyltrichloroethane

A historically important organochlorine insecticide is DDT (dichloro-diphenyltrichloroethane). Introduced commercially in 1945 for control of malarial mosquitoes, the insecticide achieved immediate success as a major factor in the reduction of malaria following World War II.

Dichloro-diphenyltrichloroethane is a contact poison highly effective against the insect nervous system yet is relatively non-toxic to humans. A dose of at least 10 mg/kg is required for toxic effects. The persistence of DDT in the environment and the contribution of the insecticide to reduction of wildlife populations prompted the reevaluation of the utility of DDT and related chlorinated hydrocarbons. Heavy use of DDT in the US before 1966 was responsible for a previously undetected epidemic of premature births. Epidemiological studies since then suggest some human reproductive toxicity of DDT. The pesticide is still widely used and highly effective in areas where mosquito-borne malaria is a major public health problem.

In experimental animals, large doses cause tremors, hyperexcitability and convulsions, paresthesias, irritability, and dizziness. Liver damage occurs after single large doses; **hypertrophy** and other histological changes in **liver** have been reported after chronic exposure. Toxic effects appear to involve the nervous system in mammals as in insects. The mechanism of action is unknown but the primary site of action is sensory; motor nerve fibers and the motor cortex are suspected targets. DDT alters Na^+ and K^+ *transport* across nerve membranes by interfering with energy metabolism required for this pathway.

Toxicokinetic studies show that DDT is chemically stable, highly insoluble in water, but soluble in lipids; consequently, it is persistent in biological systems and the environment, particularly in organic reservoirs (Table 11.3). It is poorly absorbed through the skin and is metabolized by several routes. Figure 11.2 shows the structure and metabolic fate, depending on the cytochrome enzymes involved. The metabolite dichloro-diphenyldichloroethylene (DDE), however, is more persistent in organic tissue than the parent compound (Table 11.3, half-life), but the dichloro-diphenyldichloroethane (DDD) metabolite has persisted in soil sediments for more than 20 years after the banning of DDT (Table 11.3, Maximum concentrations). Of the other metabolites, an acidic derivative [2,2-bis(4-chlorophenyl)acetic acid (or dichlorodiphenyl acetic acid; DDA)] is water-soluble but this conversion is a minor pathway. There is also microbial and environmental degradation of DDT metabolites.

Table 11.3 Persistence of the Insecticide DDT and Its Metabolites

Compound	Half-Life in Pigeon (Days)	Maximum Concentrations[a] (μg/kg)	Half-Life in Soil (Years)
DDT	28	35	2.5–15
DDD	23	151	NA
DDE	250	34	NA

Source: From: (ATSDR, 2002).
Abbreviations: DDD, dichloro-diphenyl-dichloroethane; DDE, dichloro-diphenyl-dichloroethylene; DDT, dichloro-diphenyl-trichloroethane; NA, not available.
[a] Maximum concentrations in soil sediment from 168 sites sampled along the southeastern coast of the US in the mid-1990s.

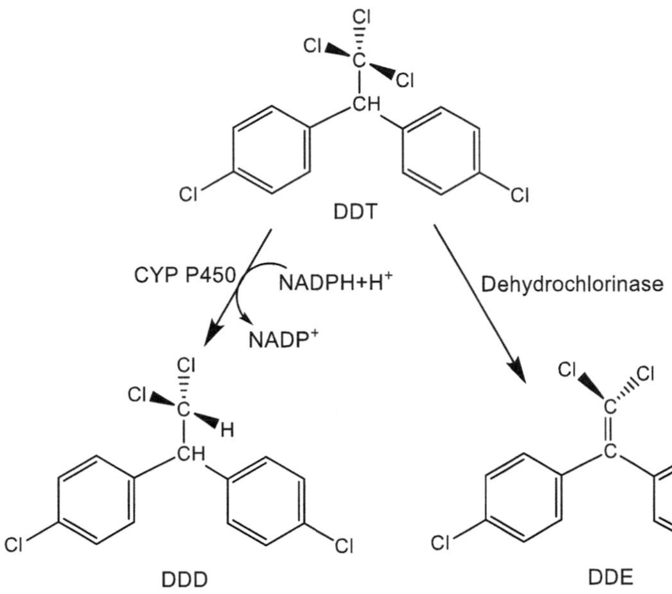

Figure 11.2 Two of the pathways of metabolism of the insecticide dichloro-diphenyl-trichloroethane (DDT). (DDD, dichloro-diphenyl-dichloroethane; DDE, dichloro-diphenyl-dichloroethylene.)

The persistence of DDT in the environment has contributed to increasing levels since it was first used. Furthermore, DDT concentrations in some exposed organisms increase at each higher trophic level of the food chain. For example, small organisms such as plankton, or *Daphnia*,[1] absorb DDT passively via filter feeding from running river or lake water. The pesticide enters fat stores of the organism, reaching concentrations in these tissues several hundred- or thousand-folds greater than the concentrations in the surrounding water. The path of the food chain follows with consumption of contaminated plankton by insects or small fish, promoting the transfer of DDT to their lipid deposits (Table 11.4). The food chain continues with the passage of fat-laden DDT in animals and humans. This continuous process of amplification or biomagnification ensures that relatively high concentrations of DDT progress in higher evolutionary animals despite initial appearance of low DDT concentrations in the water table.

Biodiversity of this toxic phenomenon was illustrated in California, US, where plankton were measured to contain 4 ppm of DDT, while bass fish found in the same area contained 138 ppm; the grebes[2] feeding on them contained 1,500 ppm. Thus what appears to be negligible concentrations of DDT in river or lake waterbeds has significant biological consequences.

Toxic concentrations of DDT also affect birds and fish in the production of eggs, particularly the eggshells. Starting in the 1940s and continuing into the 1960s, the eggs of peregrine falcons and pelicans were discovered to develop thinner shells which were liable to break. A correlation was later found between the development of the fragile eggs and the level of DDE, a metabolite

Table 11.4 Example of the Food Chain Biology and Ultimate Consequences in the Persistence of Organic Pesticides (DDT) in the Environment

Organism	Trophic Level
Pine trees	First producers
Aphids	Second herbivores
Spiders	Third insectivores
Warblers	Fourth insectivores
Hawks	Fifth carnivores

of DDT, in birds of prey such as the kestrel (Lincer, 1975). The cause was ascribed to the effect of DDE on disposition of calcium in the shell gland which is involved in the production of the eggshell.

More recently, the presence of many birds of prey in New York City in recent decades is in large part a testament to the success of nationwide environmental regulation and restoration efforts. The Bald Eagle, Peregrine Falcon, and Osprey were all brought back from steep population declines as a result of US 1972 ban on DDT, which caused eggshell thinning and reproductive failure. The species have also benefited from passage of the US Endangered Species Act (1973), expansion of the Migratory Bird Treaty Act, and dedicated conservation and restoration programs over many decades (NYC Audubon, 2022).

In humans, as in other animals exposed to the pesticide, most of the herbicide is situated in body fat, where the concentration is proportional to intake, reaching a plateau with a half-life of 6 months. The estimated intake for humans in the US in 1969 was around 35 mg/year, but the level in food is declining with a corresponding decrease present in human adipose tissue. This leads to a guideline value for DDT and metabolites in drinking water of 1 µg/L.[3] The Occupational Safety and Health Administration (OSHA) states that workers may not be exposed to amounts of DDT greater than 1 mg DDT/m³ of air (1 mg/m³) for an 8-hour workday, 40-hour work week. The Environmental Protection Agency (EPA) estimates that drinking 2 liters of water per day containing 0.59 ng of DDT/L of water and eating 6.5 g of fish and shellfish per day (from waters containing 0.59 ng DDT/L) would be associated with an increased lifetime cancer risk of $1:10^6$. Fish and shellfish tend to concentrate DDT from the surrounding water in their tissues. FDA has set action levels for DDT/DDE/DDD, at or above which FDA will take legal action to remove products from the market (ATSDR, 2002). Consequently, humans are exposed to DDT either from eating food of contaminated animal origin, fish, vegetables, or fruit which have been the exposed.

Interestingly DDT in fat depots does not appear to be harmful to animals and there is no correlation between adipose tissue levels and signs of poisoning. Circulating blood and nervous system concentrations are more relevant for toxic effects. Also, reductions of fat content of the body translate to higher DDT blood levels. Animal experiments have shown that this increase in the blood leads to toxicity.

DDT has also been detected in human milk where a concentration effect occurs. For example, lactating mothers exposed to 0.5 µg/kg/day produced milk containing 0.08 ppm DDT, exposing the suckling infants to 11.2 µg/kg/day – an exposure is twenty times greater than the mothers.

There is no evidence that DDT under chronic exposure conditions is toxic for humans although evidence of its carcinogenic potential exists in mice. Chronic exposure precipitates microsomal enzyme induction involved in the metabolism of foreign compounds, which has been implicated in hormonal imbalance seen in birds.

The history of DDT illustrates the problems of commercial use of chemicals in the environment and the corresponding assessment of risks and benefits. DDT is an inexpensive and effective insecticide. Unfortunately, it was exploited indiscriminately in agriculture in the US for years after its introduction, resulting in a marked decrease in wild bird populations. This was partly a result of a decrease in the number of insects on which the birds fed but was also a direct toxic effect of DDT. Advancements in chemical analysis improved detection of DDT residues in bird autopsies as well as in other animals.[4]

However, several points of disagreement were raised that scientifically refuted the findings. For instance, detectable levels of DDT in bird carcasses do not necessarily confirm it as the cause of death, nor does it suggest that DDT is toxic in the absence of signs or symptoms. Although it is hazardous to insects when used as an insecticide, insect biochemistry and physiology are significantly different from human metabolism.

Banning of DDT, however, resulted in development of more toxic insecticides resulting in a significant number of human deaths. In addition, control of malarial mosquitoes for which DDT is very effective, has been hampered, allowing for continued prevalence of malaria in many countries. Furthermore, there is a lack of public health data linking the chemical with human toxicity or fatalities. The risk-benefit argument for DDT, when used *responsibly* for control of *disease-carrying* insects, outweighs the risks to humans. Unfortunately, indiscriminate use and negative public perception have confounded the rational scientific arguments.

11.3 Organophosphorus Compounds

Organophosphorus (OP) insecticides were originally developed as nerve gases as possible chemical warfare agents during World War II, the first compound of which was tetraethyl pyrophosphate (TEPP). The biological action of the nerve gases, such as sarin, tabun, and soman, is similar to, but more toxic than the OPs.

The use of organochlorine insecticides has decreased recently because of their persistence in the environment and concerns with long-term effects. While the case against DDT is mainly due to its environmental impact on wildlife rather than its toxicity to humans, OP compounds have been replaced by organochlorines with significantly *more toxicity* to mammals albeit less persistent in the environment.

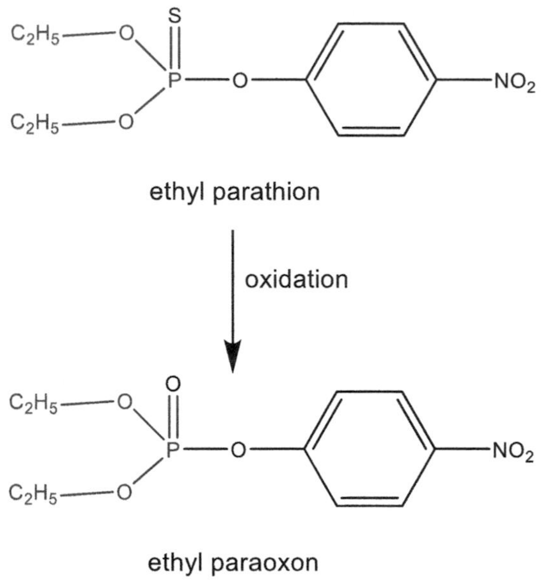

Figure 11.3 Oxidation of the insecticide parathion.

There have been a significant number of human poisonings from OP compounds particularly among agricultural workers throughout the world. Malathion (Figure 11.1) is selectively toxic because of differences in metabolism between mammals and insects, accounting for several large human poisoning cases (Table 11.1). Malathion was formulated as a water-dispersible powder, the components, and storage of which resulted in a change of the molecule. The high storage temperature in some facilities converted some of the parent compounds into *isomalathion*, rendering malathion more toxic to exposed humans.

Many OP compounds in current use as insecticides have similar modes of action and toxicity. Parathion was synthesized in 1944 (Figure 11.3) and marketed as an alternative OP insecticide. It is documented in a number of mass human poisonings (Table 11.1). Because of its high mammalian toxicity parathion was replaced for certain applications by less toxic OP chemicals (Table 11.1). However, the effects of OP compounds are qualitatively similar and their toxicity is considered collectively.

Poisoning with OP compounds is an example of an uncontrolled pharmacological effect rather than a direct toxic action. Toxicity occurs either *cumulatively* following chronic exposure or acutely after single exposures. Acetylcholine (Ach) is a neurotransmitter present at neuronal synapses (nerve endings) throughout the nervous system. Figure 11.4 illustrates the reaction of the enzyme, acetylcholine esterase (AchE) with its substrate, acetylcholine (Ach). The enzyme hydrolyzes Ach yielding a choline molecule; meanwhile, the enzyme becomes acetylated. Further hydrolysis releases the enzyme and produces acetic acid, which is readily excreted.

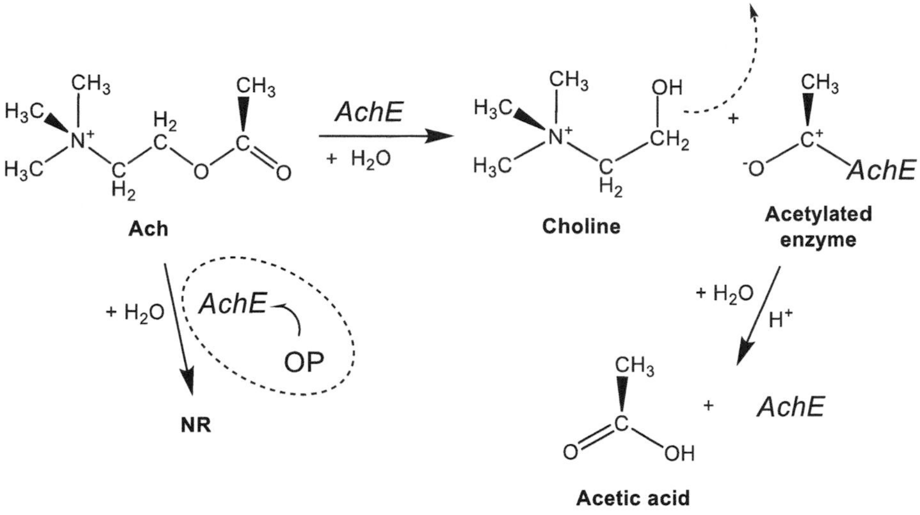

Figure 11.4 Mechanism of hydrolysis of acetylcholine (Ach) by acetylcholinesterase (AchΣ). OPs inhibit the action of the enzyme by forming an irreversible OP—Σ complex (dashed oval) rendering the enzyme incapable of hydrolyzing circulating Ach. Accumulation and over-stimulation from the action of naturally occurring Ach at synapses account for OP toxicity. NR=no hydrolysis reaction.

OP chemicals act as substrates for AchE because of similarities with the natural substrate, Ach. OPs inhibit the action of the enzyme by forming an irreversible OP – enzyme (Σ) complex, rendering the enzyme incapable of hydrolyzing circulating Ach. Hence, inhibition of the enzyme results in accumulation and over-stimulation from the action of naturally occurring Ach at synapses. The near-irreversible nature of the complex requires days to weeks for disassembly, and the excess Ach (cholinergic overload) accounts for the toxic manifestations of OP.

Similar toxicity occurs in humans and other mammalian species. However, OP insecticides are devised so that metabolism differs in mammals and insects such that the compounds are detoxified in the former. However, this is only efficient at low exposure levels; at higher insecticide concentrations humans suffer similar consequences as insects. In the Pakistani poisoning case (Table 11.1), the normal low-level detoxification route of metabolism was overwhelmed by the impurity, thus rendering humans susceptible.

Various types of OP compounds inhibit cholinesterase enzymes resulting in a spectrum of similar toxic effects, including headaches, hallucinations, salivation, increased tear formation, diarrhea, and constriction of pulmonary airways. The symptoms are part of the *cholinergic syndrome* resulting from increased levels of *Ach*. Depending on the OP compound, inhibition is occasionally *reversible*. Acetylcholinesterases differ between plasma and nerve terminals and are not equally inhibited by OP compounds. Degrees of inhibition of total body acetylcholinesterase occur in mammals; 50% inhibition leads to untoward effects whereas 80–90% is lethal. Accordingly, the mechanism of toxicity of OP compounds relies on its similarity to the normal substrate Ach (Figure 11.4). The chemical is also a substrate for the enzyme but unlike Ach, the product remains bound to the active site and the resulting complex is *slowly hydrolyzed*. Consequently, OP compounds that cause *irreversible inhibition* require an inducible but slower process of enzyme *resynthesis*.

Malathion is not a substrate for cholinesterase but requires metabolism to **malaoxon** which takes place readily in insects. In mammals, however, hydrolysis is the preferred route for forming a readily excreted diacid (Figure 3.9), and thus the basis of selective toxicity.

As noted above, noxious effects of OP compounds center around *excessive* **cholinergic stimulation** with death resulting from neuromuscular paralysis and central nervous system (CNS) depression. Also, *unrelated* to the ability to inhibit cholinesterase, a few of the chemicals also cause peripheral neuropathy, with ensuing paralysis of nerves in the arms and legs. In particular, triorthocresyl phosphate (TOCP), used as an industrial solvent, is responsible for several large-scale poisoning episodes generally in relation to food preparation and storage (see Chapter 10).

11.4 Paraquat

This notorious **herbicide** is of importance in human toxicology particularly since it has been featured in several hundred cases of fatal human poisonings over decades of industrial applications. Paraquat (PQ) and its chemically related derivative diquat are non-selective bipyridyl herbicides used widely in agricultural and commercial residential applications (lawn maintenance) to eradicate broadleaf plants and shrubs.

Unlike OP compounds, PQ toxicity is not associated with accidental contamination of food nor has it been linked to environmental impact. PQ poisoning is associated with unintentional or deliberate ingestion, usually orally. It is a contact herbicide that binds strongly to soil and plant leaves, does not leach out of soil when sprayed onto plants, and does not have diffuse environmental effects either on other plants or animals. The herbicide restricts plant photosynthesis by interfering with nicotinamide adenine dinucleotide phosphate (NADPH/NADP⁺) redox cycling; its toxicity in animals is related to similar mammalian mechanisms. When ingested, PQ produces extensive lung and kidney damage. The herbicide *selectively* accumulates in pulmonary alveolar type I and II cells. The concentration in lungs reaches a level *several times* that in plasma as the latter concentration decreases. PQ preferentially accumulates in lungs because of structural similarity with diamines and polyamines (putrescine and spermine; Figure 11.5). The intramolecular distance between the two nitrogens in PQ enables its incorporation into a selective active transport system in alveolar cells for which polyamines are the normal substrate. Only CNS cells with a similar uptake mechanism for polyamines do not accumulate PQ because of the inability of the herbicide to penetrate the polarized membrane of the blood-brain barrier (BBB).

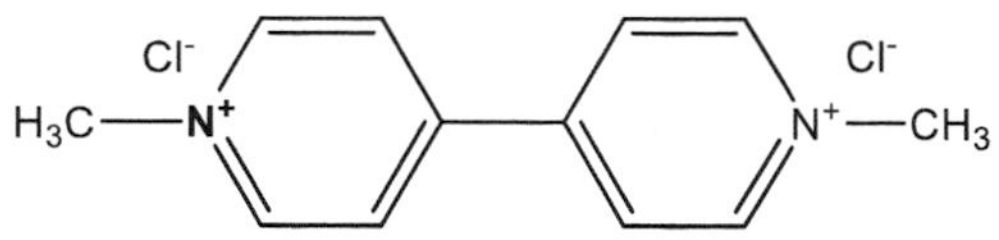

Paraquat hydrochloride

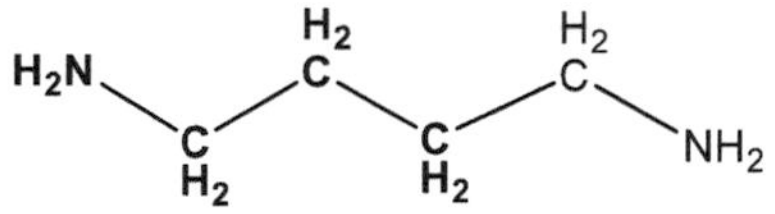

Putresine

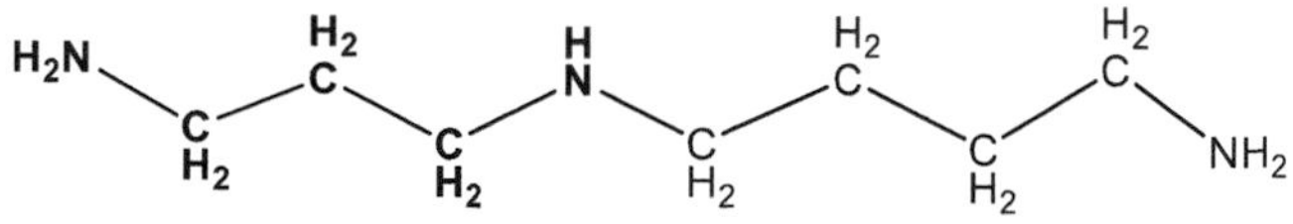

Spermidine

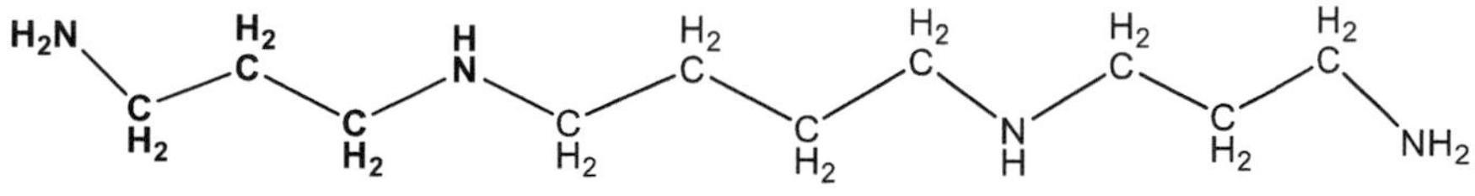

Spermine

Figure 11.5 Structure of the herbicide, paraquat, showing structural similarities to naturally occurring polyamines, putrescine, spermidine, and spermine (bold).

Paraquat is extremely toxic to humans and laboratory animals, the mechanism of which is illustrated in Figure 11.6. The oxidized compound accumulates in lungs and kidneys and undergoes redox cycling reactions (*single electron reduction*). The *oxidized* form of PQ interacts with NADPH, catalyzed by the enzymatic reaction with NADPH-cytochrome P-450-dependent reductase, resulting in the production of PQ *reduced* intermediate free radical. Redox cycling regenerates the oxidized form of PQ with oxygen forming a **superoxide anion**. This cycling continues to produce superoxides with depletion of NADPH, thus depriving the cells of the protective role of reducing equivalents. Generation of superoxide radicals also yields production of hydrogen peroxide and hydroxyl radicals – highly reactive molecular species which stimulate lipid peroxidation and metabolic disruption. The abundant supply of oxygen in the lungs is an important factor in the pathogenesis of pulmonary lesions, toxicity of which is a direct result of active uptake and distribution of the reactive chemical into lung cells.

Paraquat causes progressive fibrosis of the lungs and kidneys. In general, since there are no specific antidotes for PQ exposure, poisoning is managed aggressively with symptomatic and supportive care. Activated charcoal,

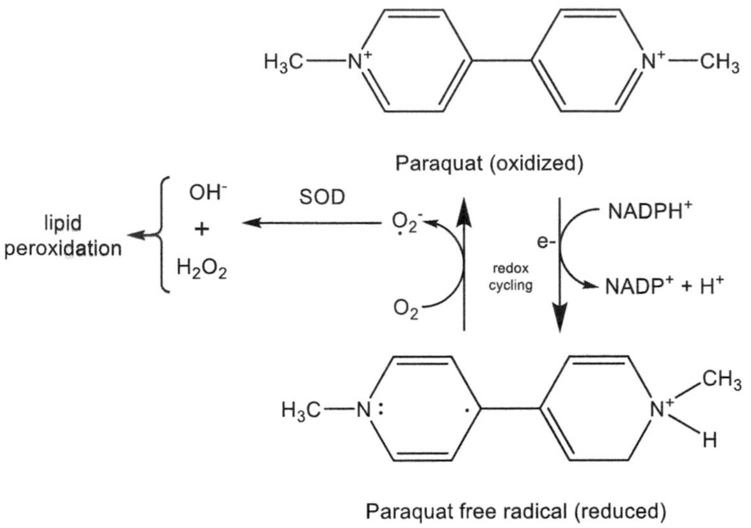

Figure 11.6 Illustration of redox cycling of PQ in the lungs. Oxidized PQ compound undergoes redox cycling reactions (*single electron reduction*). It is metabolized by nicotinamide adenine dinucleotide phosphate (NADPH) to the reduced PQ intermediate free radical. In turn, the reaction catalyzes the oxidation of NADPH to NADP+, resulting in a depletion of the reducing equivalent. An eventual decrease in the NADPH/NADP + ratio deprives the cells of the protective role of reducing equivalents. The reduced PQ free radical intermediate reacts with molecular oxygen to reform the oxidized PQ species (*single electron reduction of oxygen*). The intracellular product of oxygen reduction is the superoxide anion radical (O_2^-). Through a subsequent series of catalyzed reactions involving superoxide dismutase (SOD), O_2^- forms hydroxyl radicals (OH^-) and peroxides (H_2O_2) capable of triggering lipid peroxidation and damage to vital cell membranes and organs.

gastric lavage, and/or administration of a cathartic may prevent further absorption. Forced diuresis and hydration are effective only if intervention is attempted soon after ingestion and in the presence of lower doses of the herbicide. High-flow oxygen is generally used to counteract poor respirations, but its use risks further acceleration of oxidative lung damage. Other interventions such as whole bowel irrigation, forced diuresis, **hemodialysis, hemoperfusion,** surgical approaches, and most pharmacological interventions, do not appear to delay or amend the consequences. PQ toxicity is slow and often painful, occurring over several days to weeks with progressive lung fibrosis culminating in suffocation. The situation is associated with a poor prognosis.

11.5 Fluoroacetate

Monofluoroacetate is a natural product rodenticide pesticide and is found as a component of plants in Australia, Africa, and South America. Indigenous animals in Australia, especially the **skink** and emu, have developed tolerance. However, newly introduced, unadapted, and wandering animals, such as rats, mice, cats, and dogs, are more susceptible to fluoroacetate toxicity.[5] Interestingly, the pesticide is known as 1080 and used to eliminate possums considered pests.

Fluoroacetate is highly toxic due to the specific blockade of the Krebs (tricarboxylic acid) cycle. It is a pseudosubstrate and successfully substitutes into the Krebs cycle for acetyl-coenzyme A (CoA) as fluoroacetyl-CoA. The resulting product, fluorocitrate, binds to the enzyme aconitase, which is subsequently *blocked* and incapable of removing the fluorine atom. The net effect is the inability of the Krebs cycle to function resulting in cell death through a deficiency of metabolic intermediates and energy production.

11.6 Summary and Learning Objectives

Pesticides are chemicals that are *specifically designed* as noxious and lethal to organisms such as **insects** (as *insecticides*), plants (*herbicides*), or rodents (*rodenticides*). Some pesticides demonstrate *selective toxicity* and only affect target organs while others are non-selective and therefore are toxic to many mammalian organisms. Widespread and early indiscriminate use of the insecticide *DDT* resulted in the death of large numbers of birds and wildlife and led to its banning in several countries. Although relatively non-toxic to mammals, DDT is an effective insecticide for the control of mosquitoes carrying malarial parasites. Insect nerve fibers are a pharmacological target for the insecticide, while its metabolites are lipophilic and undergo bioaccumulation in the food chain. Consequently, animals at the top of the evolutionary chain, such as birds, are exposed to higher concentrations of the pesticide. Destruction of non-target insects also reduces the natural food supply for fowl. Chronic toxicity in humans and animals occurs particularly from pesticides that replaced DDT, such as *organophosphates* (parathion and malathion). Following metabolic transformation, the OP chemicals inhibit acetylcholinesterase. However, in mammals, alternative detoxification pathways are available. Depending on the degree of enzyme inhibition, the reaction is reversible. In mammals, however, accumulation of acetylcholine is responsible for the deleterious effects including salivation, diarrhea, bronchoconstriction, and respiratory failure (cholinergic overload). Some organophosphates, such as TOCP, also cause peripheral neuropathy.

Pesticides are toxic to humans, such as the herbicide *PQ*. Lung damage from PQ is a result of selective uptake and accumulation in lung cells with concomitant production of reactive oxygen species. Naturally occurring pesticides, such as *fluoroacetate*, are found in toxic plant species, which block the Krebs cycle. The lethal compound produces heart failure, except those wild mammalian species that developed tolerance.

Review Questions

1. Indicate which of the following statements are true and which are false: DDT is: (a) an organophosphate; (b) lipid soluble; (c) toxic to mammals; (d) metabolized by loss of HCl; (e) inhibits cholinesterase.
2. Indicate which of the following statements are true and which are false: Parathion is an insecticide that: (a) has low toxicity to humans; (b) is not metabolized; (c) acts by inhibiting Na-K ATPase; (d) causes excessive cholinergic stimulation; (e) results in bronchoconstriction.
3. Indicate which of the following statements are true and which are false: Paraquat: (a) is an organochlorine insecticide; (b) is metabolized to diquat by SOD; (c) causes lipid peroxidation; (d) is concentrated in lung tissue; (e) causes liver fibrosis.

Short Answer Questions

4. Describe the underlying mechanism of toxicity of fluoroacetate.
5. Describe the mechanism of paraquat toxicity. Draw formulas to support the answer.

Notes

1. Genus of small planktonic crustaceans, a.k.a. common water fleas..
2. Aquatic diving birds in the order *Podicipediformes,* widely distributed in freshwater as well as marine habitats.
3. As for all pesticides, the recommended guideline value for DDT in drinking-water is set at a level to protect human health; it may not be suitable for the protection of the environment or aquatic life (USEPA).
4. These findings were highlighted in the bestseller *Silent Spring,* Rachel Carson (1962), which subsequently was responsible for the regulatory ban of DDT in many countries.
5. A.K.A. 'chemical warfare' between plants and animals, where plants produce disagreeable compounds as deterrents to animals' inclination to feed upon them.

Bibliography

Agency for Toxic Substances and Disease Registry (ATSDR). *Toxicological Profile for DDT, DDE, and DDD*, U.S. Department of Health and Human Services, Public Health Service, Atlanta, GA, 2002.

Barile, F.A., Chapter 29. Herbicides in: Barile, F.A. *Barile's Clinical Toxicology: Principles and Mechanisms*, (pp. 467–476), 3rd edition, CRC Press, Taylor and Francis, New York, 2019.

Bismuth, C., Garnier, R., Baud, F.J., Muszynski, J. and Keyes, C., Paraquat poisoning. An overview of the current status, Drug Safety, 5, 243, 1990. Doi: 10.2165/00002018-199005040-00002

Bjørling-Poulsen, M., Andersen, H.R. and Grandjean, P., Potential developmental neurotoxicity of pesticides used in Europe, *Environmental Health*, 7, 50, 2008. Doi: 10.1186/1476-069X-7-50

Gangemi, S., Miozzi, E., Teodoro, M., Briguglio, G., De Luca, A., Alibrando, C., Polito, I. and Libra, M. Occupational exposure to pesticides as a possible risk factor for the development of chronic diseases in humans, *Molecular Medicine Reports*, 14, 4475, 2016. Doi: 10.3892/mmr.2016.5817.

Moriarty, F., *Ecotoxicology: The Study of Pollutants in Ecosystems*, 3rd edition, Academic Press, London, 1999.

Narahashi, T., Zhao, X., Ikeda, T., Nagata, K. and Yeh, J.Z., Differential actions of insecticides on target sites: basis for selective toxicity, *Human Experimental Toxicology*, 26, 361, 2007. Doi: 10.1177/0960327106078408.

New York City (NYC) Audubon, Urban Raptors, https://www.nycaudubon.org/our-work/conservation/urban-raptors. Last accessed November 2022.

Patnaik, P., Chapter 44. Pesticides and Herbicides: Classification, Structure, and Analysis, in: Patnaik, P., *Comprehensive Guide to the Hazardous Properties of Chemical Substances*, 3rd edition,, John Wiley and Sons, Hoboken, NJ, 2007.

Sadasivaiah, S., Tozan, Y. and Breman, J.G., Dichlorodiphenyltrichloroethane (DDT) for indoor residual spraying in Africa: How can it be used for malaria control? *American Journal Tropical Medicine Hygiene*, 77, 249, 2007. PMID: 18165500.

Shaw, I.C. and Chadwick, J., Chapter 2. Effects of Pollutants on Ecosystems, in: *Principles of Environmental Toxicology*, Shaw, I.C. and Chadwick, J., (Eds.), CRC Press, Taylor & Francis, Boca Raton, FL., 1998.

Twigg L.E., King, D.R., Bowen, L.H., Wright, G.R., Eason, C.T., Fluoroacetate content of some species of the toxic Australian plant genus, Gastrolobium, and its environmental persistence. *Natural Toxins*, 4(3), 122–127, 1996. Doi: 10.1002/19960403nt4.

U.S. Evironmental Protection Agency (USEPA), Chapter 5. Organophosphates, in: *Recognition and Management of Pesticide Poisonings*, 6th edition, Roberts, J.R. and Reigart, J.R. (Eds.), National Pesticide Information Center (NPIC), 2013. http://npic.orst.edu/rmpp.htm. Last accessed November 2022.

U.S. Environmental Protection Agency (USEPA), *Report of the Secretary's Commission on Pesticides and Their Relationship to Environmental Health*, National Service Center for Environmental Publications (NSCEP), U.S. Department Health, Education & Welfare, 1969. https://nepis.epa.gov/Exe/ZyNET.exe/94002CXI. TXT?ZyActionD=ZyDocument&Client=EPA&Index=Prior+to+1976&Docs=& Query=&Time=&EndTime=&SearchMethod=1&TocRestrict=n&Toc=&TocE ntry=&QField=&QFieldYear=&QFieldMonth=&QFieldDay=&IntQFieldOp=0 &ExtQFieldOp=0&XmlQuery=&File=D%3A%5Czyfiles%5CIndex%20Data%5C7 0thru75%5CTxt%5C00000030%5C94002CXI.txt&User=ANONYMOUS&Passw ord=anonymous&SortMethod=h%7C-&MaximumDocuments=1&FuzzyDegr ee=0&ImageQuality=r75g8/r75g8/x150y150g16/i425&Display=hpfr&DefSee

kPage=x&SearchBack=ZyActionL&Back=ZyActionS&BackDesc=Results%20 page&MaximumPages=1&ZyEntry=1&SeekPage=x&ZyPURL. Last accessed November 2022.

Weselak, M., Arbuckle, T.E. and Foster, W., Pesticide exposures and developmental outcomes: The epidemiological evidence, *Journal Toxicology Environmental Health B. Critical Reviews*, 10, 41, 2007. doi: 10.1080/10937400601034571.

Suggested Readings

Ecobichon, D.J., Chapter 8. Biological Monitoring: Neurophysiological and Behavioral Assessments, in: *Occupational Hazards of Pesticide Exposure: Sampling, Monitoring, Measuring*, Ecobichon, D.J., (Ed.), Hemisphere, Washington, DC, 2020.

Lincer, J. L., DDE-induced eggshell-thinning in the American kestrel: a comparison of the field situation and laboratory results, *Journal of Applied Ecology*, 12, 781, 1975.

Mirmigkou, S. and de Boer, J., DDT and metabolites, in: *Dioxin and Related Compounds*, Mehran Alaee, E.P. (Ed.); *The Handbook of Environmental Chemistry Book Series* (HEC, volume 49, pp. 355–378), Springer-Verlag, Netherlands, 2016.

Rainbow, P., Luoma, S.N., Vignette 4.2. Bioavailability of metals to Aquatic Biota, in: *Fundamentals of Ecotoxicology: The Science of Pollution*, M.C. Newman, (Ed.), 5th Edition, CRC Press, Boca Raton, FL, 2016.

Walker, C.H., Hopkin, S.P., Sibly, R.M. and Peakall, D.B., *Principles of Ecotoxicology*, 4th edition, CRC Press, Boca Raton, FL., 2012.

Chapter 12

Environmental Pollutants

Chapter Outline

This chapter discusses toxicology of environmental pollutants and explores some specific examples.

12.1	Introduction	163
12.2	Air Pollution	165
12.3	Particulate Matter	167
12.4	Acid Rain	168
12.5	Metals	170
	12.5.1 Lead Pollution	170
	12.5.2 Arsenic	172
	12.5.3 Mercury and Methylmercury	174
12.6	Water Pollution	177
12.7	Food Chains	178
12.8	Endocrine Disruptors	180
12.9	Summary and Learning Objectives	184
	Review Questions	185
	Short Answer Question	185
	Notes	186
	Bibliography	186
	Suggested Readings	188

12.1 Introduction

Environmental pollution is an increasing problem over the last century with the development of industry, agriculture, and societal advancements, especially with demands of an increasing population. Pollution of the environment has existed before the 20th century, to note legislation enacted in Britain during the 13th century to control smoke from household fires in London. Pollution on a current scale

DOI: 10.1201/9781003188575-12

started during the Industrial Revolution, particularly from 19th-century factories that used coal for fuel, generating large volumes of smoke as a major pollutant. Blast furnaces, wood-burning chimneys, and chemical plants added other types of noxious substances from fumes. As many industrial processes used water for power, factories were often situated near rivers where effluent was discharged, contaminating both rivers and atmosphere. More recently land pollution from agricultural use of fertilizers and pesticides has increased, as well as from dumping of toxic wastes from factories and industrial effluents. Consequently, air, water, and earth have all suffered from excessive waste products released into the environment.

Despite appalling working and living conditions which existed during the Industrial Revolution in the Western world during the 19th century and in heavily industrialized areas throughout the planet, it was not until the 20th century that a serious attempt was made to curb pollution. One event which precipitated an awareness of the magnitude of the problem was the "**great smog**" in London in the winter of 1952. A combination of weather conditions and smoke from domestic coal fires, factories, and power stations resulted in thick smog, with the release of high concentrations of sulfur dioxide, which contributed to the deaths of over 4,000 people (Figure 12.1).

As a result of the smog event, the British Parliament passed the Clean Air Act which initiated a reduction in production of smoke in major cities. Legislation throughout the world targeted at pollution of rivers allowed gradual clean-up of waterways. Such events necessarily trigger responses from the public and governments but subsequent enactment and realization of corrective measures require many years for development. However, not all regulatory acts result in successful outcomes for the environment. For example, air pollution from coal-burning power stations still occurs, pollution of which travels hundreds of miles from Britain to Norway, Sweden, and Germany, and from the US to Canada. Gases and concomitant acid rain cause damage to trees and or plant

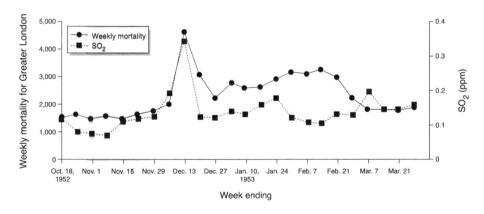

Figure 12.1 Approximate weekly mortality and sulfur dioxide concentrations for Greater London, 1952–1953. Peak death rates correlated with the toxic gas elevations. (From: Bell and Davis, 2001.)

life, as well as to aquatic organisms. It is now well documented that pollution is an *international* problem.

Pollution of the environment is a continuous, deliberate process although industrial and other accidents also contribute to the phenomenon in an acute rather than chronic manner. More specific examples are discussed below.

12.2 Air Pollution

The field of study for air pollution encompasses many disciplines from chemistry, engineering, epidemiology, zoology, botany, ecology, toxicology and meteorology to economics and political sciences.

The most visible form of air pollution is smoke which contains many constituents depending on the source and is accompanied by various potentially toxic gases. Burning of fossil fuels, coal, wood, and oil, as well as other natural resources, produces toxic gases such as sulfur dioxide, carbon dioxide, carbon monoxide (CO), and nitrogen oxides. Other chemicals are also spewed into the atmosphere as a result of burning fossil fuels. Toxic products of combustion (TCPs), such as ammonia, acids, aldehydes, cyanide, isocyanates, halogenated hydrocarbons, and styrene, are known to accompany smoke inhalation. Smoke inhalation from these substances initiates toxic responses from the heat in gases, vapors, and fumes (thermal damage), or act as simple asphyxiants and pulmonary irritants. In the UK, this amounts to millions of tons per year; discharge of sulfur dioxide from burning fuel has reached at least 4 million tons/year. In the US, the five major pollutants account for 98% of all air pollution, including CO (52%), sulfur oxides (18%), hydrocarbons (12%), particulate matter (PM; 10%), and nitrogen oxides (6%). These volatile products arise from the combustion of fuels from power stations, engine exhaust, industrial coal-burning processes, and waste disposal and burning.

Composition and dispersion of air pollutants are also influenced by climate conditions and lead to 'smog'. Originally coined to describe the combination of fog and smoke that hovered over industrial cities under damp atmospheric conditions, it now also includes air pollution from sources known to be modified by climate change.

Two types of smog are categorized: (1) reducing smog which has a high level of PM and sulfur dioxide and originates from coal burning, resulting from a combination of incomplete combustion, fog, and cool temperatures; (2) photochemical-oxidant smog has a high concentration of ozone (O_3), nitrogen oxides, and hydrocarbons and acts as an oxidizing pollutant mixture arising particularly from the interaction of constituents of car exhausts in bright sunlight. Meteorological inversion, as occurs in the US southern California basin, not only promotes this interaction but also traps pollutants near the ground.

Constituents of air pollution are subsequently altered in the atmosphere. For instance, hydrogen sulfide and nitrogen dioxide are oxidized to sulfuric and nitric acids, respectively. O_3 arises from a cyclic reaction between nitrogen dioxide and oxygen, with ultraviolet light and hydrocarbons as requisite catalysts, as noted in equation (12.1):

$$NO_2 \xrightarrow{uv} NO + O^-$$

$$O_2 + O^- \rightarrow \bullet O_3$$

$$\bullet O_3 + NO \rightarrow NO_2 + O_2 \tag{12.1}$$

where NO_2=nitrogen dioxide, NO=nitrous oxide, O_2=diatomic oxygen, O^-=**singlet oxygen**, and O_3=ozone.

Some acute effects on human and mammalian health are known from several episodes occurring within the last 100 years. Three major episodes, in the Meuse Valley, Belgium (1930), Donora, Pennsylvania (1948), and London (1952), have led to significant mortality and morbidity. In each case the areas were heavily polluted; the same meteorological conditions (inversion) prevailed which allowed a stagnant mass of polluted air to accumulate and pollution levels to rise.

Sixty-five deaths in Belgium, 20 in Donora, and 4,000 in London were attributed to smog; they occurred predominantly in the elderly, and individuals with pre-existing respiratory or cardiac disease. Daily average contaminant levels were determined: sulfur dioxide 1.34 parts per million (**ppm**) and smoke 4.5 mg/cc.[1]

Epidemiological studies have shown higher incidences of death from smog in association with pulmonary and cardiovascular disease. Air pollution is also a suspected factor in lung cancer, the incidence of which is higher in urban areas. A correlation also exists between heart disease and higher pollution levels, particularly indoor air pollution. Chronic air pollution aggravates existing respiratory diseases including the common cold.

Air filtration relieves symptoms for some susceptible individuals. Correlations are noted between levels of reducing pollutants and degrees of respiratory discomfort in patients with chronic bronchitis. In addition, mortality from chronic bronchitis is correlated with increasing amounts of sulfur dioxide and dust levels.

Data on effects of photochemical-oxidant and smog on human health are less understood. Many studies have examined the performance of athletic teams, particularly during the Olympic Games in Los Angeles (1984), Atlanta (1996), and Athens (2004) and monitored photochemical-oxidant and other air pollutant levels on performance (Shephard, 1984; Peel et al., 2010; Pierson et al., 1986; Florida-James et al., 2004). The authors conclude that CO, O_3 levels, and smog encountered in these cities affected the athletes' performance in endurance events at the Olympic Games. CO also impairs psychomotor abilities. The only likely physiologic consequence from the effects of 'reducing' smog is an increase in the workload of the respiratory system and thus a decrease in endurance performance.

Nitrogen dioxide and O_3 are *more toxic* than sulfur dioxide and are lower respiratory tract (LRT) irritants. Nitrogen oxides arise principally from car exhaust and cause respiratory symptoms at 5–10 ppm. O_3 causes damage to sensitive plants and affects humans suffering from asthma at levels of 50 parts per billion (**ppb**).

Experimental exposure of animals or human volunteers to individual pollutants confirms the toxic effects noted on human pulmonary airways such as constriction and subsequent increased airway resistance. Synergistic effects occur between pollutants when present in mixtures. For example, the reaction between sulfur dioxide, water, and O_3 yields sulfuric acid, which is facilitated by the presence of hydrocarbons and particulates. Sulfur dioxide is an irritant, but its lethal concentration is far greater than the amount normally encountered in air pollution. Levels of sulfur dioxide greater than 0.05 ppm are reported to cause an increase incidence of respiratory illness; chronic exposure to levels above 0.2 ppm increases mortality. Exposure to levels of 1–5 ppm triggers acute discomfort. Smoke has a synergistic effect on sulfur dioxide toxicity; that is the *combination* has a *greater* undesirable effect than the individual constituents alone.

Carbon monoxide is another component of pollution especially that derived from car exhausts, cigarette smoking, and natural gas and coal burners. Although the chronic toxic effects of CO are uncertain, acute effects are well understood. CO binds strongly to hemoglobin with an affinity 200 times greater than oxygen, so as to reduce the oxygen to tissues. The decreased oxygen-carrying capacity of blood risks critical organ damage, particularly to cerebral and respiratory control centers. Decreases in blood pressure, pulse (heart) rate, and cardiac output occur after 30% saturation of blood with CO, which is achieved at an ambient concentration of 75 ppm. Urban air concentration measures about 10–20 ppm resulting in about 4%–8% saturation. Exposure levels as high as 100 ppm are demonstrated in high-traffic areas, responsible for dizziness, headache, and lassitude. Levels of 120 ppm for 1 hour or 30 ppm for 8 hours are considered serious. CO present in cigarette smoke results in levels greater than 7% carboxyhemoglobin in blood of heavy smokers. Associations between chronic CO exposure in the environment and significant health hazards have not been established. However, as noted above, individuals with pre-existing cardiac, respiratory, or blood disorders appear to be more sensitive to CO.

Power stations, car exhaust, and gas and coal burners emit volatile substances containing hydrocarbons with known or suspected carcinogenic or other toxic effects. PM presents in smoke, deposits in lungs depending on particle size. However, conclusive data on effects of these pollutants on human health are currently under investigation.

12.3 Particulate Matter

Particulate matter (aka *particle pollution*) is defined as a mixture of solid particles and liquid droplets in the air. Some particles, such as dust, dirt, soot, or smoke, are large or dark enough to be seen without a microscope (others are only visible with an electron microscope). PM from smoke is present in the air along with airborne gases as mentioned above.

Particle pollution includes PM_{10}, inhalable particles with diameters that are generally 10 μm (micrometers) and smaller, and $PM_{2.5}$, fine inhalable particles with diameters that are generally 2.5 μm and smaller. There is currently concern about macroscopic-sized small particles, particularly up to 10 μm diameter (PM_{10}). These airborne particles vary in chemical composition but are primarily carbon-laden molecules emitted from automobile exhaust, construction sites, unpaved roads, open fields, smokestacks, or fires. Increasing evidence has demonstrated a significant correlation between levels of PM_{10} in the air with morbidity and mortality. The smallest of particles, $PM_{2.5}$ (fine particles), penetrate the LRT and pose the most significant risk to lung diseases. A strong association has also been established between levels of particulates and hospital admissions of asthmatic patients.

12.4 Acid Rain

Acid rain describes the wet precipitation of sulfuric and nitric acids and dry deposition of sulfur dioxide, nitric acid, and nitrogen oxides. It results from burning of fossil fuels and industrial processes which produce sulfur dioxide and nitrogen oxides. The equation below illustrates reactions that produce acid rain:

$$H_2O + SO_2 \xrightarrow{O_2;\ uv} H_2SO_4$$

$$+ \text{hydrocarbons}$$

$$NO_2 + H_2O \xrightarrow{H_2O;\ uv} HNO_3$$

$$+ \text{ozone}$$

where H_2O = water, SO_2 = sulfur dioxide, H_2SO_4 = sulfuric acid, NO_2 = nitrogen dioxide, and HNO_3 = nitrous acid.

These acids are present and are removed during rain formation (i.e. **washout**). Alternatively, the acids are removed in the upper atmosphere from the atmosphere by falling rain (i.e. **rainout**).

The effects of acid rain have been particularly noticeable in Scandinavia, partly because of the type of soil present. Sweden for example received about 472,000 tons of sulfur dioxide in 1980 but only produced 240,000 tons, some of which were deposited in neighboring countries. Consequently, Sweden suffered a net gain of 230,000 tons of acid deposit despite reducing its own production from 300,000 tons in 1978.

Acid rain is a universal problem whereby pollution is transported internationally. Increased acidity is now recognized in most EU countries as well as the US. The effects of acid rain depend on the type of deposition, the nature of the soil, and *buffering* capacity of soil. The latter is particularly important, since thin soils found in parts of northern EU have poor buffering capacity.

Consequently, the effects of acidity are greater. Acidity in soil also accumulates with time in some areas so that reducing acid deposition will not have an immediate effect.

Sulfur and nitrogen oxides are primarily responsible for causing rain, snow, and mist to become acidic. Rain and snow acidify soil and groundwater to an extent depending on buffering capacity. The volume of rain or snow melt is also important since excessive water accumulation saturates and overwhelms natural buffers in soil. Water then empties into waterways with little contact with bicarbonate and humus present in soil which would buffer the acidity. Consequently, rivers and lakes will become more acidic. Modern farming techniques, such as use of ammonium sulfate fertilizers, also exacerbate acidification. Other consequences affect the *balance* in the **ecosystem**. For example, the acid environment creates a hostile setting for microorganisms. Water of *low* pH *leaches* metals such as cadmium (Cd) and lead (Pb) from the ground and triggers the dissolution of aluminum (Al) salts. Plants that absorb the metals are damaged; ingestion by foraging animals becomes toxic. Cd is highly toxic to mammals; chronic exposure precipitates **kidney damage** and replaces calcium in the skeleton. The condition of the brittle bone syndrome (Japanese Itai-Itai disease) is associated with Cd exposure. Al leached out of the soil and dissolved in local waterways is believed to be responsible for the death of fish in Scandinavian lakes and rivers. The extent of damage to forest land, farms, and domestic vegetation resulting from wet deposition of acid is not clear. However, dry deposition of sulfur dioxide damages leaves directly. In addition, acidic groundwater not only leaches toxic metals which are absorbed by vegetation but also allows outflow of essential nutrients essential for plant and tree survival. Consequently, acidification of soil and release of toxic metals directly or collaterally impairs herbal environments.

Acid rain directly interacts with leaves on contact and infiltrates roots following seepage into soil. The altered water washes or displaces essential elements from soil leading to a deficiency in these nutrients. For instance, loss of magnesium from soil due to acidification is an important contributor in the **ash dieback** of trees that occurred in Germany. Ash dieback is a severe disease that currently devastates the EU populations of *Fraxinus excelsior L.* and *Fraxinus angustifolia Vahl.* The causal agent is the ascomycete (mold) *Hymenoscyphus fraxineus.* German research about *Hymenoscyphus fraxineus* and the compounds produced by this fungus is currently offering recommended management options for its control (Enderle et al., 2017).

Increased acidity also increases the mobility of metals in soil resulting in migration to lower levels inaccessible to the roots. However, effects of acidification vary due to different buffering capacities of soil in a variety of geographical settings.

The pH of lakes and rivers is affected directly by acid rain and indirectly by changes in the microorganisms and surrounding plants. Many species are adversely affected by low pH. For example, from 1954 to 1973, the decrease in the number of Atlantic salmon in several rivers in Nova Scotia was attributed to a drop in riverbed pH, from 5.7 to 4.9. During this period, there was also a fall in numbers of Atlantic salmon. The upset of the delicate balance among the species of fish, animals, or plants as a result of acidification, contributed to the reduction in biologic diversity.

It is universally agreed that all contributors to pollution, from industrial, commercial, and domestic sources, be reduced as much as possible, albeit it is not clear which ones are most important. Investing in the reduction of sulfur dioxide only, for example, has little effect if the important determining factor is the level of O_3 or hydrocarbons which catalyze the conversion of sulfur dioxide and nitrogen oxides to sulfuric and nitric acids, respectively. It is possible, however, to remove some of the sulfur dioxides from smoke derived from fossil fuels before, during, and after burning. Similarly, output of CO, nitrogen oxides, and hydrocarbons from mechanical exhaust systems (transportation vehicles, heating processes) have already been reduced with catalytic converters, the substitution of which has reduced carbon emissions of CO and hydrocarbons from new cars by 90% and nitrogen oxides by 75%. The latter pollutants are involved in the production of O_3 in the atmosphere.[2] Removal of chlorofluorocarbons (CFCs) from **aerosol** propellants is also responsible for *reductions* in atmospheric O_3.

12.5 Metals

12.5.1 Lead Pollution

Inorganic and organic lead (Pb) is a major environmental pollutant and a known poisonous compound for centuries. Its toxicity was recognized by Hippocrates in 300 b.c. in his description of a case of lead poisoning. For centuries workers involved in lead mining and smelting have been occupationally exposed. Pb poisoning contributed to the decline of the Roman Empire as high Pb levels were detected in Roman skeletons during the ancient period. Pb pollution arises mainly from car exhausts but industrial processes, batteries, minerals, paints, and lead-containing insecticides also contribute.[3] Use of cooking vessels with lead glaze or lead components was another source in ancient, recorded history. Industrial poisoning was common during the Industrial Revolution, where *1,000 cases a year* were noted in the UK at the end of the 19th century.

Lead is readily absorbed orally particularly from food or water, or via the lungs; although concentrations from oral intake is greater than that in air, absorption is greater from lungs than from the gastrointestinal tract. Children are more susceptible to Pb toxicity than adults as the rate of oral absorption is greater in adolescents, as well as the rate of incorporation of the metal into growing bones and nerves.

It is estimated that 98% of airborne lead globally is derived from leaded gasoline, and levels in air correlate with the amount of traffic. Pb in car exhausts is derived from tetraethyl Pb, an anti-knock compound added to gasoline and petroleum products which are converted to lead in the engine. Thus the situation becomes a particular occupational hazard for individuals employed in high-traffic conditions, such as crossing guards and highway workers, as a result of greater exposure to car exhausts.

At the beginning of the 20th century, large-scale lead poisoning in children (condition known as *plumbism*) was reported, especially in those living in poor conditions in cities in the US. The source of lead was mainly from industrial and household paints containing relatively large amounts of the additive, as well as children's toys and household furniture. The paint was ingested by children through contamination of food or water, and by an experimental tasting of deteriorating flakes of paint.[4]

The nervous system is a primary target for lead and young children are particularly susceptible. During adolescence, the most serious effect of lead poisoning is **encephalopathy** with a risk of poor neural and brain development, seizures, and cerebral palsy. Chronic exposure to lead during early childhood development is a major concern.

After absorption, 97% of Pb is absorbed by red blood cells (RBC) and incorporated into heme. The half-life ($t_{1/2}$) of Pb in RBCs is 2–3 weeks. Redistribution to liver and kidney occurs slowly, followed by excretion into bile or deposition in bone where it is eventually incorporated into hydroxyapatite crystals. Freely circulating Pb is uncommon, thus the measurement of blood Pb levels is often poor or inaccurate. This is principally because blood Pb is found mainly in RBCs, which distribute chiefly to soft tissue, and account for the high levels occurring in the liver, lung, spleen, and kidneys. Redistribution to Ca^{+2}-containing structures also explains the high Pb concentrations found in bone.

Acceptable blood lead levels (BLL) in the US for asymptomatic children are recorded between 0.20 and 0.24 µg/mL. Table 12.1 shows the suggested protocols and chelation therapy for children in NYC according to BLL. Levels greater than 45 µg/mL require aggressive treatment protocols.

Table 12.1 Recommended Management of Children with Possible Lead Exposure

BLL (µg/dL)	Recommended Action	Chelation Therapy
5–<20	Provide education, risk assessment, reporting BLL to NYCDOHMH; follow-up with appropriate agencies in 3 months.	No chelation therapy
20–<45	Provide recommended actions as above PLUS: evaluate for iron deficiency anemia, X-rays if needed. Follow-up with appropriate agencies in 1–3 months as per BLL test.	No chelation therapy
≥ 45	As above, PLUS: confirm BLL with venous sample, perform FEP test + medical exams; follow-up 1–3 months as per BLL test.	Chelation therapy: DMSA, $CaNa_2EDTA$ and/or BAL depending on BLL

Source: From: the New York City Department of Health and Mental Hygiene (NYCDOHMH). Lead poisoning: Prevention, identification and management, *City Health Information,* 2020, https://www1.nyc.gov/assets/doh/downloads/pdf/lead/lead-guidelines-children.pdf. For chelation therapy: http://www1.nyc.gov/assets/doh/downloads/pdf/lead/lead-chelation.pdf.
Abbreviations: BAL, British anti-Lewisite, dimercaprol; BLL, blood lead level; $CaNa_2EDTA$, calcium disodium edetate, calcium disodium versenate; DMSA, succimer; FEP, free erythrocyte protoporphyrin.

Toxic effects occur at lower levels, however, and are explained by the mechanism of toxicity. Lead interferes with heme and porphyrin synthesis and its effects on enzymes in this pathway are demonstrated in Figure 12.2. Lead binds to enzymes at several steps in heme synthesis: enzymes ferrochelatase, aminolevulinate synthetase (ALAS), and aminolevulinic acid dehydratase (ALAD) are involved with uptake of iron into RBCs. Increased excretion of aminolevulinic acid (ALA) in urine is one marker for lead exposure. Net effects on porphyrin synthesis include reduction in hemoglobin levels, appearance of coproporphyrin, and ALA in urine. Free erythrocyte protoporphyrin (FEP) is increased and ALAD is inhibited.

In 1970, 10% of children in New York City and Chicago had BLL of $0.6 \mu g/mL$, many of which could not be accounted for by living conditions. Thus, iron deficiency anemia is a common result from lead exposure partly due to inhibition of hemoglobin synthesis and destruction of RBC.

While most children show no clinical symptoms, lead exposure can result in learning and behavior problems. Exposures at higher levels present with anemia, abdominal pain, colic, vomiting, seizures, symptoms of encephalopathy, hypertension, or kidney problems and can lead to organ damage and death. Iron deficiency anemia and central nervous system (CNS) effects appear with continuous and prolonged exposure.

As well as affecting the CNS and heme synthesis, lead also triggers skeletal changes in children following chronic exposure. Lines of discoloration at the growing ends of long bones, and at the base of nail cuticles and gingiva (Burtonian lines) are due to deposits of lead. Bone shape is also affected. Acute exposure to lead also causes kidney damage, while chronic exposure precipitates interstitial **nephritis**.[5]

The discussion above relates primarily to the actions of exposure to inorganic lead, yet organic lead is *more toxic* since it is lipid-soluble and well absorbed. For example, triethyl lead, which results from the combustion of petroleum-containing tetraethyl lead, is readily absorbed through skin and into brain and is a primary cause of lead encephalopathy. This accounts for the toxic effects apparent in occupational workers exposed in chemical plants where tetraethyl lead is manufactured. Symptoms occur rapidly and include delusions, hallucinations, and ataxia.

Much of the ambient lead pollution has abated principally due to the removal of lead from gasoline products without major deleterious consequences on costs or automobile performance. The highly toxic effects of lead are well understood and exposure to biochemical pathways has been well studied. The regulations that have been instituted to reduce lead exposure are a success story in identification, prevention, and treatment of a major environmental pollutant.

12.5.2 Arsenic

Among the chemical compounds notorious for contributing to earth and water pollution are heavy metals, particularly arsenic (As). This element is widely distributed in the earth's crust and is associated with mining, used for zinc, copper, gold, and lead extraction, and pesticides. Also seafood, particularly shellfish, accumulate organic As which is less toxic than the inorganic form. Also water

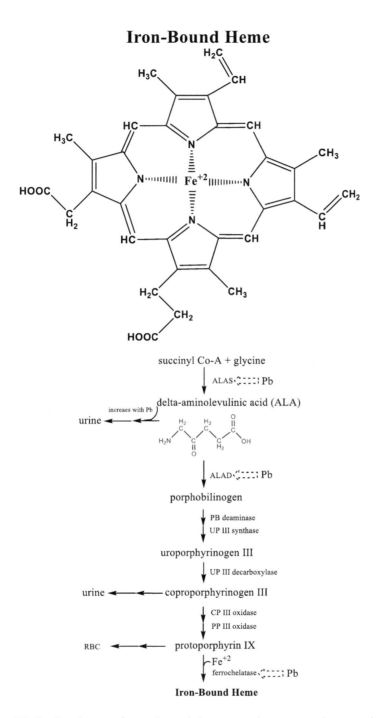

Figure 12.2 Synthesis of iron-bound heme in the mammalian erythrocyte. Pb interferes with proper functioning of enzymes necessary for heme synthesis (dashed arrows) and incorporation of iron into the complex. (ALAS, aminolevulinate synthetase; ALAD, aminolevulinic acid dehydratase.)

173

from groundwater wells and hot springs shows trace amounts of naturally present AS.

Groundwater is a significant source of As poisoning and in some parts of the world, levels are especially high. Significant contamination of water sources was reported in Bihar, India, where AS concentrations in groundwater were detected above the permissible limit. Hand pumps in the district of Buxar were used to replace wells containing bacteria. The same wells were contaminated with AS from groundwater, and subsequently found to present severe AS poisoning with concentrations above 1,500 ppb. The World Health Organization (WHO) guidelines state that the permissible limit of AS in drinking water is 10 ppb, while the Indian government states it to be 50 ppb, five times higher. These districts show far higher concentrations than either limit (CNN Health, 2017).

In this and other countries with high levels of contamination, chronic exposure to AS causes hyperpigmentation of skin, keratosis, and cancer. It is also responsible for the development of black-foot disease, a peripheral vascular disorder, and skin cancer.

12.5.3 Mercury and Methylmercury

Mercury is 'the hottest, the coldest, a true healer, a wicked murderer, a precious medicine, and a deadly poison, a friend that can flatter and lie' (Woodall, 1639).

Like lead and other metals, mercury is highly toxic, the properties of which have been known for centuries. The phrase 'Mad as a Hatter' has its origins from the effects noticed in exposed workers to mercury salts used in industries to cure felt for hats. Historically, Hg has also been used therapeutically to treat syphilis and as a stimulant.

Mercury exists in three chemical forms: elemental, inorganic, and organic, each of which has its own toxic features. Elemental mercury (Hg^0), often used in scientific instruments and formerly incorporated in commercial thermometers, renders toxicity by absorption in vapor form. Hg^0 readily vaporizes even at room temperature and exposure damages the CNS. Inorganic mercury (Hg^+ and Hg^{2+}), in mercury salts, is soluble in water and ingestion results in kidney damage. Organic mercury compounds ($R\text{-}Hg^+$) readily penetrate intact membranes of living organisms and, therefore, are more hazardous than inorganic mercury. As with elemental mercury, the target is the brain and CNS.

Different forms of mercury have similar mechanisms of action involving the reaction of the metal or its ions with sulfhydryl groups, which are part of proteins, such as enzymes. Hence mercury is a potent inhibitor of enzymes where the SH group has an important role. Differences in toxicity of the three forms of the metal are due primarily to distribution in the body. *Elemental mercury* readily penetrates pulmonary alveoli and accesses the capillaries where it is oxidized in RBC to Hg^{2+}. The elemental form also penetrates the blood-brain barrier (BBB) in adult and fetal cells where it is metabolized to Hg^{2+}. Mercury is then trapped in these sites in the ionized form. *Inorganic mercury* alternatively does not cross the BBB but reaches the kidney where it promotes its toxic actions. *Organic mercury* is sufficiently lipid-soluble to distribute to the CNS where it is oxidized to Hg^{2+}

and causes neurological damage. Although the three forms are toxic as a result of binding to sulfhydryl groups in proteins, *differences in distribution* lead to the selective types of toxicity. This is an important illustration of the influence of distribution on the toxicity of xenobiotic compounds.

Exposure to mercury used to be mainly an occupational hazard rather than an environmental one. More recently, however, the metal has gained access to critical environmental paths. This has occurred through the use of organomercury fungicides and in the industrial manufacture of plastics, paper, and batteries, with the resultant discharge of contaminated effluents into lakes and rivers. High levels of the pollutant have been detected in the waters near a battery plant in Michigan, where levels of 1,000 ppm were discovered, well above permissible levels of 5 ppb. Mercury has been detected in air presumably arising from industrial processes.

Dumping of inorganic form of the metal used to be tolerated because it was thought that this chemical entity was relatively innocuous and easily dispersed. Illegal dumping is now controlled and organomercury fungicides are phased out.

Availability of mercury-containing fungicides has led to water contamination via run-off from fields. Other sources of the environmental pollutant are wood pulp factories and chloro-alkali chemistry plants, which were presumably responsible for contamination of freshwater fish detected in Sweden. As with other lipid-soluble contaminants present in the environment, bioconcentration in the food chain also occurs.

A tragic and infamous event occurred in Japan in the 1950s that highlighted the dangers of inorganic mercury as a water pollutant (Harada, 1972). In 1956, a newly built factory on Minamata Bay began commercial production of vinyl chloride and acetaldehyde. Mercuric chloride was used as a catalyst, after which it was discharged into the bay with the rest of the effluent from the factory. Within the year a novel but mysterious illness appeared among local fishermen and their families, later known as Minamata disease. Household pets also suffered similar symptoms. It was eventually recognized in 1959 that the sickness was due to contaminated seafood poisoning with mercury. By 1960, methylmercury was detected in samples of seafood and in sediments derived from the factory. Apparently edible crustaceans, readily consumed by local populations, ingested and absorbed methylmercury. A food chain developed with lipid-soluble organic mercury concentrated by the aquatic organisms. Further investigation revealed that inorganic mercury discharged into rivers, lakes, or waterways was not inert but could be *biomethylated* to methylmercury by microorganisms (Figure 12.3). This occurred especially under *anaerobic* conditions, as in the effluent sludge collected at the bottom of Minamata Bay. This chemical sequence of events showed that inorganic mercury discarded into rivers and lakes is not innocuous, as previously assumed, and is not necessarily dispersed.

Contamination at Minamata Bay led to 700 cases of poisoning and over 70 deaths for several unsuspecting years. Identification and diversion of effluent by the factory eliminated the disease. Other mass poisonings also occurred throughout the world as a result of organomercury compounds applied as fungicides to treat seed grain. A large-scale poisoning incident

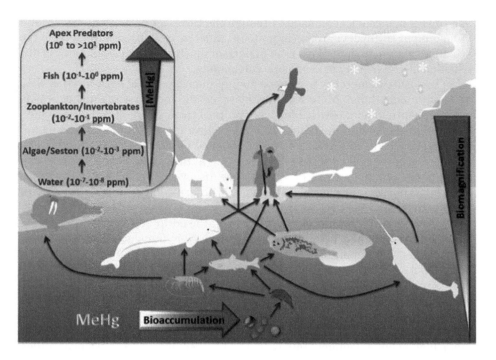

Figure 12.3 Methylmercury (MeHg) bioaccumulation and biomagnification in a typical marine food web. The inset shows the range of MeHg concentrations in aqueous compartments of the food chain. Note how MeHg concentrations increase with each trophic level because of biomagnification (arrow, left), from 10^{-8}ppm in water to 10^1 in higher organisms. (From: Lehnherr, 2014.)

Note: Seston refers to minute material moving in water and including both living organisms (plankton and nekton) and nonliving matter (plant debris or suspended soil particles).

occurred in Iraq (1971) when alkylmercury fungicides were used to treat cereal grain, eventually fed to livestock, resulting in 6,000 cases of poisoning and 500 deaths (Skerfving and Copplestone, 1976).

In 1969, a New Mexico family fed treated grain to their farm pigs, which were then consumed. Three of ten children exposed experienced behavioral abnormalities and neurological disorders. A child exposed *in utero* was born with brain injury where the urinary level of mercury was *15 times* that of the mother.

Symptoms of methylmercury poisoning reflect the entry of the compound into the CNS, beginning with memory loss, paresthesias, ataxia, narrowing of the visual field, and progression to loss of muscle coordination, emotional instability, and development of **cerebral palsy**. Children and newborn infants were most severely affected and those exposed *in utero* were born with severe cerebral palsy even when mothers were symptom-free – classic characteristic of a **teratogen**. Methylmercury crosses the placenta and *concentrates* in fat tissue and brain of the fetus. In addition, fetal RBCs concentrate methylmercury at a rate 30% greater than adult RBCs, total damage of which is irreversible.

Methylmercury that enters brain is demethylated; the inorganic mercury released then binds to sulfhydryl groups of enzymes, inactivating them. Methylmercury has a *long half-life* in biological systems, approximately 70 days. It is localized particularly in liver and brain, which constitutes 10%–20% of the body burden. From this information it is possible to calculate known toxic concentrations and allowable daily intake (ADI) of 0.1 mg/day, allowing for a safety factor of 10. This ADI corresponds to eating 200 g of fish with a mercury level of 0.5 ppm. Seafood in Lake Michigan and in waterways around Sweden have been found to contain as much as *ten times* more mercury.

Like mammals, birds and other biological creatures ingest mercury. For example, studies of the Crested Grebe and Goshawk show that tissue mercury levels have steadily increased since 1870 (Bradley et al., 2017; Wallace et al., 1971).

Chemical substances, such as pesticides and fungicides, which have the potential to contaminate environments, are screened for toxicity. Ecotoxicity testing requires determination of the **biochemical and chemical oxygen demand (BOD** and **COD)**, respectively. BOD designates the ability of microorganisms to metabolize an organic substance. COD is the amount of oxygen required to oxidize a substance. The ratio of COD to BOD is an indication of *biodegradability* of the substance. There are other test systems that suggest the persistence of the compound in the environment, such as determination of abiotic degradation (see U.S. Environmental Protection Agency (U.S. EPA) and U.K. Health and Safety Executive (U.K. HSE) for further reading).

12.6 Water Pollution

Rivers, lakes, and oceans are polluted directly by discharge of effluent from factories and industrial processes, sewage, and domestic waste. Water becomes contaminated also by chemicals on land including pesticides and fertilizers applied to crops and washed by rain into estuaries. Rain also accumulates substances from the atmosphere. Industrial companies dump waste material into underground storage tanks where leakage has been known to contaminate the water table, which risks the domestic water supply in adjacent areas.

Some water pollutants, such as fertilizers from agricultural run-off, sewage, and organic waste products from the food industry, lead to overgrowth of algae and other undesirable aquatic plants which eventually choke local environments and deplete available nutrients. In the process of **eutrophication, aerobic bacteria** accelerate decaying algae which then consume available oxygen in the water. This is soon followed by appearance of **anaerobic bacteria** that continue to feed from decaying plant matter in lakes and riverbeds. The bacteria produce toxic compounds which, along with the lack of oxygen, cause the water to stagnate, threatening other aquatic life.

Humans, animals, and plants are exposed to toxic pollutants in water either through direct oral ingestion or by consuming organisms that have become contaminated by it. The problem is exacerbated in developing countries where toxic substances, such as heavy metals, are not effectively cleared by normal water treatment procedures.

Water pollutants affect organisms within the environment in different ways. High concentrations of toxic compounds kill most or all the organisms within a particular area where concentrations are sufficiently high. More insidious pollutants damage reproductive cycles of organisms. For instance, fish eggs are very susceptible to toxic compounds at low levels which lead to decline in vulnerable fish populations.

Another way in which a pollutant interacts with the environment is by entering the food chains without causing damage to lower organisms. As with the vulnerable populations, reproductive cycles of predators at the top of the chain are affected, contributing to an imbalance with prey. Persistent compounds such as methyl mercury and dichlorodiphenyltrichloroethane (DDT) enter food chains and affect relationships between predator and prey.

Pollutants however may remain in the environment unaltered or will undergo metabolism by biochemical processes. Consequently, two contributing factors to the changing consequences of environmental pollution are the involvement of food chains and alteration of the compound within the setting.

12.7 Food Chains

For a terrestrial animal, the likely route of exposure to a toxic compound is via food. The food chain is one method by which animals and humans are exposed to persistent pollutants. Substances may be persistent in one environment or species but not in another, depending on the characteristics of the system. The food chain incorporates water-borne, soil, and airborne pollutants. Two main types of food chain pathways function according to the method of ingestion; (1) Grazing food chain is a sequence in which one organism, such as a plant, is eaten by another, an herbivore, which is eventually consumed by a carnivore (see Chapter 11, Table 11.4); (2) **Detritivore food chains** involve decay and death of organisms, the latter of which are generally small where there is no difference in size between lower and higher trophic levels. Both types of evolutionary processes, as well as other minor pathways, contribute to environmental toxicology affecting the overall system of the food web.

The amounts of contamination in species at each trophic level are measured and compared yielding computation of a concentration factor. However, several factors contribute to the interpretation of this calculation. For example, the mode of sampling of a population has inherent bias. Ideally, sampling should be random, without the observer's partiality. If animal carcasses are sampled, the levels of a particular chemical pollutant vary widely depending on the cause of death, such that the concentration of pollutant in live animals is as important as the concentration in animals dead of unknown causes. This is due to the subtle population effects of the pollutant, as the breeding behavior or production of eggs, which affects the whole population. In addition, the presence of a chemical in the environment does not necessarily indicate establishment of significant contamination and similarly, identification of a chemical in an organism does not automatically suggest a toxic effect. Advanced technological methods for detecting trace quantities of toxic compounds should not immediately lead to the most obvious statements, where reasonable assessments and *interpretation* of those data are required to achieve appropriate conclusions. Unlike controlled laboratory experiments, environmental exposure is often intermittent – pollutants do not always reach steady state but fluctuate continuously. As previously mentioned, the persistence of a chemical varies between species and ecosystems. For example, low levels of organochlorine insecticides in small mammals is not reflected at the same levels in birds feeding on them. This common occurrence is explained by differences in the toxicokinetic factors associated with the chemical between the two species.[6]

Thus, sampling is an important feature of the study, such that predators carry prey from a wide area in which there are great variations in exposure. Consequently, environmental toxicology interprets the interaction of complex systems where prediction, interpretation, and conclusion must be carefully evaluated.

Ecological and biological population effects of pollutants are considered public health concerns while individual effects fall within the medical realm. Consequently, a pollutant that reduces or stops reproduction of species at some stage is of greater consequence than a pollutant that is more acutely toxic but causes toxicity of older, more susceptible members of that species. However, distress in the latter members has *less effect* on the population if the victims were past significant reproductive capacity, since the toxic compound is classified as a contributor to the cause of death. Since not all individuals in a population reproduce, the effect on that population is diminished in comparison to the consequences of a toxic chemical which leads to death of a broad proportion within the same group.

An example that illustrates this effect on the reproductive cycle and the problems of persistent pesticides in food chains is the effect of organochlorine insecticides on eggshells in predatory birds. At the top of the food chain, predatory birds have the highest concentrations of some pesticides. For example, the peregrine falcon population in the UK declined precipitously between 1955 and 1962. At the same time, the frequency of egg breakage increased because of a decrease in eggshell thickness, demonstrating a linear relationship between eggshell strength and thickness index. Peregrine falcon eggs studied later between 1970 and 1974 had a lower thickness index and strength than those studied in 1850–1942 (Peakall et al., 1976). Dichlorodiphenyldichloroethylene (DDE), the metabolite of DDT, was investigated as one cause of decreased thickness, while direct toxicity from the insecticide dieldrin was suggested as another cause of the decline in population. Areas north of Scotland had higher eggshell thickness indexes and lower levels of DDE than eggs from southern areas. Similarly, data from the US for kestrels showed a correlation between eggshell thickness and DDE concentrations (Wiemeyer and Porter, 1970).

Pollutants also dissolve in water if they are ionized/water-soluble chemicals or are miscible (Figure 12.3). Alternatively, hydrophobic compounds form suspensions or aggregates and remain undispersed in water, as with oils and hydrocarbons. Although water-soluble substances reach sufficient toxic concentrations to be toxic to aquatic organisms, in an enclosed system they eventually disperse. These compounds are not likely to accumulate in organisms. Hydrophobic substances, however, are not polar, are lipid soluble, and are well absorbed by aquatic organisms which filter water over gills to extract oxygen and nutrients. Consequently, when small organisms such as *Daphnia* and zooplankton become contaminated with lipophilic pollutants such as DDT, they are ingested by larger organisms such as small fish, where the contaminant enters its fatty tissue. In addition, small creatures ingested in large numbers concentrate on the compounds that they carry and are not readily excreted after consumption. As noted above, the food chain continues until humans, at the top of the food chain, accumulate sufficient components to suffer toxic effects (Figure 12.3).

Food chains occur in aquatic environments with water pollutants, or in terrestrial organisms with airborne, soil, water, or food-born pollutants. An important aspect of conserving food chains, therefore, is the scope for biomagnification of the substance as it moves through the sequence.

Important characteristics of a chemical substance that enters a food chain are its lipid solubility and its metabolic stability in biological systems – representing important physico-chemical characteristics. These factors determine the extent to which compounds are incorporated by organisms and their ability to localize in adipose tissue, while remaining until the organism is ingested by a predator. Polar and ionized, hydrophilic, compounds, are captured by organisms but are readily excreted. Lipophilic pollutants which are absorbed and then *rapidly metabolized* to *polar metabolites* similarly are inclined for rapid *excretion* and hence will not persist in the organism or transfer to predators.

Although some environmental pollutants are not lipophilic initially, they are *metabolized* by microorganisms, plants, or higher animals, to fat-soluble metabolites which are more persistent. As evidenced by DDT, its metabolite, DDE, is more lipophilic and more persistent (see Chapter 11, Figure 11.2 and Table 11.3).

12.8 Endocrine Disruptors

'**Endocrine disruptors** are exogenous compounds which cause adverse health effects in an intact organism or its progeny as a result of interaction with hormonal systems' (WHO, 2013).

Recently several coincident observations have led scientists to conclude that chemical substances in the environment are interfering with the endocrine systems of humans and animals. These endocrine disruptors (ED) have since been noted to activate a range of dysfunctions in human and animal (domestic and feral) reproductive, glandular, and hormonal systems. The wildlife effects are well documented and are reproducible experimentally. Human effects are more difficult to definitively associate with environmental chemicals while some studies are controversial. However, there is considerable interest in the effects of EDs which is potentially of great importance (Autrup et al., 2020; Barile et al., 2021).

It is widely accepted that chemicals, capable of causing endocrine disruption, have been released into the environment and are capable of mimicking estrogen, testosterone, and its antagonists (estrogen mimics, anti-estrogens, anti-androgens). The net effects are changes in physiological hormone balance which result in a variety of physiological and pathological anomalies. The debate, however, is whether concentrations of the chemicals are sufficient to contribute to the effects observed in animals and suspected in humans.

There is a variety of chemicals believed to be responsible, most of which are synthetic. Some naturally occurring compounds from plants or fungi are also included. These chemical groups consist of organochlorine insecticides (e.g. DDT), industrial compounds such as polychlorinated biphenyls (PCBs) and alkylphenols, and therapeutic drugs such as contraceptive hormones. Much of the waste products and metabolites from the synthetic compounds are eliminated through urine and appear in bodies of water via sewage. Natural products include fungal products, zearalenone, and plant-derived agents, such as **genistein**. Most are lipophilic and persistent, undergoing bioaccumulation and biomagnification in the environment.

Wildlife effects. Evidence for EDs in wildlife is derived from studies that incorporate a variety of animal species ranging from rodents to molluscs to alligators. Changes in fish were first noticed in rainbow trout (UK) and winter flounder (US) in rivers polluted with sewage outfall or industrial effluent, including hermaphroditic mutations. The incidence of androgynous occurrence was up to 100% of the fish in the Aire River (UK). Male fish were also producing vitellogenin, a protein produced by females in response to estrogen, which was reproduced experimentally when fish were exposed to sewage. Vitellogenin was subsequently used as a biomarker of response for the effect of EDs on fish.

Some substances that cause male fish to produce vitellogenin, such as alkylphenols, octylphenol, and nonylphenol, have now been identified. These compounds also decrease testicular growth in males and bind to estrogen receptors. However, nonylphenol is less potent than natural estrogen, establishing a controversial issue (Autrup et al., 2020; Barile et al., 2021). However, ethynylestradiol, a synthetic estrogen, has been shown to induce vitellogenin in males and retards testes growth, at concentrations found in effluent from sewage treatment plants.

A well-documented effect of an environmental ED on the reproductive system of aquatic organisms is the action of tributyl tin on molluscs. Tributyltin oxide (TBTO) is a biocide in wood preservatives and incorporated in paints for hulls or recreational boats to retard fouling by algae and barnacles. Tributyl tin concentration in crowded harbors and marinas is sufficient to affect molluscs such as the dog whelk. Molluscs appear to be especially sensitive to tributyl tin concentrations less than 1 ng/L. The results are labeled as imposex, a type of sexual abnormality wherein male sex organs, such as the penis, develop in the genetic female. The effect is universally observed with different species of marine snails, results of which were reproduced in several laboratories (Birchenough et al., 2002; Davies et al., 1987).

The mechanism of toxicity involves inhibition of aromatase, an enzyme involved in metabolism of sex hormones. Tributyl tin also affects the thymus gland in mammals, leading to depletion of lymphocytes with consequential repercussions on the immune system. However, this occurs at concentrations several orders of magnitude higher than those which induce imposex in molluscs.

The widely known example of endocrine disruption is that caused by organochlorine compounds in alligators in Florida, US. When it was reported that the population of alligators in Lake Apopka in northern Florida was declining, the immediate conclusion was deemed poor reproductive success. Male animals had small phalli, poorly organized testes, and low testosterone levels. In contrast, females had high blood estrogen levels but abnormal ovarian morphology. The mechanism was attributed to an effect of pollutants on metabolism of steroid sex hormones. The high level of organochlorine compounds such as the DDT break-down product, DDE, was well documented, which has been experimentally determined to alter reproductive and hormonal functions in alligators.

Human effects. Many studies involving effects on human reproduction are well documented and established, yet some are contentious. Endocrine-disrupting chemicals (EDCs) commonly appear as additives in commercial products such as pesticides, herbicides, plasticizers, and as contaminants in processed foods, potable water, and personal care goods. A list of commonly encountered EDCs and their probable disease links are summarized in Table 12.2.

Testicular and breast cancers have increased since 1945 – sperm counts and sperm quality has also declined over the same period. This is particularly apparent in Scandinavian countries but is not supported by data from other nations. There is also an increase in other male reproductive disorders such as cryptorchidism and hypospadia.

In contrast to the consequences of EDs observed and reproduced in animals, documented effects on human reproductive function are not clearly associated with exposure to particular chemicals. A notable exception to this is diethylstilbestrol (DES) which was used therapeutically in the 1950s to prevent miscarriages in women. This synthetic estrogen was the basis of reproductive anomalies in male and female offspring of women who received the drug. These

Table 12.2 List of Common EDCs, Applications and Probable Disease Links

EDC	Applications	Disease Links
Alkylphenols	Detergents, fuel additives, lubricants, phenolic resins	Breast cancer
Atrazine	Herbicide	Delayed puberty, carcinogenesis
Bisphenol A (BPA)	Plastic manufacture, epoxy resins in food contact materials	Breast and ovarian cancers, neurobehavioral anomalies, altered pubertal development
DDT[a]	Pesticides	Breast cancer, among other cancers
Dioxin	Byproducts of fuel combustion	Cancer, testicular damage, diminished sperm quality, oligospermia infertility
Ethinyl estradiol	Synthetic steroid for oral contraception	Endometrial cancer, hepatotoxicity
Phthalates	Plastics, fragrances, medical tubing	Metabolic syndrome, birth defects, oligospermia, asthma, neurobehavioral abnormalities
PCBs[b]	Electrical coolant, in building materials	Cancer, immunosuppression, thyroid atrophy, porphyria

[a] Dichlorodiphenyltrichloroethane; possible disease link.
[b] Polychlorinated biphenyls.

findings support the hypothesis that estrogenic compounds are responsible for some of the observed effects. The effect of DES was also reproduced in some experimental animals with similar results.

Dysfunction of reproductive organs, disruption of menstrual cycle, and production of abnormal pregnancies were noted in a significant proportion of girls born to mothers who had been prescribed DES. In a small cohort of that population, adenocarcinoma of the vagina developed when girls reached puberty. Male offspring exhibited increased incidence of cryptorchidism and microphallus, as well as some evidence of decreased sperm count and motility. These effects, along with testicular cancer, were reproduced in experimental animals. Since DES does not bind to available globulin, as with other sex hormones, it is able to enter cells freely and produces a greater effect than an equivalent blood concentration of endogenous estrogens.

DES was also used as a growth promoter in cattle, suggesting that unnecessary human exposure results from consumption of residues in meat. Human exposure to other synthetic estrogens used in hormone contraception occurs via drinking water. For instance, ethynylestradiol (EES) has been detected in drinking water in the UK. Metabolites of estrogenic compounds, synthetic and naturally occurring, are excreted into urine and detected in sewage systems.

Although DDT is implicated as a possible xenoestrogen, neither the chemical nor its persistent metabolite, p, p′-DDE, interacts significantly with the estrogen receptor (ER). However, the latter interacts with the androgen receptor (AR) and therefore could conceivably be interpreted as an anti-androgen. DDE levels have been measured in breast adipose tissue in an attempt to correlate levels with the incidence of breast cancer; results however have been equivocal. An association of DDE with the hormone-responsive type of breast cancer only is suggested. However, it is important to note that the current exposure of the human population to DDT is relatively low and continually decreasing. Furthermore, studies of humans exposed to higher levels of DDT when first introduced into the manufacturing industry reveal little correlated toxicity. The organochlorine compound chlordecone, however, has estrogen-like activity in humans. Male workers exposed to high levels during its manufacture were discovered with changes in reproductive capacity, including abnormal sperm with decreased motility and low counts. Although some polychlorinated biphenyls (PCBs) possess weak estrogenic activity, others are anti-estrogenic. Similarly, dioxin (TCDD) shows significant anti-estrogenic activity. In both cases, the activity is correlated with binding to the AR receptor. Dioxin has several effects on male and female reproductive systems of mammals, such as adverse effects on spermatogenesis, sexual behavior, and reproductive capability. Rier et al. (1993) report that the effects of dioxin on the reproductive system occur at doses as low as 0.001 µg/kg/day in primates.

Octylphenol, an alkylphenol, demonstrates estrogenic activity mediated via the estrogen receptor. However, activity is three orders of magnitude less than estradiol suggesting that the probable effect on humans is low.

Finally, it is important to note that many naturally occurring estrogens, many times less potent than estradiol, have greater potency than some of the synthetic chemicals often cited. Thus, the plant products isoflavone, coumestans, lignane, and the fungal product zearalenone, bind to the estrogen receptor. Other plant-derived products, including indole-3-carbinol present in vegetables, have anti-estrogenic activity.

The data suggest that human exposure to a wide variety of compounds in the environment has varied estrogenic (xenoestrogens) and anti-estrogenic activity. It is not clear whether exposure at environmental concentrations poses a threat to human reproductive health. Alternatively, the environment contains many compounds which in combination have the potential to promote synergistic estrogenic effects – an area currently receiving considerable attention (Autrup et al., 2015).

Xenoestrogens act through other pathways via the estrogen receptor. For example, the compounds interact with other structures such as the Ah receptor or growth factor receptor. In fact, there exists an association between binding to Ah receptors and anti-estrogenic activity. Alternatively, some xenoestrogens act by altering hormonal metabolism. For example, 17β-estradiol is metabolized to 2-hydroxyestrone and 16α-hydroxyestrone. The former has low activity and low genotoxicity whereas 16α-hydroxyestrone is genotoxic and is a potent estrogen. Muti et al. (2000) report in a breast cancer study that levels of 16α-hydroxyestrone are higher than in control patients and that the ratio of 16α-hydroxy to 2-hydroxyestrone is associated with breast cancer. Some polycyclic aromatic hydrocarbons for instance also inhibit formation of 2-hydroxyestrone and divert the metabolism of estradiol toward the more potent 16α-hydroxyestrone.

12.9 Summary and Learning Objectives

Exposure of biological systems to chemicals via skin contact, oral intake, or breathing occurs through environmental pollution of atmosphere, water, or soil. Contamination results from industrial, agricultural and human activities which have increased since the advent of the industrial age of the 19th century. Human, animal, and plant morbidity, mortality, and injury result from the consequences of environmental damage. The atmosphere is polluted by gases such as sulfur and nitrogen oxides, O_3, CO, hydrocarbons, and PM that contribute to reducing and photochemical smog. Some of these pollutants promote acid rain, damaging trees acidify lakes and rivers, and affect organisms. The consequences of acid rain also destroy leaves and plants which eventually leach essential minerals from soil. Heavy metals such as lead, from car exhausts and industrial activity, pollute air, soil, and water, the consequences of which are a known cause of damage to kidneys, RBC, skeletal, and nervous systems. Wastewater from industrial, domestic, or agricultural sources triggers overgrowth of algae, resulting in the development of *eutrophication*[7] and direct toxic effects. Groundwater in many countries is polluted with AS, a known cause of cancer and skin diseases. Various pollutants (alkylphenols, DDT, and PCBs) and fungal products are suspect EDs which are presumably responsible for reproductive dysfunction in animals (alligators, dog whelks, and fish) and humans by virtue of their estrogenic, anti-estrogenic or anti-androgenic activities, although the latter causal relationship is not well documented.

Environmental lipophilic pollutants, particularly if DDT and dieldrin, accumulate in organisms and animals at the top of the food chain (predators), where exposure is higher concentrations than that which bioaccumulates in the environment. Mercury, an important contributor to pollution, exists in three toxic forms – organic, elemental, and inorganic). The unregulated mercury-laden factory effluent polluted Minamata Bay, Japan, which bioaccumulated in fish and caused death and disease in exposed humans. Subsequent legislation from this disastrous event now requires testing for the potential impact of chemicals on the environment and organisms (*Daphnia*, earthworms).

Review Questions

1. Indicate which of the following are true and which are false: Lead: (a) is toxic because it inhibits mitochondrial respiration; (b) is present in cigarette smoke; (c) damages red blood cells; (d) is not toxic to the nervous system; (e) is absorbed via the lungs.
2. Indicate which of the following are true and which are false concerning mercury poisoning? (a) metallic mercury is non-toxic; (b) organic mercury is toxic to the kidney; (c) inorganic mercury is toxic to brain cells; (d) inorganic mercury binds to SH groups; (e) methylmercury has a half-life of 70 days.
3. Indicate which of the following statements is true and which are false: (a) the great smog in London occurred in 1852; (b) photochemical smog contains only nitrogen oxides; (c) O_3 is a non-toxic gas that promotes good health; (d) PM10 represents a concentration of oxidants of $10 \, \mu g/m^3$; (e) acid rain is formed from chlorinated hydrocarbons interacting with the O_3 layer; (f) reducing smog has a high level of sulfur dioxide and particulates.
4. Indicate which of the following statements are true and which are false: Effect of DDT on the bird population was due to: (a) toxicity of DDT to chicks; (b) loss of tree cover due to its herbicidal action; (c) damage to eggs by the metabolite DDE; (d) migration (e) disappearance of insects.

Short Answer Question

5. Define the terms **bioaccumulation** and **biomagnification**; in your answer discuss their importance in toxicology. Use appropriate examples to support your statements and describe the properties that chemicals must possess for bioaccumulation.

Notes

1. NOEL for sulfur dioxide and smoke are 0.25 ppm and 0.75 mg/cc, respectively.
2. It is important to note that a minimum level of ozone in atmosphere is necessary in order to protect against the damaging effects of UV light on skin.
3. Elimination of lead-based gasoline to unleaded form has greatly diminished environmental dispersion of the metal.
4. An abnormal craving for placing unnatural, non-nutritive substances in the mouth is known as *pica,* although it has been associated with lead ingestion in children.
5. Which also explains the nephritis associated with drinking 'moonshine' whiskey where alcohol still used for the production of the 'bootleg' alcohol contained lead piping or lead solder.
6. ADME: absorption, distribution, metabolism, elimination.
7. Excessive plant and algal growth due to increased availability of one or more limiting growth factors needed for photosynthesis such as sunlight, carbon dioxide, and nutrient fertilizers (Schindler 2006).

Bibliography

Arora, M., Arsenic-polluted water linked to cancer in India. *CNN Health*, 2017. https://www.cnn.com/2017/04/28/health/arsenic-water-pollution-cancer-india/index.html.

Autrup, H., Barile, F.A., Berry, C., Blaauboer, B.J., Boobis, A., Bolt, H., Borgert, C.J., Dekant, W., Dietrich, D., Domingo, J.L., Batta Gori, G., Greim, H., Hengstler, J., Kacew, S., Marquardt, H., Pelkonen, O., Savolainen, K., Heslop-Harrison, P. and Vermeulen, N.P., Human exposure to synthetic endocrine disrupting chemicals (S-EDCs) is generally negligible as compared to natural compounds with higher or comparable endocrine activity. How to evaluate the risk of the S-EDCs? *Environmental Toxicology and Pharmacology,* 78, 103396, 2020. Doi: 10.1016/j.etap.2020.103396.

Autrup, H., Barile, F.A., Blaauboer, B.J., Degen, G.H., Dekant, W., Dietrich, D., Domingo, J.L., Gori, G.B., Greim, H., Hengstler, J.G., Kacew, S., Marquardt, H., Pelkonen, O, Savolainen, K. and Vermeulen, N.P., Principles of pharmacology and toxicology also govern effects of chemicals on the endocrine system, *Toxicological Sciences*, 146, 11–15, 2015. Doi: 10.1093/toxsci/kfv082.

Barile, F.A., Berry, C., Blaauboer, B.J., Boobis, A., Bolt, H., Borgert, C.J., Dekant, W., Dietrich, D., Domingo, J.L., Galli, C.L., Gori, G.B., Greim, H., Hengstler, J., Heslop-Harrison, P., Kacew, S., Marquardt, H., Mally, A., Pelkonen, O., Savolainen, K., Testai, E., Tsatsakis, A. and Vermeulen, N.P. The EU chemicals strategy for sustainability: in support of the BfR position, *Archives of Toxicology*, 95, 3133–3136, 2021. Doi: 10.1007/s00204-021-03125-w.

Bell, M.L. and Davis, D.L., Reassessment of the lethal London fog of 1952: Novel indicators of acute and chronic consequences of acute exposure to air pollution, *Environmental Health Perspectives*, 109 (3), 389–394, 2001, http://ehpnet1.niehs.nih.gov/docs/2001/suppl-3/389-394bell/abstract.htm.

Birchenough, A.C., Barnes, N., Evans, S.M., Hinz, H., Krönke, I. and Moss, C. A review and assessment of tributyltin contamination in the North Sea, based on surveys of butyltin tissue burdens and imposex/intersex in four species of neogastropods, *Marine Pollution Bulletin*, 44, 534–543, 2002. Doi: 10.1016/s0025-326x(01)00275-2.

Davies, I.M., Bailey, S.K. and Moore, D.C. Tributyltin in Scottish sea lochs, as indicated by degree of imposex in the dogwhelk, Nucella lapillus (L.). *Marine Pollution Bulletin* 18, 400–404, 1987.

DiGuilio, R.T. and Newman, M.C., Chapter 30. Environmental Toxicology, in: *Casarett and Doull's Toxicology, Basic Science of Poisons*, Klaassen, C.D. (Ed.), 9th edition, McGraw-Hill, New York, 2019.

Enderle, R. Fussi, B., Lenz, H. D., Langer, G., Nagel, R. and Metzler, B., Ash dieback in Germany: research on disease development, resistance and management options, in: *Dieback of European Ash (Fraxinus spp.): Consequences and Guidelines for Sustainable Management*, Vasaitis, R. and Enderle, R. (Eds.), (pp. 89–105), Swedish University of Agricultural Sciences, 2017. https://www.slu.se/globalassets/ew/org/inst/mykopat/forskning/stenlid/dieback-of-european-ash.pdf. Last accessed November 2022.

Florida-James, G., Donaldson, K. and Stone, V., Athens 2004: the pollution climate and athletic performance. *Journal Sports Sciences*, 22, 967–980, 2004. Doi: 10.1080/02640410400000272.

Harada, M., *Minamata Disease*, Kumamoto Nichinichi Shinbun Centre & Information Center/Iwanami Shoten Publishers, 1972. ISBN 4-87755-171-9 C3036.

Lehnherr, I., Methylmercury biogeochemistry: a review with special reference to Arctic aquatic ecosystems, *Environmental Reviews*, 22, 1–15, 2014. Doi: 10.1139/er-2013-0059.

Muti, P., Bradlow, H.L., Micheli, A., Krogh, V., Freudenheim, J.L., Schünemann, H.J., Stanulla, M., Yang, J., Sepkovic, D.W., Trevisan, M. and Berrino, F., Estrogen metabolism and risk of breast cancer: a prospective study of the 2:16α-hydroxyestrone ratio in premenopausal and postmenopausal women. *Epidemiology*, 11, 635–640, 2000.

Peakall, D.B., The role of biomarkers in environmental assessment. Introduction, *Ecotoxicology*, 3, 157–160, 1994. Doi: 10.1007/BF00117080.

Peakall, D.B., Reynolds, L.M. and French, M.C., DDE in eggs of the peregrine falcon, *Bird Study*, 23(3), 181–186, 1976. Doi: 10.1080/00063657609476499.

Peel, J.L., Klein, M., Flanders, W.D., Mulholland, J.A. and Tolbert, P.E. Impact of improved air quality during the 1996 Summer Olympic Games in Atlanta on multiple cardiovascular and respiratory outcomes, *Research Report Health Effects Institute*, 148, 3–23, 2010.

Pierson, W.E., Covert, D.S., Koenig, J.Q., Namekata, T. and Kim, Y.S., Implications of air pollution effects on athletic performance, *Medicine Science Sports Exercise,* 18(3), 322–327, 1986. Doi: 10.1249/00005768-198606000-00012.

Rier, S.E., Martin, D.C., Bowman, R.E., Dmowski, W.P. and Becker, J.L. Endometriosis in rhesus monkeys (Macaca mulatta) following chronic exposure to 2, 3, 7, 8-tetrachlorodibenzo-p-dioxin, *Fundamental and Applied Toxicology*, 21(4), 433–441, 1993.

Shaw, I.C. and Chadwick, J., Chapter 2. Effects of Pollutants on Ecosystems, in: *Principles of Environmental Toxicology*, Shaw, I.C. and Chadwick, J., (Eds.), CRC Press, Taylor & Francis, Boca Raton, FL, 1998.

Shephard, R.J., Athletic performance and urban air pollution, *Canadian Medical Association Journal*, 131(2), 105–109, 1984.

Skerfving, S.B. and Copplestone, J.F., Poisoning caused by the consumption of organomercury-dressed seed in Iraq, *Bulletin of the World Health Organization*, 54, 101–112, 1976.

Wallace, R.A., Fulkerson, W., Shults, W.D. and Lyon, W.S. *Mercury in the Environment: The Human Element.* U.S. Department of Energy, Office of Scientific and Technical Information, 1971. https://www.osti.gov/biblio/6217966.

WHO, UNEP, Endocrine Disrupting Chemicals, 2012; Bergman, A., Heindel, J.J., Jobling, S., Kidd, K.A., Zeller, R.T., (Eds.), U.N. Environment Programme and the WHO, 2013.

Wiemeyer, S. and Porter, R. DDE thins eggshells of captive American Kestrels, *Nature*, 227, 737–738, 1970. Doi: 10.1038/227737a0.

Woodall, J., *The Surgeons Mate or Military & Domestic Surgery,* 1639, http://name.umdl.umich.edu/A66951.0001.001; last accessed November 2022.

Suggested Readings

Bradley, M.A., Barst, B.D. and Basu, N. A review of mercury bioavailability in humans and fish. *International Journal of Environmental Research and Public Health*, 14, 16, 2017. Doi: 10.3390/ijerph14020169.

Chintalapati, A.J. and Barile, F.A. Chapter 26, Metals, in: *Barile's Clinical Toxicology: Principles and Mechanisms*, 3rd edition, CRC Press, Taylor and Francis, New York, 2019.

Walker, C.H., Sibly, R.M., Hopkin, S.P. and Peakall, D.B., *Principles of Ecotoxicology*, 4th edition, Taylor & Francis, London, 2012.

Chapter 13

Natural Products

Chapter Outline

This chapter discusses a variety of specific examples of naturally occurring toxins, including:

13.1	Introduction	190
13.1	Plant Toxins	190
	13.1.1 Pyrrolizidine Alkaloids	190
	13.1.1.1 Case Study	190
	13.1.2 Pennyroyal Oil	191
	13.1.3 Ricin	192
	13.1.4 Bracken	192
13.2	Animal Toxins	193
	13.2.1 Snake Venoms	195
	13.2.2 Tetrodotoxin	195
13.3	Fungal Toxins	196
	13.3.1 Death Cap Mushroom	196
	13.3.2 Aflatoxins	197
13.4	Microbial Toxins	197
	13.4.1 Botulism and Botulinum Toxin	197
	13.4.2 *E. coli* Infections and Exotoxins	197
13.5	Summary and Learning Objectives	198
	Review Questions	199
	Short Answer Questions	199
	Notes	199
	Bibliography	199
	Suggested Readings	200

DOI: 10.1201/9781003188575-13

13.1 Introduction

Many of the chemicals that find their way into the environment are synthetic and are of major concern to the public. There are, however, hundreds of naturally occurring compounds of animal, plant, fungal, and microbial origin that also have toxic potential. In fact, some of the most toxic substances are natural poisons, such as botulinum toxin, contrary to marketing and popular culture that imply that organic and herbal products are intrinsically harmless and safe. For example, allergies to natural constituents of food are known to occur just as with synthetic additives. Some of these substances have been known for centuries and have also been used for illegitimate activities or unregulated medical treatments.

Since the vast classifications of natural toxins are of diverse structures and mechanisms of action, the following discussion focuses on some representative and important examples of toxic substances derived from plants, animals, fungi, and microorganisms.

13.1 Plant Toxins

There are many well-studied plant toxins ranging from the irritant formic acid found in nettles[1] and ants to more poisonous compounds, such as atropine, isolated within the notorious berries of the deadly nightshade (*Atropa belladonna*), as well as cytisine, in laburnum and coniine (hemlock). Some examples of natural plant, herbal, mammalian, fungal, and aquatic toxins are discussed below.

13.1.1 Pyrrolizidine Alkaloids

Pyrrolizidine alkaloids are a large group of structurally related compounds found in more than 6,000 plants in the *Leguminosae*, *Compositae*, and *Boraginaceae* families, many of which occur as weeds throughout the world. About half of the pyrrolizidine alkaloids have been identified as toxic and the constituents are the most common cause of poisoning for humans and animals, both livestock and domestic. Contamination occurs in cereal crops or with plant use in herbal remedies.

13.1.1.1 Case Study

In Austria, an 18-month-old boy presented with **veno-occlusive disease**. He had been given herbal tea since he was 3 months old. The herbal tea was intended to include the component Coltsfoot[2] but was in fact made with Alpendost.[3] The boy had congestion of the **sinusoids** of the liver and necrosis and bleeding from the small veins (Sperl et al., 1995).

A study in South Africa in two hospitals identified 20 children suffering from veno-occlusive disease which was thought to be due to the use of traditional remedies. Most of the children had fluid in the abdominal cavity and enlarged livers. There was high morbidity and mortality; the disease progressed to liver cirrhosis in the survivors. In four cases, pyrrolizidine alkaloids were detected in the urine (Chen and Huo, 2010).

Poisoning occurs in various parts of the world, especially where agricultural conditions are poor and the indigenous population is forced to use contaminated crops. For example, in 1930s South Africa, the poor white population suffered the toxic effects of these alkaloids because their staple diet was wheat, which became contaminated. Their Bantu neighbors however ate maize as part of their staple diet which was not contaminated – consequently, they were not affected. More recently, poisonings have occurred in Tashkent, Central India, and Northern Afghanistan. In one incident 1,600 poisoning cases were reported where the threshed wheat was found contaminated with *Heliotropium popovii* seeds yielding an alkaloid concentration of at least 0.5%. In the West Indies especially, these plants are also used in traditional medicine as components of herbal teas.

Toxicity depends on the particular alkaloid. One of the most studied pyrrolizidine alkaloids is monocrotaline, a component of *Heliotropium*, *Senecio*, and *Crotolaria* species. The chemical causes an unusual type of liver injury, particularly following acute exposure to herbal teas. The injury targets the liver sinusoids leading to veno-occlusive disease.

Monocrotaline produces veno-occlusive disease in laboratory animals and damages lungs. Overall the effect of chronic exposure to low herbal doses is liver cirrhosis, evident in members of the West Indian population, estimated to account for ⅓ of the cirrhosis seen at autopsy in the island nations. The constituent alkaloids, such as monocrotaline (Figure 13.1), undergo metabolic activation to a reactive metabolite which damages cells and hepatocytes that line liver sinusoids, leading to **hemorrhagic necrosis** and eventually veno-occlusive disease. This blockage of hepatic blood vessels alters the vasculature, diverting liver blood supply and stimulating development of new unaccounted circulatory pathways.

Animals are also exposed to the toxic effects of natural vegetation. In abundant areas of grazing land, animals discount plants such as ragwort (*Senecio jacobaea*) which contain alkaloids. In Australia, however, widespread losses of horses, cattle, and sheep occur from *Heliotropium* poisoning. This is also another route of human exposure since the alkaloids are detected in the milk of cows grazing on such plants.

13.1.2 Pennyroyal Oil

The Pennyroyal plant and its derivative oil have been used to terminate pregnancies in countries where it is possible to buy the oil. The plant is used to make tea or the oil is ingested orally, both methods of which trigger liver damage as well as induce miscarriages. The oil contains several terpenoid compounds; metabolic activation is required for toxicity.

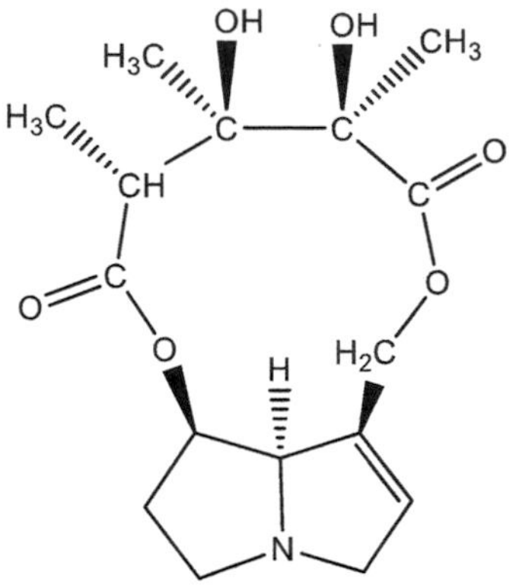

Figure 13.1 Structure of monocrotaline, a pyrrolizidine alkaloid.

13.1.3 Ricin

Ricin is one of the most toxic chemical substances known, derived from the seeds of the castor oil plant. It is notorious in the international media when it was claimed that the Bulgarian secret police used minute quantities of the powder on the tip of an umbrella to kill the Bulgarian journalist Georgi Markov in London in 1978. Although no trace of any poison was found in the victim's body, it was suspected that a potent chemical was perpetrated, the symptoms of which were consistent with those of ricin poisoning. A tiny metal pellet was recovered from a wound on the victim's leg, apparently inflicted with the pointed instrument. The pellet was described as appropriate to contain a reservoir for a powdery substance, albeit only a few micrograms could fit within the chamber. It was later confirmed that ricin was discovered when the Bulgarian secret police files were unlocked.

Ricin is a small protein consisting of two **polypeptides** – a short A chain and a longer B chain – linked via a disulfide bridge. The B chain attaches the ricin molecule to the outside of the mammalian cell by binding to the galactose molecule of a **glycoprotein**. The cell membrane invaginates and the ricin is absorbed into the cell through an endosome. The molecule is then released from the glycoprotein and the chains are cleaved at the disulfide bridge. The B chain proceeds through the Golgi and endoplasmic reticulum, allowing the A chain to reach the **ribosomes** where it blocks protein synthesis. One molecule of ricin is sufficient to kill one cell (Figure 13.2).

13.1.4 Bracken

Bracken is a genus of large, coarse ferns in the family *Dennstaedtiaceae*. Ferns are vascular plants that have alternating generations – large plants that produce spores and small plants that produce sex cells. Brackens are noted for their large, highly divided leaves (Figure 13.3).

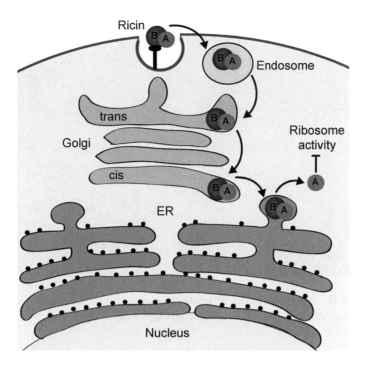

Figure 13.2 Intracellular uptake of ricin and ribosome inactivation. Ricin is internalized through clathrin-dependent and -independent endocytosis. Inside the cell ricin proceeds from the early endosome into the *trans*-Golgi network. The chemical then progresses from the Golgi into the endoplasmic reticulum (ER) through retrograde trafficking; its catalytic A chain is released into the cytosol where it inactivates the ribosome. (From: Bozza et al., 2015; Creative Commons © license, https://doi.org/10.1016/j.biotechadv.2014.11.012.)

The bracken fern contains the chemical **ptaquiloside**, which produces a carcinogenic compound upon degradation. In Japan, the shoots of the young bracken fern are eaten; consumption correlates with the high incidence of esophageal cancer among the native population. Animals that eat the fern as fodder suffer from bladder and intestinal cancer. The metabolic product of ptaquiloside reacts with the adenine nucleotide base of DNA resulting in loss of integrity of the DNA chain.

13.2 Animal Toxins

As with plant toxins, animal toxins comprise a diverse range of structures (Figure 13.4) and mechanisms of action. A typical familiar example is formic acid[4], found in ants. Other examples include tetrodotoxin, a chemical component of the puffer fish, and saxitoxin, located in shellfish and fish that consume **dinoflagellates**. Animal toxins

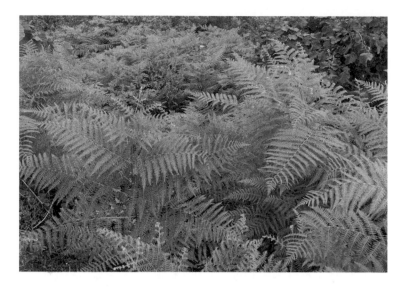

Figure 13.3 Bracken ferns (*Pteridium aquilinum*). (Creative Commons ©
license, https://commons.wikimedia.org/wiki/File:E%C4%9Frelti_otu_-_Bracken_
Fern_1.jpg.)

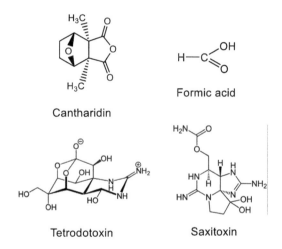

Figure 13.4 Structures of representative animal toxins showing the diversity of
the molecular structures of cantharidin, formic acid, tetrodotoxin, and saxitoxin.

are mixtures of complex proteins, precipitating different forms of toxic exposure,
ranging from bee stings or allergic reactions to dietary components. Throughout
the world, death and illness due to exposure to animal toxins represent an important proportion of poisoning cases.

13.2.1 Snake Venoms

Snake bites represent universal forms of poisoning from natural toxins. Many snake venoms are similar in their protein or polypeptide components and their mechanisms of action. The proteins are hydrolytic enzymes, including the proteinases, phospholipases, ribonucleases, deoxyribonucleases, phosphomonoesterases, phosphodiesterases, and ATPases. Table 13.1 lists the comparative toxicities of some snake venoms, the complex mixtures of which cause a variety of effects. For example, the presence of foreign proteins in the venom produces allergic reactions and fatal **anaphylactic reactions**. The enzyme components *digest* various tissue constituents either at the site of action, causing local necrosis, or at distal sites creating systemic effects. For example, the bite of the diamondback rattlesnake, the most poisonous snake in the US, produces a very painful swelling within minutes. Nausea, vomiting, and diarrhea occur, and cardiac effects, including a decrease in systemic arterial blood pressure and development of a weak, rapid pulse. Control of central nervous system respiration results in respiratory paralysis. Hemolytic anemia and **hemoglobinuria** are occasionally noted, resulting in thrombosis and hemorrhage. Vascular permeability and nerve conduction change, accompanied by cerebral **anoxia**, pulmonary edema, and heart failure. Phospholipases found in snake venom cause intravascular hemolysis by direct action on red cell membranes.

13.2.2 Tetrodotoxin

Almost all pufferfish, as well as the Californian newt, contain tetrodotoxin, a chemical that makes them foul tasting and often lethal to other fish. In humans, tetrodotoxin is lethal up to 1,200 times more poisonous than cyanide. Fish is eaten as a delicacy in Japan provided it is properly and expertly prepared. However, fatalities have occurred which resulted from incorrect preparation of the fish; about 60% of poisoning cases are fatal. Tetrodotoxin and accompanying ichthyocrinotoxin are found in roe, liver, and skin of pufferfish.

Table 13.1 Comparative Toxicities of Representative Snake Venoms, in Order of Increasing Toxicities

Snake Venom	Yield (g)	LD_{50} i.v. mg/kg
Copperhead	40–72	10.92
African puff adder	130–200	3.68
Mojave rattler	50–90	0.21
Russell's viper	130–250	0.08
Sea snake	7–20	0.01

Source: From: Ciembor and Oehme (1981) and Watkins (2019).

Tetrodotoxin is a potent sensory and motor nerve poison. It *selectively blocks* sodium channels along the axon, preventing the inward action potential current. Lethal doses occur at about 10 µg/kg body weight (bwt). Initial effects include tingling of the oral mucous membranes followed by muscular incoordination, salivation, skin numbness, vomiting, diarrhea, and convulsions within 10–25 minutes. Respiratory arrest results from skeletal muscle paralysis.

13.3 Fungal Toxins

Many fungi produce toxins of a variety of chemical types with potential for acute or chronic poisoning. Poisonous mushrooms are often confused with edible varieties resulting in accidental acute poisoning. Intentional ingestion of identifiable and characterized chemicals, derived from fungal sources, containing psychoactive substances, has led to untoward toxic reactions. Noxious effects vary from relatively mild gastrointestinal disturbances to severe organ damage. The psychoactive constituents, mescaline, and psilocin for example, affect the central nervous system, while the aflatoxins are potent carcinogens.

13.3.1 Death Cap Mushroom

The "Death Cap" mushroom, *Amanita phalloides* is the most poisonous mushroom known and one of the easiest to succumb to its allure. Although rare in the Western world, poisoning is occasionally encountered when accidentally ingested.

The fungus contains several toxins: the phallotoxins, including phalloidin, phalloin and phallolysin, and the amatoxins (α, β, and γ amanitin). The phallotoxins cause violent gastroenteritis which occurs rapidly within 4–8 hours after ingestion.

When eaten the victim typically won't experience symptoms for at least 6–24 hours. Eventually, signs and symptoms of abdominal cramps, vomiting, and dehydrating diarrhea ensue. The delay in onset obscures the cause as associated with mushrooms, often leading to the more benign diagnosis of illness such as stomach flu. In addition, if the patient is hydrated, the symptoms may lessen and the condition enters a latent phase, where signs and symptoms appear to abate (a.k.a. *honeymoon phase*).[5] Hallucinations, liver and kidney failure, coma, and death are probable.

The amatoxins have a delayed toxic effect on the liver and kidney as target organs; liver necrosis and destruction of renal tubular cells result. Both the phallotoxins and the amanitins are strongly bound to plasma proteins yet are toxic in this conjugated form.

Antidotes are currently not available; treatment is symptomatic and supportive care is necessary. The most favorable treatment approaches include early detection and identification of the cause, maintenance of airway, breathing, and cardiac integrity (ABCs of emergency procedures).

13.3.2 Aflatoxins

The aflatoxins are thoroughly discussed in Chapter 10, Food Additives and Contaminants. Briefly, high doses of aflatoxin B_1 are responsible for liver damage; exposure to lower doses through the diet produces chronic toxicity, notably induction of liver tumors. The toxin is most likely to occur in stored food products contaminated with the mold *Aspergillus flavus* or when prepared food or ingredients are infected.

13.4 Microbial Toxins

Several well-known bacterial toxins infect human and animal populations universally, a few of which are discussed below.

13.4.1 Botulism and Botulinum Toxin

Botulinum toxin is derived from spore-forming anaerobic bacteria, *Clostridium botulinum*, capable of growing in home-canned vegetables, smoked or salted meats and fish, cheeses, and poorly canned tuna. Infant botulism is commonly associated with ingestion of honey.

The organism produces a mixture of six neurotoxic proteins responsible for the syndrome, botulism, accompanied by high mortality rates. The bacterial chemical is one of the most toxic substances known with a human LD_{50} of 0.001–0.003 µg/kg (or 1–3 nanograms/kg, by inhalation). Although the spores are resistant to high heat the toxin is denatured at 80°C. The onset of symptoms is 18–36 hours after ingestion with a typical range as short as 4 hours or as long as 4 days.

The mechanism underlying the effect of botulinum toxin is the irreversible blockade of motor nerve terminals at the skeletal neuromuscular junction, thus preventing the release of acetylcholine at the terminal synapse. Consequently, the muscle lacks innervation and the subject responds with skeletal muscle paralysis. The symptoms manifest as weakness of limbs, difficulty in breathing, convulsion, coma, and death if severe. A mixture of immune globulin (antibody) fragments (BAT, Botulism Antitoxin Heptavalent, Equine) is available for treatment of symptomatic botulism following documented or suspected exposure to botulinum neurotoxin serotypes A, B, C, D, E, F, or G in adults and pediatric patients.

13.4.2 E. coli Infections and Exotoxins

This gram-negative enteropathogenic bacterium is an emerging cause of food-borne illness. The *Escherichia* genus consists of five species of which *E. coli* is the most common and clinically important. Infections are common in the US and the EU. *E. coli* possesses a broad range of toxic factors, exotoxins, and adhesion molecules allowing the organisms to attach to the GI and urinary tracts.

Many enteropathogenic groups of *E. coli* inhabit the small and large intestines of healthy cattle and are further classified according to their serologic serotypes. Most *E. coli* strains are part of the normal human bacterial flora. *E. coli* serotype O157:H7, however, is not. In fact, it is one of the most virulent strains, responsible for producing fatal enterotoxins.[6]

E. coli is the most common microorganism responsible for sepsis and urinary tract infections, as well as a prominent cause of neonatal meningitis and gastroenteritis in developing nations.

The organism's ability to invade intestinal epithelial cells, its capacity to release exotoxins, and its ability to express adhesion molecules, confers the properties necessary for producing gastroenteritis. During infection, the toxin binds to receptors on intestinal epithelial cells, stimulating hypersecretion of water and electrolytes. The disease is characterized by acute dysentery accompanied by abdominal cramps with little or no fever.

Infection is acquired through ingestion of poorly cooked ground beef, consumption of unpasteurized milk and juice, leafy vegetables, salami, and contact with cattle. Waterborne transmission occurs through swimming in contaminated lakes, pools, or drinking inadequately chlorinated water. The organism is easily transmitted from person to person and has been difficult to control in child day-care centers.

Stool cultures and serology confirm the presence of *E. coli* O157:H7 in suspected infections. Except for severe complications, most infections are self-limiting in 5–10 days. Antibiotic treatment is unwarranted and may precipitate kidney infections. Antidiarrheal agents, such as loperamide, should also be avoided.

13.5 Summary and Learning Objectives

There are many toxic chemicals found naturally in the environment among plants, fungi, bacteria, and mammals. Pyrrolizidine alkaloids, such as monocrotaline, found in *Senecio* and *Heliotropium* plant species, cause liver damage in humans and animals as a result of contamination of crops and incorporation into herbal remedies. Pennyroyal oil from the Pennyroyal plant induces miscarriages and precipitates liver damage. Ricin, derived from the castor oil bean, is the most potent toxic protein. Ptaquiloside found in the bracken fern is a carcinogen in both humans and animals. Animal toxins such as snake venoms generally consist of a variety of hydrolytic enzyme toxins (e.g. proteinases, phosphoesterases) which produce anaphylactic shock and tissue necrosis. From the puffer fish and select bacteria, tetrodotoxin is a potent nerve poison. Phalloidin the active chemical poison in the death cap mushroom, impairs liver and kidneys. From the uncontrolled growth of the fungus *Aspergillus flavus* comes the liver-damaging poison aflatoxin. Botulinum toxin a product of the bacterium *Clostridium botulinum* consists of neurotoxic proteins which cause irreversible blockade of the neuromuscular junction, with resultant paralysis and fatal respiratory failure.

Review Questions

1. Indicate which of the following are true and which are false: (a) pyrrolizidine alkaloids are found in mushrooms; (b) *Amanita phalloides* is a poisonous snake; (c) botulinum toxin is produced by bacteria; (d) ricin is derived from the puffer fish; (e) fluoroacetate is a plant toxin.
2. Which of the following statements are true and which are false concerning tetrodotoxin? (a) it is found in blue green algae; (b) causes paralysis of muscles in humans; (c) affects calcium channels; (d) blocks nervous transmission; (e) poisonous effects are instantaneous.

Short Answer Questions

3. What is the mechanism underlying the toxicity of botulinum toxin?
4. What is the mechanism of action of tetrodotoxin?

Notes

1. Herbaceous plant with jagged leaves covered with stinging hairs.
2. Recently introduced to North America, Coltsfoot is a plant native to Europe and parts of Asia. The leaf, flower, and root are used to make medicine. Despite serious safety concerns, coltsfoot is used for asthma, cough, sore throat, swelling of the airways, and other conditions, but there is no valid scientific evidence to support these uses.
3. Alpendost is a perennial plant of the *Asteraceae* family (Daisy). Alpine pasture leaves were often used like coltsfoot since they looked similar and the effect was roughly the same. The plant was used both internally and externally as tea or in the form of baths for pleurisy, skin ulcers, and cough. Today internal use is not recommended due to the liver-damaging ingredients.
4. The name is derived from the Latin, *formica*, for 'ant'.
5. Interestingly, cooking doesn't make a poisonous mushroom safe. In fact, poisoning can occur by breathing in the cooking fumes from poisonous mushrooms.
6. The serotype designation (O:, H:) refers to the expression of surface and fimbrial antigens, respectively, that uniquely characterize this genus.

Bibliography

Bozza, W.P., Tolleson, W.H., Rivera-Rosado, L.A. and Zhang, B. Ricin detection: Tracking active toxin, *Biotechnology Advances*, 33, 117–123, 2015.

Chen, Z. and Huo, J.R., Hepatic veno-occlusive disease associated with toxicity of pyrrolizidine alkaloids in herbal preparations, *Netherlands Journal Medicine*, 68(6), 252–260, 2010.

Ciembor, P. and Oehme, F.W., A literature review of snakes and snakebite therapy, *Veterinary Human Toxicology*, 23(2), 97–100, 1981.

Sperl, W., Stuppner, H., Gassner, I., Judmaier, W., Dietze, O. and Vogel, W., Reversible hepatic veno-occlusive disease in an infant after consumption of pyrrolizidine-containing herbal tea, *European Journal Pediatrics*, 154, 112–116, 1995. Doi: 10.1007/BF01991912.

Twigg, L.E. and King, D.R., The impact of fluoroacetate-bearing vegetation on native Australian fauna: A review, *Oikos*, 61, 412–430, 1991.

Suggested Readings

Barile, F.A. Chapter 34, Chemical and biological threats to public safety, in: *Barile's Clinical Toxicology: Principles and Mechanisms*, 3rd edition, CRC Press, Taylor and Francis, Boca Raton, FL, 535, 2019.

Harris, J.B. (Ed.) *Natural Toxins, Animal, Plant and Microbial*, Oxford University Press, Oxford, 1987. ISBN-13: 978-0198541738.

Mebs, D., Toxicity in animals: Trends in evolution? *Toxicon*, 39, 87, 2001. Doi: 10.1016/s0041-0101(00)00155-0.

Watkins III, J.B., Chapter 26, Toxic effects of plants and animals, in: *Casarett and Doull's Toxicology*, Klaassen, C.D. (Ed.), 9th edition, McGraw-Hill, New York, 2019. ISBN-13: 978-1259863745.

Commercial and Domestic Products

Chapter Outline

This chapter includes examples of toxic events that occur with commercial and domestic products, often used every day at home or in the workplace. Treatment of poisoning is also discussed.

14.1 Introduction   201
14.2 Carbon Monoxide   202
14.3 Ethylene Glycol (Antifreeze)   204
14.4 Cyanide   206
14.5 Alcohol (Ethanol, Ethyl Alcohol)   208
14.6 Glue Sniffing and Solvent Abuse (Hydrocarbons)   208
14.7 Summary and Learning Objectives   209
Review Questions   210
    Short Answer Questions   210
Notes   210
Bibliography   211

14.1 Introduction

This group of potentially poisonous substances comprises many diverse chemicals and drugs, some of which have been previously discussed. For example, the herbicide dichlorvos is widely used in commercial gardening as well as in industrial farming, and consequently is often found in households.

Household products feature in poisoning cases usually after accidental ingestion by children and in unintentional circumstances. Most inquiries relating to childhood poisoning, especially in children between 2 and 5 years old, involve ready access to therapeutic and non-medicinal household products, and have

DOI: 10.1201/9781003188575-14

potential to become toxic substances in the home or workplace. However, over the last 50 years, the number of deaths due to chemical exposure in the home has decreased, mainly as a result of consumer product safety regulations and greater awareness of these potentially fatal products. Many deaths however in children and adults are due to carbon monoxide (CO) exposure, discussed in detail below.

The scope of potentially toxic substances ranges from corrosives to chemicals that injure upon ingestion. Bleach is commonly involved in poisoning cases because of its ubiquitous use around the house. Other substances include strong detergents such as dishwasher cleaners, and caustic substances[1] such as drain cleaners, abrasive agents, and descalers.[2] When ingested orally bleach produces a burning sensation in the throat, mouth, and esophagus. The tissue damage results in *edema*[3] in the pharynx and larynx. In the stomach, the presence of endogenous hydrochloric acid generates hypochlorous acid which is an *irritant*, and chlorine gas which is inhaled causing toxic effects in the lungs. Although not necessarily fatal, serious injury from ingestion of bleach results in permanent gastrointestinal (GI) scarring often requiring surgical intervention.

Hydrocarbon solvents such as turpentine substitute and white spirit are often used for cleaning paint brushes. Inhalation or aspiration of sufficient quantities precipitates chemical **pneumonitis**. Because of their low viscosity and volatility, the solvents spread through the upper and lower airways easily affecting large pulmonary areas.

14.2 Carbon Monoxide

This highly toxic gas is a major universal cause of several hundred poisoning deaths annually despite the fact that a major source, fossil fuels (coal), has been replaced by natural gas. CO is produced from a variety of sources including automobile exhaust, cigarette smoking, gas stoves, and boilers, especially with poor ventilation. Many cases appear in local news headlines primarily as a result of unattended gas burners with poor ventilation or automobiles whose engines have been running, many with fatal outcomes.

Chemically CO is a simple molecule whose mechanism of action is well studied. In addition, treatment of accidental poisoning is effective if the victim is attended in time. In 1895, Haldane conducted experiments with CO using himself as a subject. He carefully documented the effects as the concentration of CO in his blood rose toward lethal levels. The earlier work of Claude Bernard (1865) also contributed to our current knowledge of CO toxicity.

Similarly, as with oxygen, CO reacts with hemoglobin in red blood cells by binding to the iron atom of heme (Figure 14.1). CO binds to heme *with greater avidity*[4], about 220 times that of oxygen, rendering the resultant product, carboxyhemoglobin, unable to transport oxygen. This competitive binding phenomenon between oxygen and CO for the hemoglobin molecule depends on the relative concentrations of the gases and is a crucial factor in the poisoning sequelae. Since CO binds more avidly to the iron atom, the concentration of toxic gas necessary to saturate hemoglobin is much less than that of oxygen in air. The $CO::O_2$ was determined by Haldane and is shown by the equation:

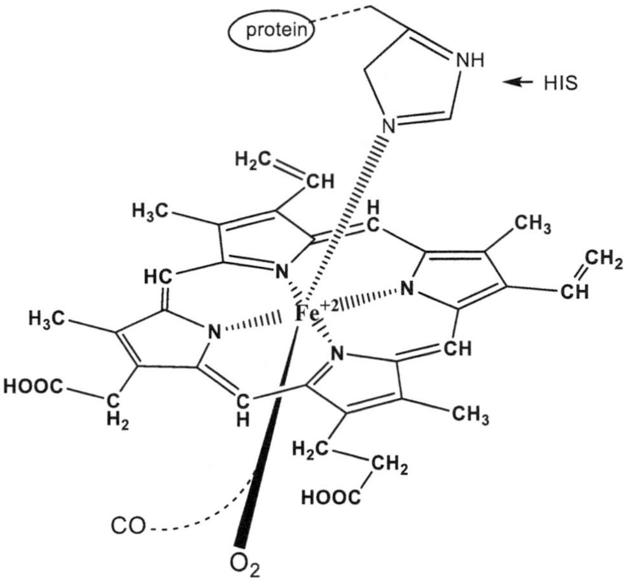

protein

NH

← HIS

N

H_2C=CH

H_3C

H
C

CH_3

HC

N

CH_2
CH

H_3C

Fe^{+2}

N

N

N

N

=CH

HOOC
C
H_2

C
H

=CH

CH_3

H_2C
CH_2
HOOC

CO

O_2

Figure 14.1 The heme moiety of hemoglobin illustrating binding of oxygen to the iron atom. The iron center (Fe^{+2}) coordinates six bonds total and is at the center of a large, complex porphyrin ring. The iron center binds four nitrogens in one plane; the nitrogen of a histidine (HIS) group forms the fifth bond. The histidine is a proximal amino acid residue in the protein portion of hemoglobin, while oxygen forms the sixth bond of the coordinates. CO competes with oxygen for the same site but is more tightly bound.

$$\frac{[COHb]}{[HbO_2]} = \frac{M[P_{CO}]}{[P_{O_2}]}$$

where $M = 220$, at pH 7.4. [COHb] and [HbO_2] = concentration of carboxyhemoglobin and hemoglobin, respectively. [P_{co}] and [P_{O_2}] are the partial pressures of CO and oxygen, respectively.

Consequently, when 50% saturation of hemoglobin with CO is converted to carboxyhemoglobin, the ratio of CO to oxygen required for toxicity is *1/220* in the air or about *0.1% – a lethal level*. Since CO is also *odorless* and *tasteless*, it remains undetected in ambient air and, as such, is known in toxicology as a *Silent Killer*. The net pathologic effect of CO poisoning is oxygen deprivation and ischemic damage. Energy production is reduced, anaerobic respiration dominates, and accumulation of lactic acid causes systemic acidosis.

The symptoms of CO poisoning depend on the concentration to which the victim is exposed. Headache, mental confusion, agitation, nausea, and vomiting are typical symptoms, while the skin becomes characteristically pink due to carboxyhemoglobin accumulating in blood. The victim hyperventilates, loses consciousness, and suffers respiratory failure. Brain and cardiac damage results from hypoxia, and cardiac arrhythmias complicate the situation.

Treatment for mild to moderate exposure involves immediate removal of the victim from the source of the gas or allows fresh uncontaminated air to enter into the environment. As the concentration of CO in the ambient and inspired air falls, carboxyhemoglobin dissociates and CO is expired. The rate of loss of toxic gas from the blood can be *increased* by treating the patient with 100% oxygen at atmospheric pressure, where the half-life is reduced from 250 to 50 minutes. (Treatment of patients with 100% oxygen at *elevated pressures* [above 2.0 atmospheres] reduces the half-life of elimination but is associated with serious oxygen toxicity and is not recommended.)

14.3 Ethylene Glycol (Antifreeze)

Antifreeze liquid contains toxic compounds which feature in poisoning, either unintentional or deliberate. The major constituent of antifreeze is ethylene glycol (EG) which is sometimes combined with methanol.

Ethylene glycol is sweet-tasting, dihydric alcohol, with effects similar to those of ethanol. On occasion, it is consumed instead of potable alcohol by alcoholics. However, it is toxic; fatalities occur with as little as 30–120 mL antifreeze. The chemical requires *metabolism* to cause toxicity. There are various intermediate metabolic products terminating in oxalic acid (Figure 14.2). Acidosis results from the reaction of the intermediate acidic metabolites and also from increasing levels of nicotinamide adenine dinucleotide reduced (**NADH**), which is incorporated in the production of lactic acid. Besides its acidic nature, oxalic acid damages brain neurons by crystallization. Calcium oxalate crystals also precipitate in, and damage, kidney tubules.

The first step in the metabolism of EG involves the enzyme alcohol dehydrogenase (ADH). The competitive inhibition for the enzyme serves as the basis for the treatment of EG poisoning. Fomepizole and ethanol are specific antidotes for EG (and methanol) intoxication. Fomepizole is an ADH inhibitor that effectively blocks the metabolism of EG and reduces the conversion of the glycol to the corresponding aldehyde and oxalic acid. Administration of fomepizole and ethanol also forces the competition of the alcohols for ADH, thus diverting the metabolism away from EG and methanol. Caution is in order for ethanol administration since it may cause central nervous system (CNS) depression and hypoglycemia, as the dose is not easily manipulated. However, fomepizole has great efficacy and fewer side effects than ethanol, hence it is the favored antidote in the treatment of EG intoxication.

Hemoperfusion or hemodialysis is only used in severe poisoning cases and when other treatment options have been exhausted.

The Austrian wine scandal of 1986 involved the use of EG as a wine sweetener. The amounts used however were not acutely toxic although the chronic toxic effects of EG – deposition of calcium oxalate and formation of kidney stones – was a cause for concern. The fact that wine also contains ethanol raises the interesting possibility that the toxicity would be reduced by the continued presence of the antidote!

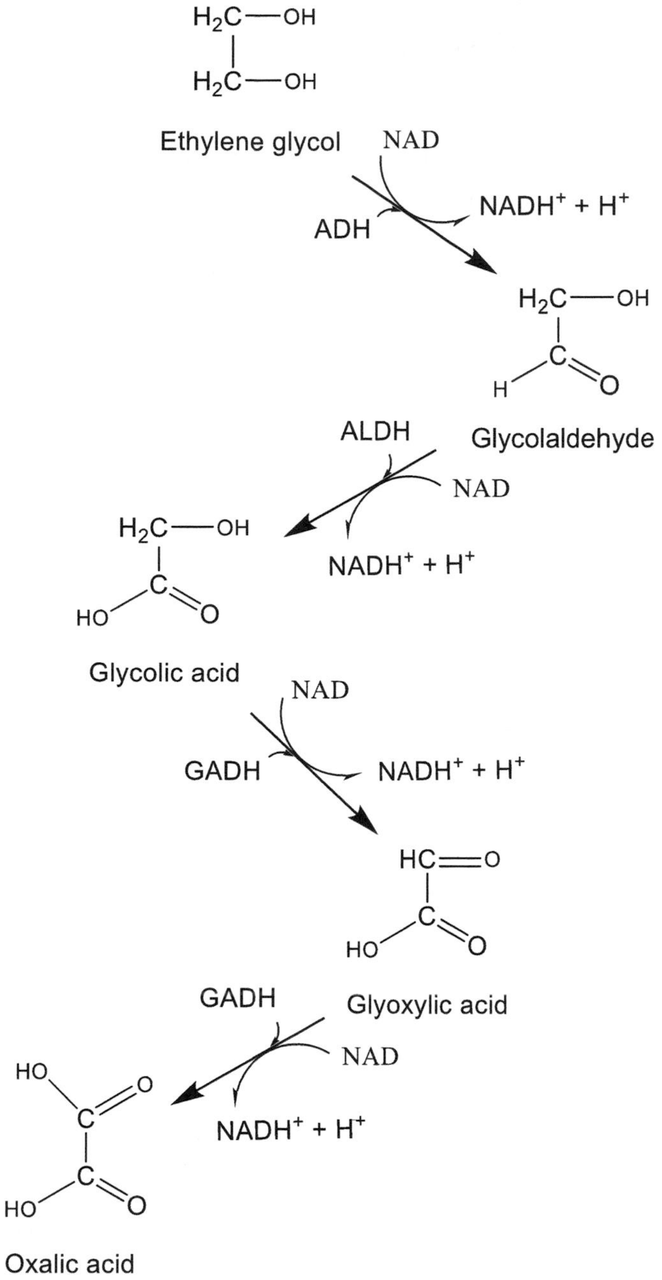

Figure 14.2 Oxidative metabolism of EG requires the enzymes ADH and aldehyde dehydrogenase (ALDH), which yield the corresponding aldehyde and glycolic acid, respectively. Further reduction progresses with glyceraldehyde dehydrogenase (GADH) producing the final acidic products, glyoxylic and oxalic acids.

Methanol (CH_3OH), which is sometimes present in antifreeze, is also found in methylated spirits (industrial spirit), toxicity of which results from metabolism to formaldehyde (HCHO) and formic acid (HCOOH), according to the following equation:

$$CH_3OH \rightarrow HCHO \rightarrow HCOOH$$

The aldehyde is responsible for blindness. As with EG poisoning, methanol is metabolized by ADH, and treatment of poisoning requires administration of fomepizole or ethanol for correction of metabolic acidosis, as noted above.

14.4 Cyanide

Various chemical entities of cyanides are found both naturally in the environment and formed from human activity, including hydrogen cyanide (HCN), arsenous acid (H_3AsO_3), and potassium (KCN) and sodium (NaCN) cyanides. Cyanide is often associated with homicidal or suicidal poisoning as the chemical is historically associated with dramatic crime stories. However, the ubiquitous nature of cyanide invites several methods of exposure. For example, fatalities in fires result from inhaling vaporized cyanide, when plastics, rubber, or chemical liquids generate HCN gas in smoke. Cyanides are extensively used in the metal industry and mining for extraction of metals, as well as commercial pesticides, presenting a potential for occupational and environmental poisoning. Many cases of pollution of waterways and soil are documented from mining processes. In February 2000, cyanide from a mining operation leaked into the river Tiza, Romania, poisoning most of the fish. The chemical flowed down the river devastating many fish in rivers and tributaries of neighboring Hungary.

Naturally occurring cyanides, such as amygdalin, a cyanogenic glycoside, are found in kernels and pits of fruits, including apricots, peaches, and apples. Cassava is a natural source of cyanide, an important food crop native to Africa. The Cassava plant must be prepared carefully to avoid cyanide poisoning, usually done by soaking and then washing the plant in water. This allows the enzymes in the plant to degrade the cyanogenic glycoside, linamarin, allowing the water-soluble cyanide ion to be washed out. Without proper preparation, the cyanogenic glycosides are degraded by the stomach and intestinal enzymes, releasing sufficient quantities of poisonous cyanide ions. Poorly prepared cassava eaten regularly in deficient diets can lead to chronic toxicity, characterized by muscle paralysis, goiter, and cretinism.

Hydrogen cyanide is rapidly fatal when inhaled as a vapor; 200 mg NaCN or KCN ingested orally requires several minutes for activity depending on the presence of food in the stomach and intestinal tract.

Cyanide's mechanism of action involves inhibition of the mitochondrial respiratory chain. Cyanide binds to cytochrome aa_3 blocking the movement of electrons to the final electron acceptor, O_2 (Figure 14.3). Cellular metabolism is subsequently compromised and ATP production is considerably reduced. The brain, heart, and lungs are affected initially since they require ATP and have

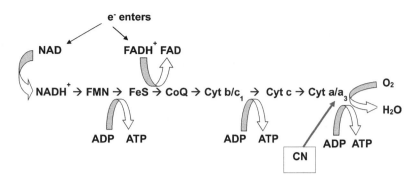

Figure 14.3 Site of action of cyanide (CN) in the mitochondrial electron transport chain. Continuous redox reactions promote electron transport along the pathway. Reactions proceed with formation of ATPs. The final electron acceptor is oxygen (O_2) with the formation of water. CN interferes with the transfer of electrons to O_2 and blocks the formation of ATPs, by binding to **cytochrome a/a3**. (Cofactor FMN, flavin mononucleotide; CoQ, coenzyme Q).

limited capacity to cope with a deficit. Unlike CO, cyanide does not compete with oxygen's ability to bind to hemoglobin. Although the lungs have enough oxygen, cyanide prevents the utilization of oxygen as an electron acceptor in the respiratory chain. Consequently, the cause of death is respiratory failure due to its inability to use oxygen.

There are several antidotes to cyanide poisoning. The goal of treatment is to immediately decrease CN binding to cytochrome enzymes with the specific antidote available. The cyanide antidote package consists of amyl nitrite inhalant, sodium nitrite, and sodium thiosulfate. Detoxification involves the conversion of CN to the cyanomethemoglobin, with amyl nitrite and sodium nitrite. Nitrites convert reduced Hb-Fe^{+2} ([H]) to oxidized methHb ([O]). The sequence is outlined in reaction 14.1:

$$Hb\text{-}Fe^{+2} + NO_2 \rightarrow Hb\text{-}Fe^{+3} + NO$$

$$\left[H\right] \qquad \left[O\right] \; methHb\left[O\right] \; \left[H\right]$$

(14.1)

MethHb[O] has a greater affinity for CN than cytochrome oxidase a/a_3. The CN transfers from the cytochrome enzyme complex to methHb[O], forming cyanomethemoglobin (CN-Hb-Fe^{+3}) and regenerating the enzyme complex, according to reaction 14.2:

$$Hb\text{-}Fe^{+3} + CN\text{-}cytochrome\text{-}Fe^{+3} \rightarrow CN\text{-}Hb\text{-}Fe^{+3} + cytochrome\text{-}Fe^{+3}$$

$$methHb[0] \; \left[CN::a/a_3\right] \qquad cyanomethhemoglobin$$

(14.2)

Lastly, sodium thiosulphate is administered; it induces formation of water-soluble thiocyanate (SCN) which is excreted, while regenerating methemoglobin.

Chronic, non-fatal exposure to cyanide such as that which occurs because of eating cassava, results in paralysis of spinal cord nerves – a common toxic effect in African nations where Cassava is a staple diet.[5] A secondary effect is **goiter** (enlarged thyroid) due to thiocyanate detoxification products stimulating interference in uptake of iodine essential for proper thyroid function.

14.5 Alcohol (Ethanol, Ethyl Alcohol)

Ethanol is the most ubiquitous drug and features in more cases of poisoning or adverse effects than most substances. In general, society does not view alcohol as a drug or chemical notwithstanding its *pharmacological* and *toxic* actions. The effects of ethanol vary with dose; it is rapidly absorbed from the GI tract and distributes into all physiological compartments. About 90% is metabolized to acetaldehyde, acetic acid, and eventually to carbon dioxide and water at a rate of 10–20 mL/hr.

Following acute doses ethanol produces central nervous system (CNS) depression. The effects are related to the plasma level (blood alcohol concentration [BAC]) and range from mild intoxication at 50–100 mg/dl[6] to cardiovascular collapse and respiratory arrest above 500 mg/dl. The pharmacological desirable effects occur at low doses; following higher concentrations however the effects are pronounced, progressing from visual impairment, muscular incoordination, and slowed reaction times through unconsciousness, coma, and death. At this level respiratory depression, hypotension, hypothermia, and hypoglycemia are life-threatening, largely due to inhibition of gluconeogenesis by alcohol.

After chronic exposure to ethanol, the liver is the main target organ although the brain also suffers. Continuous chronic drinking of moderate to excessive amounts precipitates fatty liver as a result of accumulation of triglycerides in hepatic cells. **Cirrhosis** occurs after chronic abuse distorting the architecture of the liver by replacement of normal hepatic tissue with collagen, preventing efficient function. The biochemical basis of hepatic effects of ethanol involves alterations in the level of cofactor NADH and disturbances in intermediary metabolism. Thus, a *shift* in redox potential with an increased NADH+/NAD ratio leads to impaired mitochondrial oxidation of fatty acids such that more triglyceride is synthesized. Ethanol causes various other metabolic effects which contribute to its toxicity.

Chronic ethanol intoxication is associated with an increased risk for liver cancer as well as GI carcinogenic pathologies.

14.6 Glue Sniffing and Solvent Abuse (Hydrocarbons)

Glue sniffing and solvent abuse became common among teenagers during the 1970s and 1980s. Different types of solvents and *inhalants* are still commonly used with correspondingly different effects. Solvents, chemically characterized as hydrocarbons (HC) are found in many household products including glues, spray paints, paint strippers, aerosols, varnishes, cleaning fluids, nail polish removers, lighter fluids, deodorants, hair sprays, and whipped cream canisters. Their widespread availability in consumer products renders them easily accessible and inexpensive, and a source of toxicity and fatality from accidental or deliberate inhalation, ingestion, or dermal exposure.

In the U.S., surveys indicate that nearly 21.7 million Americans aged 12 and older have used inhalants at least once in their lives. The U.S. National Institute of Drug Abuse (NIDA) Monitoring the Future (MTF) survey reveals that 13.1% of 8th-graders have used inhalants.[7] However, the percentage of adolescents reporting substance use decreased significantly in 2021, representing the largest one-year decrease in overall illicit drug use reported since the survey began in 1975. The decrease also includes vaping for both marijuana and tobacco products which follow sharp increases in use between 2017 and 2019, which then leveled off in 2020 (NIDA, NIH, 2021).

The vapors of the organic chemicals are usually inhaled providing a quick "desirable" sensation of euphoria, although quickly accompanied by serious toxic sequelae. Acute effects of solvents are narcosis or anesthesia notwithstanding serious sensitization of the heart. Chronic effects are generally unknown but include changes in personality, behavior, and general morbidity. Additional symptoms from some substances include loss of consciousness, hallucination, stupor, and seizures. GI effects involve nausea and vomiting. Hematological consequences of HC toxicity result in mild hemolysis. Toluene for example is commonly found in glues and responsible for narcosis.[8] Halogenated solvents such as aerosol propellants are more hazardous, as inhalation produces *sensitization of the myocardium* to catecholamines[9] precipitating ventricular arrhythmias – a common lead-in to heart attacks and sudden death. Trichloroethane exposure is also associated with chronic cardiac toxicity.

14.7 Summary and Learning Objectives

There are many chemicals considered as household items that are potentially poisonous, including pesticides, organic solvents, detergents, and acids. A frequent toxic offender, often leading to fatalities in the home, is *CO* resulting from poor ventilation of gas stoves, smoke and fires, gas heaters, and automobile exhaust. The gas binds strongly to hemoglobin thereby competing with and depriving the tissues of oxygen. Symptoms include severe headache, confusion, acidosis, unconsciousness, and death from respiratory and/or cardiac failure. When ingested *EG* a component of auto antifreeze produces acidosis, kidney and brain damage due to metabolism to toxic aldehydes and acids. *Cyanide* is a universal chemical found in domestic (e.g. cassava) and commercial settings. Cyanide binds to cytochrome aa_3 in the mitochondrion thereby preventing flow of electrons and preventing further synthesis of ATP. Death is usually rapid because of cardiac or respiratory failure.

Alcohol (ethanol) is a ubiquitous but potentially toxic substance that accounts for many cases of liver damage (cirrhosis).

Solvents and other volatile substances are inhaled[10] leading to unconsciousness which is also associated with premature heart failure.

Review Questions

1. Indicate which of the following are true and which are false. Fomepizole and ethanol are specific antidotes for the treatment of EG poisoning because they: (a) facilitate the excretion of EG; (b) block the metabolism of EG; (c) increase detoxification of EG; (d) chelate EG; (e) none of the above.
2. Carbon monoxide is poisonous because it: (a) binds to cytochrome aa_3 in the mitochondria; (b) binds to hemoglobin; (c) causes respiratory alkalosis; (d) causes respiratory failure; (e) forms methemoglobin.
3. Indicate which of the following are true and which are false with reference to EG: (a) is an alcohol; (b) causes metabolic acidosis; (c) is metabolized to lactic acid; (d) crystallizes in the brain (e) is metabolized by aldehyde dehydrogenase.
4. Indicate which of the following are true: (a) solvents cause death by sensitization of the myocardium; (b) alcohol is toxic because it stimulates the CNS; (c) alcohol is metabolized to formic acid; (d) the major target organ for methanol toxicity is the liver; (e) large doses of alcohol cause blindness; (f) high doses of alcohol lower blood sugar.
5. Which of the following are used as antidotes for poisoning?: (a) methanol; (b) disodium EDTA; (c) thiocyanate; (d) N-acetylcysteine (NAC); (e) pralidoxime (2-PAM).

Short Answer Questions

6. Discuss the basis of treatment for cyanide poisoning.
7. Discuss the basis of treatment for CO poisoning.

Notes

1. Corrosive agents.
2. Strongly acidic descaling agents are usually corrosive to the eyes and skin, and also attack and degrade clothing fibres; appropriate protection such as rubber gloves and plastic aprons should be used in cleaning operations.
3. Swelling of the area due to accumulation of water and inflammatory fluids.
4. Refers to the strength of bonding to a molecule
5. Interestingly, reliance on Cassava as a major part of the diet in African countries precipitates a deficiency in sulphur amino acids, low levels of thiosulphate, and decreases the ability to detoxify cyanide.
6. dl = deciliter or 100 mL.
7. According to the U.S. National Institute of Drug Abuse (NIDA), *inhalant* refers to various substances that can only be inhaled, including solvents (liquids that become gas at room temperature), aerosol sprays, gases, and nitrites (prescription drugs for chest pain).

8. A state of stupor, drowsiness, or unconsciousness produced by drugs or chemicals.
9. Blood levels of naturally occurring neurotransmitters epinephrine, norepinephrine, dopamine, rise from stressful situations or from chemical intake.
10. The practice of inhaling vapors of volatile organic liquid agents is known as "glue sniffing".

Bibliography

Barile, F.A., Chapters 25. Gases; and, Chapter 27. Aliphatic and aromatic hydrocarbons, in: *Barile's Clinical Toxicology: Principles and Mechanisms*, Barile, F.A. (Ed.), CRC Press, Taylor and Francis, Boca Raton, FL, 2019. ISBN-13: 978-1498765305

Ellenhorn, M.J. and Barceloux, D.G., *Medical Toxicology. Diagnosis and Treatment of Human Poisoning*, Elsevier, New York, 1988.

Flanagan, R.J., Widdop, B., Ramsey, J.D. and Loveland, M., Analytical toxicology, *Human Toxicology*, 7, 489–502, 1988.

Gossel, T.A. and Bricker, J.D., *Principles of Clinical Toxicology*, 3rd edition, Raven Press, New York, 1994.

NIDA, *Percentage of Adolescents Reporting Drug Use Decreased Significantly in 2021 as the COVID-19 Pandemic Endured*, National Institute on Drug Abuse, National Institutes of Health (NIH), Dec. 2021; https://nida.nih.gov/news-events/news-releases/2021/12/percentage-of-adolescents-reporting-drug-use-decreased-significantly-in-2021-as-the-covid-19-pandemic-endured. Last accessed November 2022.

Rosling, H., *Cassava Toxicity and Food Security*, UNICEF, *Scientific Research*, p. 40, 1988. https://scirp.org/reference/referencespapers.aspx?referenceid=610943. Last accessed November 2022.

Saul, H., The debate over the limits, *New Scientist*, 1932, 12–13, 1994.

Vuori, E., Ojanpera, I., Forensic toxicology, in: *General and Applied Toxicology*, Ballantyne, B., Marrs, T. and Syversen, T.L.M. (Eds.), 3rd edition, John Wiley and Sons, Oxford, Hoboken. N.J., 2009. ISBN-13: 978-0470723272.

Fundamentals of Toxicity Testing

This chapter discusses testing of chemicals for toxicity and alternative methods to animal testing.

Chapter Outline

15.1 Introduction   213
15.2 Evaluation of Toxicity   214
15.3 Epidemiological Studies   215
15.4 Animal Welfare   216
15.5 Considerations for Experimental Testing   217
    15.5.1 Acute Toxicity Tests   219
    15.5.2 Sub-chronic Toxicity Tests   220
    15.5.3 Chronic Toxicity Tests   221
15.6 *In Vitro Testing as* Alternatives to Animals   223
15.7 Summary and Learning Objectives   225
Review Questions   225
    Short Answer Questions   225
Notes   226
Bibliography   226

15.1 Introduction

In most countries, human and veterinary drugs, food additives, contaminants, industrial chemicals, pesticides, and cosmetics are evaluated for their toxicity potential. The objective of *in vivo* studies is to identify potential toxicity of

DOI: 10.1201/9781003188575-15

chemicals, whether commercially available or in development. *In vitro* methods are also incorporated into pharmacology studies to identify the mechanisms of action of therapeutic drugs and chemicals. The underlying premise for using animals in acute or chronic testing is that effects of administration of a synthetic agent on an animal mimic possible outcomes that the agent may produce in humans or mammals. The system also implies that short-term tests in animals parallel acute exposure in the human population.

The term *in vitro toxicology* generally refers to handling of cells and tissues outside of intact organ systems under conditions that support their growth, differentiation, and stability. Since the initial experiments over 60 years ago established the validity of cell culture techniques in toxicology, the methods have proven fundamental for understanding and developing critical procedures in cellular and molecular biology, as well as in toxicology, pharmacology, genetics, reproductive biology, and oncology.[1] Cell culture technology has improved dramatically because of interest in methods and through its broad applications. Consequently, the discipline of cell culture and its application to *in vitro* toxicology represents a tool poised to answer questions in biomedical sciences that can only be addressed by examining proliferation of isolated cells without the influence of other organ systems.

15.2 Evaluation of Toxicity

Evaluation of toxicity of a chemical is determined according to the following objectives:

a. by observing human, animal, or plant populations exposed to existing chemicals (epidemiology);
b. by administering chemicals to animals or plants in the laboratory under controlled conditions and observing the effects (*in vivo*);
c. by exposing mammalian cultured cells, subcellular fractions, or single-celled organisms to chemicals (*in vitro*).

Exposure of humans to chemicals occurs accidentally through the environment, in the occupational setting, or intentionally, as with drugs and food additives. Similarly, exposure of humans to chemicals in the workplace, when adequately monitored and recorded, provides evidence of toxicity. Thus, monitoring of exposure by measuring substances and their metabolites in body fluids and using biochemical indices of physiological or pathological change are performed in humans. For example, monitoring of agricultural workers for exposure to organophosphorus compounds is followed by measuring the degree of inhibition of cholinesterases in blood samples. However, acquiring such data is often difficult and incomplete, and the information may not have enough validity as a stand-alone study. Of particular importance is lack of quantitative chronic exposure data for humans in prolonged occupational settings. The current development of sensitive and specific biomarkers for several pathologic conditions, including cancers, has improved acquisition of such data.

Studying populations of predatory birds and measuring unique parameters, such as eggshell thickness and pesticide level, is an ecotoxicological example of testing for toxicity in the field.

Before marketing of therapeutics, drugs are first administered to a small number of human volunteers in clinical studies (**phase 1 clinical trials**), and to progressively larger numbers of patients (**phase 2 and 3 clinical trials**), before drugs are approved by regulatory agencies and available to the public. Clinical trials and public monitoring of adverse reactions are essential for pre-clinical administration and post-marketing evaluation of drugs, respectively. Phase 1 trials yield information about metabolism and disposition. Phase 2 and Phase 3 trials provide data on adverse drug reactions (ADR) and efficacy, respectively.

For human and veterinary medicines in the UK, a system for reporting adverse reactions to drugs for human medicines is the yellow card system; for veterinary drugs, adverse reactions of animals are also reported.

15.3 Epidemiological Studies

Data obtained from human exposure or clinical trials is analyzed through epidemiological practices. Typically, effects observed are compared to those in control subjects with the objective of determining an association or difference between exposure to a chemical, a concurrent disease, adverse effect, or non-exposed group.

There are four types of epidemiological studies:

a. **Cohort studies**: individuals exposed to a chemical of interest are followed over a specified time *prospectively*.
b. **Case-control studies**: test subjects exposed to a chemical or develop a disease are compared *retrospectively*, with similar control subjects without disease.
c. **Cross-sectional studies**: prevalence of a disease in an exposed group is examined.
d. **Ecological studies**: incidence of a disease in one geographical area, where a hazardous chemical exposure exists, is compared with the incidence in another area in the absence of the same chemical.

For accidental, unintentional exposure, analysis is normally *retrospective* and is labeled as a 'case-control study'. The control population includes human subjects chosen with similar attributes such as age, sex, and/or underlying parameters. For instance, this type of design is used for studying relationships between exposure to a volatile chemical in the workplace and lung cancer. Even when the prevalence of lung cancer exists in controls, depending on their physiological and pathological status, the objective is to determine if prevalence is higher in those exposed to the chemical. Post-marketing reporting for ADRs is also followed in the population. In this type of design, the data is represented as an odds ratio – that is representing an estimate of relative risk.

Prospective studies (a.k.a. cohort study) are used in clinical trials of therapeutic agents. Controls are subjects selected from a patient population that are already diagnosed for an applicable disease for which a drug is prescribed. Control groups receive a *placebo* – an inactive similarly appearing substitute.

Epidemiological data is analyzed in various ways to yield a range of measures of effect. As noted above, data is represented as an *odds ratio*,[2] i.e., ratio of risk of acquiring disease in an exposed group compared to a control group. *Relative risk* is determined as the ratio of occurrence of disease in the exposed to unexposed population. *Absolute excess risk* is an alternative quantitative measure.[3]

Establishing and interpreting epidemiological studies for assessing their significance requires awareness of potential confounding factors such as the presence of unintentional bias and the need for proper controls.

Although human data from epidemiological studies is important, most of the information on the toxicity of chemicals is obtained from experimental studies in animals. Data so acquired is incorporated into risk assessment analysis and safety evaluation of drugs prior to human exposure. Similar information is necessary for food additives before incorporation into foodstuff, and for industrial and environmental chemicals, particularly to calculate the no observed adverse effect level (NOAEL).

Because *in vivo* tests are experimentally controlled, with factors determined in the laboratory, quality of data is valid. The number of animals used should be enough to demonstrate statistical significance. The problem of extrapolation between animal species and humans, however, is considerable; historically toxic effects occurring in animals have not always been a reliable guideline for human risk assessment.

15.4 Animal Welfare

Humane conditions and proper treatment of animals are essential for scientific and ethical reasons as this helps to ensure that the study is reliable, robust, and ethically conducted.

The U.S. Animal Welfare Act (1966) authorizes the U.S. Secretary of Agriculture to regulate, transport, sale, and handling of dogs, cats, nonhuman primates, guinea pigs, hamsters, and rabbits intended to be used in research or "for other purposes".

Research facilities are defined according to standards set by the Act. Regulations have been developed regarding record keeping and humane care and treatment of animals in or during commerce, exhibition, experimentation, and transport. The regulations also mention inspections and appropriate use of anesthetics, analgesics, and tranquilizers. An amendment to the Act (1985) clarifies what is meant by "humane care" and details sanitation, housing, and ventilation requirements, as well as institutes regulations providing exercise for dogs, and mandates provisions for establishing an adequate physical environment promoting psychological health of nonhuman primates. It specifies that pain and distress must be minimized in experimental procedures and requires that principal investigators consider alternatives to such procedures. It also defines experimental practices that are considered painful.

The 1985 Act establishes a requirement for formation of, and describes the role and composition of, the Institutional Animal Care and Use Committees (IACUCs). It prevents unintended duplication of research, provides for employee training, searches for ways to reduce, replace, or refine animal testing (3Rs), and obtains information on how to decrease pain and distress. A thorough understanding of these regulations reinforces importance of preventing and avoiding misuse, overuse, and unnecessary suffering of animals.

In the UK, controls on the use of animals in research have existed since 1876. The Animals (Scientific Procedures) Act (1986) was amended in 2012 to direct UK law to be consistent with the requirements of the EU. UK regulations are widely regarded as some of the strictest in the field and require scientists to hold personal licenses and prior approval in experiments using animals.

15.5 Considerations for Experimental Testing

The performance of *in vivo* toxicity tests depends partly on the type of substance, its expected use and national and international regulations. The amount of data necessary also requires knowledge of end-use of the substance. For instance, industrial chemicals produced in small quantities for non-therapeutic use only require minimal toxicity data while human and animal therapeutic drugs require extensive toxicological testing. Pesticides are tested on many different types of animal and plant species in the environment and examined for their persistence and behavior in food chains. Stability of such substances in actual environments is also important. Consequently, ecotoxicology involves more extensive residue analysis than does drug toxicology.

The species selected depends partly on the type of toxicity test, data anticipated, and ethical and financial considerations. For example, although primates are generally most similar to humans and desirable as appropriate species for estimating human toxicology, cost and ethical reasons often rule out this genus of mammals. The most common species used are rodents particularly because of ease of handling, size, accumulated knowledge of the species, and cost. Currently, mice have the advantage of availability in genetically modified variations.

For veterinary drugs or environmental pollutants, the target species is usually incorporated into studies, identifying young adult animals of both sexes. The exposure level of chemical application ideally spans both non-toxic and maximally toxic doses.

Examples of relevant factors that are considered *prior to establishing an experimental setup* include:

1. is the substance a novel compound (no prior commercial use)?
2. is it destined for release into the environment?
3. will it be available for human consumption?
4. is it administered as a single, repeated, or continuous dose?
5. what is the dosage level?
6. is there consideration of the age group exposed? and
7. is there a risk during pregnancy or to women of childbearing age?

Toxicity is an *intrinsic* property of many molecules that result from interaction with biological systems. Consequently, knowledge of the physicochemical properties of molecules helps toxicologists to understand potential toxicity and to predict disposition and metabolism. For example, structure–activity relationships are studied prior to experimental testing as in pharmacology, since this information is valuable in predicting toxicity of similarly structured chemicals, especially appropriate in chemical mutagenesis and carcinogenesis. This initial knowledge from preliminary studies influences the course of subsequent toxicity tests especially if there are similarities to compounds of known toxicity. Toxicokinetic parameters such as solubility, partition coefficient, melting or boiling point, vapor pressure, and purity are important indicators for prediction. A volatile industrial liquid for instance with a high-vapor pressure should be evaluated for toxicity by inhalation and dermal application.

As well as physicochemical considerations there are also biological factors including:

1. most appropriate species for study;
2. sex of animals;
3. use of inbred or outbred strains;
4. housing parameters;
5. appropriate diet;
6. use of pathogen-free animals;
7. metabolic similarity to humans;
8. route of administration;
9. duration of study;
10. number of animals in groups; and
11. vehicle, i.e., composition of drug delivery.

The route and vehicle of administration, and indicators measured, depend on the anticipated applications of the drug. For example, metabolic studies can be combined with toxicity studies so that plasma levels and urinary metabolites are coordinated and identified and applied to the clinical chemical parameters. Biochemical and pathological measurements are decided before the study starts.

Preliminary toxicity studies are carried out to determine the *approximate range of toxic dosage*. This information is gathered for a drug from previous pharmacological studies; for industrial chemicals, however, chemical and biological activity is unknown. Consequently, initial range-finding studies exploit dosage on a logarithmic or half-log scale. These initial studies are important to avoid unnecessary sacrifice of large numbers of animals in subsequent studies. Preliminary tests also involve *observation* of animals to gain insight into possible unsuspected toxic effects.

Once approximate toxic dosage ranges are determined various detailed toxicity studies are performed, including: acute, **sub-chronic** (28- or 90-day), chronic, mutagenicity, carcinogenicity, teratogenicity, reproductive, and *in vitro* studies. Irritant or corrosive compounds also require more specific types of toxicity tests such as irritancy and skin sensitization studies.

Because of varying circumstances of exposure, drugs, food additives and contaminants, industrial chemicals, cosmetics, and pesticides require different assessments. Chemicals bound for the environment, such as pesticides, also undergo ecotoxicity evaluations, including testing with invertebrates such as *Daphnia*, earthworms, fish, phytoplankton, and higher plants.

15.5.1 Acute Toxicity Tests

Acute toxicity tests are those designed to determine effects that occur within a short period of time after dosing. These protocols determine dose-response relationships and LD_{50} values. The precise method of performing studies varies depending on the compound, its ultimate use, and regulations imposed. In general, at least four dosages are used in *logarithmic progression* especially if range-finding experiments are not available. However, traditional LD_{50} determinations are currently not mandatory by most regulatory authorities. Thus, a variety of established techniques are currently used for LD_{50} determinations with the intention of minimizing the number of animals. These include the:

1. Up-and-down procedure (UDP) or staircase method (OECD #425);[4]
2. Fixed-dose approach (FDP, British Toxicology Society, OECD #420);
3. Acute toxic class method (ATCM, OECD #423 and #436);
4. Revised UDP test method (ICCVAM, NIH Publication 02-4501).[5]

In the UDP procedure, animals are dosed one at a time. If an animal survives, the dose for the next animal is increased; if it dies, the dose is decreased. Each animal is observed for 1 or 2 days before dosing the next animal.

The FDP was first proposed in 1984 by the British Toxicology Society as an alternative to the conventional LD_{50} test (OECD Test Guideline 401) for determining acute oral toxicity. The FDP used fewer animals and caused less suffering than the LD_{50} test and provided information on acute toxicology that allowed substances to be classified according to the European Union hazard classification system. In 1999, as part of an initiative to phase out Test Guideline 401, a review of the FDP was undertaken, the aim of which was to provide further reductions and refinements, and to catalog the procedures according to the criteria of the United Nations' Globally Harmonized System (GHS) of classification and labeling of chemicals (OECD #420). Animals are observed up to 14 days and for survival at 48 hours after treatment, after which preset doses are similarly administered orally. As few as six but not more than fifteen animals are incorporated per test.

The ATCM (OECD Test Guideline 423 and 436) avoids the criteria of lethality as an exclusive indicator by incorporating evident clinical signs of toxicity at one of a series of fixed-dose levels on which to base classification of the test material. Refinements to this protocol have been introduced to minimize suffering and distress of test animals. The oral ATCM incorporates considerably fewer animals and provides information on the hazardous properties of a chemical, and allows it to be ranked and classified according to the GHS classifications of chemicals that cause acute toxicology.

Lastly, the revised UDP test method includes three components: (1) a primary test providing an improved estimate of acute oral toxicology with a reduction in the number of animals used when compared to classical methods; (2) a limit test for substances anticipated to have minimal toxicology; and (3) a supplemental test to determine slope and confidence interval for the dose-response curve.

Recently the U.S. Center for Drug Evaluation and Research (CDER) of the Food and Drug Administration (FDA) published the 'Guidance for Industry' (2010) that recommends international standards and promotes harmonization of the nonclinical safety studies to support human clinical trials of a given scope and duration as well as marketing authorization for pharmaceuticals. The guidance establishes recommendations for nonclinical safety assessment for marketing approval of pharmaceuticals which usually include pharmacology studies, general toxicity, toxicokinetic and nonclinical pharmacokinetic studies, reproduction toxicity and genotoxicity studies, and an assessment of carcinogenic potential. Other nonclinical studies to assess phototoxicity, immunotoxicity, juvenile animal toxicity, and abuse liability are also conducted.

In addition, the guidance is instrumental for facilitating the timely conduct of clinical trials and for reducing the use of animals in accordance with the 3Rs (reduce/refine/replace) principles. Consideration is also given to use of new *in vitro* alternative methods for safety evaluation. These methods, if validated and accepted by all ICH[6] regulatory authorities, can be used to replace current standard *in vivo* methods.

Information obtained from acute toxicity studies is the basis of the dose-response relationship and observations on toxic effects and time required for pathologies to emerge. It is important to note that the dosage range is wide enough for observation of effects unless determined that the doses are beyond those expected for similar chemicals. The range and method of delivery are influenced by the expected or intended route of administration and exposure concentration.

Post-mortem and pathological examinations of tissues are performed during and at the conclusion of the protocols.

15.5.2 Sub-chronic Toxicity Tests

Sub-chronic toxicity tests are performed following acute toxicity studies. These involve exposing animals to test substances for longer periods, usually 30 or 90 days, frequently, continuously or daily. Sub-chronic tests provide information on target organs affected by compounds and their major toxic effects. The studies are particularly useful for detecting compounds with a slow onset, with *reversible* or *adaptive* responses. Measurements of drug levels in blood and tissue are measured and correlated with observable results. Clinical chemistry measurements during the study are correlated with development of pathological lesions. Data derived from sub-chronic toxicity experiments also help in the *design* of chronic studies. Sub-chronic toxicity protocols are also used to identify a no observed effect level (NOEL) while incorporating data from other tests.

15.5.3 Chronic Toxicity Tests

Chronic toxicity tests involve exposure of animals to compounds of interest for at least 90 days to 2 years in rodents and 6–12 months in non-rodents. The tests are combined with *in vivo* carcinogenicity studies, where exposure of rodents is for their lifetime; satellite groups are used for interim chronic toxicity information. Currently, the ICH has determined that chronic toxicity tests do not need to be as long as 2 years if shorter times yield significant information. As with sub-chronic tests, chronic studies *terminate* with a pathological examination while clinical chemistry measurements are performed at intervals throughout. Clinical chemistry measurements support development of pathological changes which are also noticed at post-mortem. Changes in other measurements such as body weight and food and water intake also suggest the presence of adverse effects. Chronic toxicity studies are important for drugs administered over *long periods of time*, for food additives present in products for *lifetimes*, and for environmental and industrial chemicals that are present in the environment at *low levels* for *longer time periods*.

For the three types of toxicity tests, selection of dosages, species, strain of animal, route of exposure, parameters measured, and other considerations are important. These factors are influenced by specific chemicals studied, by expected circumstances of exposure, and the regulations of the countries where the agents are used.

Requirements of the New Substances Notification Scheme in the EU, originally promulgated in 1994, are replaced by the New Chemical Substance Notification in the EU – REACH (Registration, Evaluation, Authorization, and Restriction of Chemicals, 2007). REACH regulation has replaced the old framework of notification of new substances (NONS) in the EU. Under this administrative agency, new chemical registration requires an inquiry dossier submitted to ECHA (European Chemicals Agency). This applies to companies who are interested in placing a new chemical substance on the EU market for the first time and companies who decide to register an existing substance without pre-registration. The regulations serve to illustrate the range of physicochemical, toxicological and ecotoxicological studies that are required. The amount of testing required depends upon the amounts of product produced. Table 15.1 details the requirements for the proper conduct of toxicology testing protocols, monitoring, and categorizations. In addition, teratology, fertility, and carcinogenicity studies may be required *depending on the amount* of compound manufactured and data presented from other tests. Further methods require repetition of studies using alternative routes of administration, different species, or *in vitro* screening. Similarly, additional ecotoxicology studies include *subacute* or *chronic* toxicity studies in *Daphnia* and fish, effects on higher plants, and determination of bioaccumulation.

Reproductive studies determine the complex interactions of compounds on fertility, fetal development, and sexual propagation. Teratogenicity tests examine specific effects of chemical agents on the development of the embryo and fetus, detecting gross anatomical or behavioral *abnormalities* in the newborn animals. Effects on fertility of male and female animals and implantation by drugs administered post-coital are evaluated, while similar agents are studied that also interfere with sexual mating and development. Pathological evidence of gonadal damage

Table 15.1 Categories of Data and Information Required for Investigation of a New Chemical Substance under the EU New Chemical Substances Notification Scheme

Category	Required Data & Information
Identity	Proprietary, Generic name Formula: empirical, structural Composition Methods of detection
Toxicology Studies	Acute toxicity: oral, inhalation, parenteral Dermal, ocular irritancy, sensitization Subacute, chronic toxicity
Precautions for:	Intended, proposed uses Production, importation, handling, storage Emergency measures
Ecotoxicology Studies[a]	Toxicity to fish, *Daphnia*, plants, fauna ADME Bioaccumulation
Physicochemical properties	Melting, boiling, freezing point Relative density Vapor pressure; surface tension Water, lipid solubility; Partition coefficient Flash point Flammability Explosive, oxidizing properties
Applications for:	Industry, occupational, public Continuous monitoring Proposed classification, labeling

[a] Absorption, distribution, metabolism, excretion studies

from drugs and chemicals is investigated for possible effects on male and female fertility in chronic studies.

Mutagenicity tests determine the ability of compounds to induce genetic damage, through mutational changes in germ cells and somatic cells – the mechanism of which is closely related to carcinogenic activity. Mutagenicity tests are traditionally performed with bacterial and cultured mammalian cells *in vitro*. *In vitro* assays include the **micronucleus test** and the **dominant lethal assay**.

Carcinogenicity tests are required when mutagenicity tests produce positive results. The compound is administered in drinking water or incorporated into the diet, for the lifetime of the animal, typically 2-year studies in rodents. Appearance of tumors during the experiments or at post-mortem is garnered from physical and histopathological examination of tissue sections from affected organs.

Toxicity tests are generally authorized by the pharmaceutical or chemical company producing the compound and performed by contract research laboratories. The conduct of the studies conforms to guidelines issued by the Organization for Economic Cooperation and Development (OECD), promulgated according to national regulatory requirements in the EU and USA. **Good Laboratory Practice (GLP)** procedures govern every aspect of conduct of studies including reporting of results. This system was introduced to ensure that toxicity tests are competently and systematically performed in accordance with acceptable standard operating (laboratory) procedures (SOP).

As well as the requirements of regulatory agencies, toxicity data lends itself to the development of clinical applications. For instance, animal studies on cyanide provided data that was useful in the treatment of poisoning with the chemical. Absence of any toxicity data on methyl isocyanate initially hampered the efforts of rescue workers and clinicians at Bhopal in India after the massive chemical plant disaster. Clinical studies with acetaminophen toxicity led to the discovery of an important and successful therapeutic antidote. Attempts to understand the mechanisms underlying the toxicity of compounds allow for investigation of chemical harm and better design of protocols to discover pathologic potential.

15.6 *In Vitro Testing* as Alternatives to Animals

It has become necessary to re-examine *in vivo* toxicology studies because of the need to find alternatives to live animal experimentation in biomedical research. Specifically, public objections and disapproval of animal testing have forced industry stakeholders, research institutions, industrial concerns, and regulatory agencies to direct their initiatives toward the development of alternative models for animal testing. As increasing pressure has mounted from scientific and public interest groups, the field of alternative *in vitro* methods has witnessed favorable transformations and development, including applications of the technology and its introduction into the regulatory arena. Some of these techniques have been rapidly adopted by pharmaceutical and cosmetic industries as preliminary toxicology screening tools, used in parallel with conventional animal testing protocols. Consequently, the past 30 years has witnessed an unprecedented development of non-genetic, systemic, and local *in vitro* methods as alternatives to animal testing.

The current philosophy is embodied in the concept of the three Rs: replacement, reduction, and refinement – replacement of animals with appropriate *in vitro* testing systems capable of obtaining equivalent data for toxicology information; reduction in the number of animals used particularly for screening protocols and in repetitive experiments where information is similarly available; and refinement in the methods of animal experimentation where pain and suffering are minimized or alleviated. The latter recommendation also refers to conditions of housing, feeding, and handling of animals before, during, and after studies are concluded.

The term *in vitro toxicology* refers to the handling of tissues outside of intact organ systems under conditions that support their growth, differentiation, and stability. Since the seminal experiments established the validity of cell culture techniques in toxicology, the methods have proven fundamental for understanding and developing critical procedures in cellular and molecular biology, as well as in pharmacology, genetics, reproductive biology, and oncology. Cell culture technology has improved dramatically because of interest in the methods and through its broad applications. The technology has also proved more economical than traditional animal handling measures.

Today, cell biologists have further developed culture techniques to aid in their understanding of cellular and extracellular interactions such as mesenchymal-epithelial relationships, epithelium-cell matrix interactions, and stem cell biology. These *in vitro* studies have materialized largely through the improvement to cell culture protocols such as chemically defined culture media, the addition of cellular substrata to culture flasks, the introduction of porous membranes and filter inserts that allow for the passage of low molecular weight soluble substances, the development of treated plastic surfaces, incubation of cells with co-cultures, and development of 3D cultures.

Prediction of chemically induced toxicity in humans from *in vitro* data continues to be a significant challenge for the biomedical community, pharmaceutical, and toxicological industries. Generally, conventional *in vitro* cell culture systems are limited by their inability to maintain phenotypic characteristics over time in culture, including stable expression of metabolic and bioactivation pathways. Even their complex adaptive responses to chemical exposure are sometimes difficult to interpret. In addition, these systems require significant advancement and improvement before long-term toxicity studies can deliver an understanding of key cellular and molecular events involved in human risk assessment. Despite these drawbacks, cell culture models have been able to explain primary and secondary adaptation to chemical exposure and have been useful for identification of important mediators of inflammation, proliferation, and apoptosis. Considerable progress has also been achieved in implementing a more effective strategy for *in vitro-in vivo* extrapolation and human risk assessment, particularly with the significant advances in tissue culture technology and the improvement in the level of biological complexity of the models. Many of the systems currently available, including 3D cultures, microchips, and microphysiological systems (MPS) describe the progress achieved with *in vitro* analysis of chemicals, as well as the need for more relevant, *in vitro* surrogate systems of human and animal organs. Other models have been incorporated into acute and chronic toxicity testing, particularly with the use of organotypic models, the ability to recreate the multicellular architecture, and strive to mimic hemodynamic properties of the intact organism using novel culture platforms. As these systems become more widely used for chemical and drug toxicity testing, there is a corresponding need to establish standardized testing conditions, endpoint analyses, and acceptance criteria. In the future, a balanced approach between sample throughput and biological relevance should provide better *in vitro* tools that are complementary with other testing models and assist in conducting more predictive human risk assessment.

As an example of the monumental progress made with dermal and ocular testing, *in vitro* screening tests for skin irritancy and sensitization have replaced *in vivo* rabbit and guinea pig studies. *In vitro* human or animal dermal cell cultures are examined for changes in membrane permeability, leakage, or morphology at doses that suggest sensitization or irritation, after which the chemical is not required to undergo further tests *in vivo*.

15.7 Summary and Learning Objectives

Toxicity testing of chemicals is a *regulatory* requirement for the protection of humans and animals. Toxicity from chemicals and drugs is determined from clinical trials, epidemiology studies, and *in vivo/in vitro* laboratory studies.

Epidemiology, cohort, case-control, cross-sectional or ecological studies, relate relative, or absolute risk. *In vivo* tests are performed with the appropriate questions posed throughout the investigation, namely dosage, frequency, physico-chemical properties, and biological considerations. The nature of the test depends on the type of chemical, its application, and its molecular characteristics. Frequency studies involve *acute, sub-chronic*, and *chronic* durations. More specific tests include those for *reproductive toxicity, teratogenicity, carcinogenicity*, and *ecotoxicity*. For industrial chemicals, only acute tests are warranted for classification. *Acute tests* help to define a dose-response relationship. *Sub-chronic* and *chronic studies* indicate target organ toxicity, blood levels, and no observed effect level. *In vitro* toxicity studies are performed as screening tools and simultaneously with *in vivo* experiments and are guided by consideration of the 3 Rs: *replacement, reduction*, and *refinement*. Replacement incorporates *in vitro test* systems as alternatives for animal experimentation, including bacteria for mutagenicity, mammalian cell cultures, high-throughput screening assays, genetic identification, DNA/RNA sequencing, and genetic/epigenetic biomarkers. Testing for cytotoxicity utilize mammalian-derived cells, mostly for screening chemicals prior to *in vivo* evaluation or for evaluation of skin toxicity, allergenicity, immunotoxicology, and for the replacement of the LD_{50} requirement. Reduction minimizes the number of animals, particularly when initiating experiments for the determination of dosage range, mechanism, or suspected pathological changes. Refinement refers to devising methods that produce the least amount of distress on the animal test subjects, such as relief of pain, length of study, amelioration of disease, housing, and handling.

Review Questions

1. Indicate which of the following are true and which are false: (a) acute toxicity studies are primarily for determination of mutagenicity; (b) sub-chronic toxicity tests measure dose-response; (c) ecotoxicity studies employ tests with *Daphnia*; (d) teratogenicity tests are part of reproductive toxicity studies.
2. Which of the following are NOT required in toxicity testing for EU new chemicals strategy?: (a) dose; (b) identity; (c) precautions; (d) application; (e) cost.

Short Answer Questions

3. List the seven questions that are asked before a toxicity study is executed.
4. List the four types of epidemiological studies.
5. Define the 3 Rs in relation to toxicity testing.

Notes

1. The terms *cell culture* and *tissue culture* are used interchangeably in this section.
2. Calculated as: A × (B/C) × D.
3. Relative risk calculated as: A/B where A = number of cases of disease in total exposed group per unit of population; B = number of cases of disease in total non-exposed control group per unit of population.

    Absolute excess risk refers to number of cases of disease per unit of exposed population minus number of cases of disease per unit of unexposed population.
4. OECD, Organization for Economic Cooperation and Development (EU).
5. ICCVAM, Interagency Coordinating Committee on the Validation of Alternative Methods (US).
6. International Conference on Harmonisation of Technical Requirements for Registration of Pharmaceuticals for Human Use.

Bibliography

Barile, F.A., Chapter 1. Cell Culture Methodology and Its Application to *In Vitro* Cytotoxicology, in: *Introduction to In Vitro Cytotoxicology: Mechanisms and Methods*, Barile, F.A. (Ed), CRC Press, Boca Raton, FL, 1994.

Barile, F.A., Chapter 14. Cell Culture Methods for Acute Toxicology Testing, in: *Principles of Toxicology Testing: Mechanisms and Methods*, Barile, F.A. (Ed), 2nd edition, CRC Press, Boca Raton, FL, 2013.

Bruce, R.D., An up-and-down procedure for acute toxicity testing, *Fundamentals Applied Toxicology*, 5, 151–157, 1985. Doi: 10.1016/0272-0590(85)90059-4.

Chan, P.K.(P.), Hayes A.W., Chapter 22. Acute Toxicity and Eye Irritancy, in: *Hayes' Principles and Methods of Toxicology*, Hayes, A.W., Kruger, C.L., (Eds.), 6th edition, CRC Press, Taylor & Francis, Boca Raton, FL., 2014.

Ecobichon, D.J., Chapter 3. Acute Toxicity Studies, in: *The Basis of Toxicity Testing*, Ecobichon, D.J. (Ed), 2nd edition, CRC Press, Boca Raton, FL, 1997.

Flynn, G.L., Chapter 4. Critique of Cell Culture Methods in Skin Permeability Assessment, in: *Advances in Animal Alternatives for Safety and Efficacy Testing*, Salem, H., Katz, S.A. (Eds.), 1st edition, CRC Press, Taylor & Francis, Boca Raton, FL, 1997.

Gad, S.C., Chapter 33, Alternatives to in vivo Studies in Toxicology, in: *General and Applied Toxicology*, Ballantyne, B., Marrs, T. and Turner, P. (Eds), 3rd edition, John Wiley & Sons, London, 2009.

Heuvel, M.J., Van Den, D.A.D. and Shillaker, R.O., Evaluation of the BTS approach to the testing of substances and preparations for their acute toxicity, *Human Toxicology*, 6, 279, 1987. DOI: 10.1177/096032718700600405.

OECD, *Test No. 420: Acute Oral Toxicity - Fixed Dose Procedure, OECD Guidelines for the Testing of Chemicals, Section 4*, OECD Publishing, Paris, 2002. Doi: 10.1787/9789264070943-en.

OECD, *Test No. 425: Acute Oral Toxicity: Up-and-Down Procedure, OECD Guidelines for the Testing of Chemicals, Section 4*, OECD Publishing, Paris, 2008. Doi: 10.1787/9789264071049-en.

OECD, *Test No. 436: Acute Inhalation Toxicity – Acute Toxic Class Method, OECD Guidelines for the Testing of Chemicals, Section 4*, OECD Publishing, Paris, 2009. Doi: 10.1787/9789264076037-en.

Salem. H and Katz, S. *Advances in Animal Alternatives for Safety and Efficacy Testing*, Salem, H. and Katz, S (Eds.), 1st edition, Taylor & Francis, 1997.

Stokes, W.S., Schechtman, L.M. and Hill, R.N., The interagency coordinating committee on the validation of alternative methods (ICCVAM): A review of the ICCVAM test method evaluation process and current international collaborations with the European Centre for the Validation of Alternative Methods (ECVAM), *Alternatives to Laboratory Animals (ATLA)*, 30, 23–32, 2002. Doi: 10.1177/026119290203002S04.

U.S. Department of Health and Human Services (DHHS), Food and Drug Administration (FDA), Guidance for industry: M3(R2) nonclinical safety studies for the conduct of human clinical trials and marketing authorization for pharmaceuticals, *Guidance for Industry* (fda.gov), January 2010. https://www.fda.gov/regulatory-information/search-fda-guidance-documents/m3r2-nonclinical-safety-studies-conduct-human-clinical-trials-and-marketing-authorization.

World Health Organization (WHO), *Hazardous Chemicals in Human and Environmental Health, IPCS,* WHO, IPCS, Geneva, 2000. https://apps.who.int/iris/handle/10665/66161.

Chapter 16

Risk Assessment

Chapter Outline

This chapter discusses the principles of assessment of risk from the use of chemicals to which humans and animals are exposed.

16.1 Introduction	229
16.2 Risk Assessment and Interpretation of Toxicological Data	230
16.2.1 Risk Assessment	230
16.2.1.1 Hazard Identification	231
16.2.1.2 Dose-Response Assessment	232
16.2.1.3 Exposure Assessment	235
16.2.1.4 Risk Characterization	236
16.3 Biomarkers in Risk Assessment	238
16.4 Summary and Learning Objectives	239
Review Questions	240
Short Answer Questions	240
Notes	240
Bibliography	240

16.1 Introduction

Regulations vary between countries for adequate and proper use of chemicals within societies. The purpose of understanding risk assessment (RA) and associated regulatory toxicology is to ensure that the benefits of chemical substances intended for use by humans outweigh the risks from that exposure.

DOI: 10.1201/9781003188575-16

16.2 Risk Assessment and Interpretation of Toxicological Data

At least 100,000 chemicals are currently produced and marketed in the US with 1,000–1,500 new chemicals added each year. The U.S. Food and Drug Administration (FDA) is responsible for the approval of therapeutic drugs only after they are determined to be safe for conditions for which they are tested. Other regulatory agencies, such as the U.S. Consumer Products Safety Commission (CPSC) and the U.S. Environmental Protection Agency (EPA) are responsible for safety, production, marketing, and overall exposure to non-therapeutic chemicals, consumer products, as well as monitoring of environmental and occupational standards associated with these commodities, respectively.

The EU divides feed and food risk analysis into RA, risk management, and risk communication, whereas the European Food Safety Authority (EFSA) and European Medicines Agency (EMA) are responsible for the processes of RA and risk evaluation, especially those surrounding genetically modified foods and pesticides, and how these characteristics affect the politicization of these processes. EFSA is responsible for RA; the Commission for Risk Management shares risk communication depending if it is an assessment or management issue (Chatzopoulou1 et al., 2020).

Consequently, modern concepts of risk management are based on the foundation that the pharmaceutical and chemical industries have a responsibility to minimize the risks associated with these products. This chapter concentrates on RA principally because this broad topic has applications to the safety and efficacy of most other consumer products, particularly those that are relevant to toxicological risk evaluation and interpretation of toxicological data. In addition, RA is involved with maintenance of environmental and occupational regulations.

16.2.1 Risk Assessment

Risk is a mathematical concept that refers to the likelihood of undesirable effects resulting from exposure to a chemical. **Risk** is the probability that a hazard will cause an adverse effect under specific exposure conditions. Risk is also calculated as follows:

$$\text{Risk} = \text{Hazard} \times \text{Exposure}$$

Hazard is the intrinsic capability of a substance to cause an adverse effect. Conversely, safety refers to 'the practical certainty that adverse effects will not occur when the substance is used in a manner and quantity proposed for its use'. As exposure to the population increases so does the probability of harm; conversely reduction in exposure reduces risk. *RA* is the process whereby hazard, exposure, and risk are calculated and estimated for human and animal populations. RA is performed on chemicals with the following objectives:

a. determine if the chemical has the potential to be a hazard to humans in the environment;
b. likelihood of persistence of the chemical in the environment and if bioaccumulation increases its hazard potential;

c. probability that sensitive human and ecological populations exposed to significant levels of the chemical are hazardous;

d. existence of an indication of hazard risk to human health; and,

e. if the likelihood of exposure via use or production poses an unhealthy situation.

An underlying concept in RA relies on determination of safe and effective doses or concentrations below which a chemical is NOT hazardous to the affected populations. Consequently, it is possible to determine a level of exposure that is without appreciable risk to human health or the ecosystem. RA is a scientific process; the next stages are risk-benefit analysis and risk management that require a different type of approach.

Risk management considers alternative policies for the most appropriate course of regulatory action based on the results of RA and social, economic, and political considerations.

Quantitative RA is an estimation of toxic exposure concentrations or doses that, within a defined probability level, lead to specific increases in lifetime incidence rates for an undesirable consequence associated with the toxic substance. The predicted models depend largely on accumulated retrospective and prospective data including applicability of scientific knowledge. RA is based on a *lack* of available data for a substance with potential for human or animal toxicity and calculation of an estimate of potential toxicity on data that are available. Consequently, gathering reliable and valid toxicity data for prediction of human and animal health risks relies on a systematic approach in the quantitative RA evaluation process. The analytical approach includes:

1. Hazard identification
2. Dose-response assessment
3. Exposure assessment
4. Risk characterization

16.2.1.1 Hazard Identification

The process of hazard identification uses qualitative methods to evaluate the potential for adverse health effects of chemicals or physical substances. The information incorporated into the database is obtained from relevant retrospective epidemiological studies and case studies. In addition, controlled animal and *in vitro* studies are also conducted.

The data gathered from these experimental studies contribute to understanding levels and routes of exposure, time of administration, multiple target organ toxicity, and combinations of chemicals. Organization of animal studies is particularly important to extrapolate data for human RA.

While chemicals constitute many threats of different severity, the *primary hazard* is set for subsequent stages of RA. For example, a chemical that is responsible for reversible liver toxicity at high doses may also produce tumors in skin at lower doses. Thus, its carcinogenicity potential is the hazard of concern.

Although human data is preferred, it is neither always reliable nor available, where the information must be supplemented with other data sources.

Epidemiological data often suggests causal relationships between exposure to the chemical and an effect in humans. Animal toxicity data generates histopathological, clinical chemistry, and biochemical information. More recently, *in vitro* data obtained using human and animal cells has been successfully incorporated into screening protocols in order to reduce and refine *in vivo* toxicity experimentation. Predictive use of structure-activity relationships is also possible and necessary to estimate toxicity based on molecular orientation of the chemical.

16.2.1.2 Dose-Response Assessment

This stage quantifies identifiable hazards and evaluates the relationship between dose and adverse effects in humans.

As relevant studies are examined for assessment of potential toxicity, the second objective of RA is the determination of the relationship between dose administered and the expected/observed response (dose-response assessment). Factors used to estimate the dose or exposure associated with the appearance of adverse effects are recognized according to the determination of the following statistical computations:

Quantal relationship: The number of test subjects or individuals in a population that demonstrates an effect. It varies with level of exposure;

Graded relationship: The severity of lesions exhibited by the test subjects or individuals; a graded relationship is proportional to dose;

Continuous relationship: Alteration of a physiological or biological indicator (e.g. body weight) with respect to dosage regimen.

Accordingly, definitive proof of a dose-response relationship is understood as a statistically positive correlation between the intensity and frequency of the effect with increasing dose. An important factor that influences interpretation of the relationship involves recognition of experimental thresholds for chemicals in animal studies and demonstration of similar thresholds in human populations. Thresholds define acceptable exposure levels within human populations.

The following criteria have historically been judged as invaluable for forecasting risks to human populations:

- selection of an appropriate animal species for testing;
- determination of a sufficient number of animals for an experimental setup;
- incorporation of a variety of chemical exposure levels;
- estimation of an adequate duration and frequency of administration of the agent that mimics human lifelike exposures; and
- use of suitable *in vitro* screening techniques[1] to calculate threshold estimates for subsequent application of the 3Rs to *in vivo* experimentation.

Although many model systems are currently available, relatively few contain adequate information to allow application of dose-response models. The EPA Gene-Tox Database, the EPA/IARC genetic activity profile (GAP) database, and the toxicological activity profile (TAP) database are examples of prototype profiles derived from a variety of test systems based on thousands of chemicals. They are used to support hazard classification of potential toxicants. The exposure-response database (ERDB) allows entry of detailed toxicologic results from experimental studies in support of dose-response assessment. These models permit a high level of automation in performance of various types of dose-response analyses.

The EPA/IARC (GAP) database applies to RA of carcinogens in a two-step process: (1) qualitative assessment of data from hazard identification, and (2) quantitation of risk for definitive or probable human carcinogens. Details of IARC classification of chemicals in relation to carcinogenicity are outlined as follows and according to Table 16.1:

Group 1: *Agent is carcinogenic to humans.* Chemical data provides sufficient evidence of carcinogenicity in humans (e.g. aflatoxin, benzene, arsenic, and tobacco smoke). Chemicals in this category generally show a causal relationship between exposure and cancer in humans.

Group 2A: *Agent is probably carcinogenic in humans.* Applied when evidence of carcinogenicity in humans is limited but convincing evidence appears from experimental animals (e.g. acrylonitrile, cadmium, and benzo[a]pyrene).

Table 16.1 IARC Carcinogenicity Classification of Chemicals[a]

Classification	Description and Examples
Group 1	Agent is carcinogenic to humans; aflatoxin, arsenic, benzene, tobacco smoke
Group 2A	Agent is probably carcinogenic in humans; acrylonitrile, cadmium, benzo[a]pyrene
Group 2B	Agent is possibly carcinogenic in humans; carbon tetrachloride, hexachlorobenzene, urethane
Group 3	Agent is not classifiable as to its carcinogenicity; aniline, dieldrin, maneb
Group 4	Agent is probably not carcinogenic in humans; caffeine

[a] See text for explanation. From: IARC (2006 and 2021).

Group 2B: *Agent is possibly carcinogenic in humans.* Only limited evidence of carcinogenicity in humans is available and less than convincing evidence is present from experimental animals (e.g. carbon tetrachloride, urethane, and hexachlorobenzene).

Group 3: *Agent is not classifiable as to its carcinogenicity.* Chemicals in this category do not demonstrate adequate evidence for carcinogenicity in humans or experimental animals (e.g. aniline, dieldrin, and maneb).

Group 4: *Agent is probably not carcinogenic in humans.* Chemical has not been found to induce cancer in experimental animals or in humans despite thorough *in vivo* and *in vitro* testing (e.g. caffeine).

Additional models used for assessing carcinogenicity include

a. **One-hit model** assumes that cancer involves only one stage and a single molecular event is sufficient to induce a cellular transformation.

b. **Linearized multistage model (EPA)** determines the cancer slope factor calculated to predict cancer risk at a specific dose; assumes a linear extrapolation to zero dose threshold, i.e. an estimate (mg/kg/day) of the probability that an individual will develop cancer if exposed to the chemical for 70 years.

c. **Multi-hit model** assumes several interactions are necessary for transformation of a normal to a tumorous cell.

d. **Probit model** assumes a log-normal distribution for tolerance in the exposed population.

In addition, physiologically based pharmacokinetic (PBPK) models utilize computerized data on absorption, distribution, metabolism, sequestration, kinetics, elimination, and mechanism to estimate the target dose for extrapolation.

The cancer risk values generated by these models vary according to the parameters inputted or incorporated. For example, the lifetime risk for chlordane for one cancer death in one million people ranges from 0.03 μg/L of drinking water for the one-hit model, 0.07 μg/L from the linearized multistage model to 50 μg/L for the probit model.

Information derived from animal carcinogenicity studies is difficult to assess since it is necessary to demonstrate an *increased frequency* of tumors in a small population such as those used in animal cancer studies, where a significant incidence of some tumors already exists. In addition, estimation of low-dose exposure levels and determining their effects in human populations are also laborious. Threshold values represent a range of the lowest possible exposures that are tolerated by humans in the environment or in an occupational setting without risk of adverse health effect. The dose-response relationship however does not always calculate with good correlations, particularly at lower concentrations. This is scientifically frustrating for the most part because experimental situations that attempt to mimic low-dose exposures, as those encountered in the environment, are not necessarily linear at low levels. Consequently, data obtained from chronic *in vivo* and valid *in vitro* studies must be carefully examined before the data is used to support the estimation of threshold values.

Consequently, doses close to the **maximum tolerated dose (MTD)** are used in carcinogenicity testing despite problems of dose-dependent metabolism, dose-dependent kinetics, and the possibility of other pathological effects influencing carcinogenicity. This approach is contentious, however, as carcinogens may show dose-dependent metabolism which is crucial to interpretation of carcinogenicity data. That is, large doses of a compound are metabolized in a quantitatively or qualitatively different manner to that of the expected dose or exposure level. Consequently, a compound is only carcinogenic under those extreme dosing conditions. For example, the industrial chemical hydrazine is a *weak* carcinogen after high exposure or dose levels. It also causes DNA methylation, a *possibly mutagenic* event which promotes cancerous changes but only occurs after *large*, hepatotoxic doses. The implications are that the acute toxic effect is involved in DNA methylation and that the acute effect is necessary for the development of cancer. For noncarcinogens where the dose response shows a threshold, a dose can be determined at which there is no adverse effect, the no adverse effect level (NOAEL) – an event which is likely to occur in humans and is the most sensitive toxic outcome observed. If a NOAEL cannot be determined, i.e. the data is insufficiently robust, then the lowest-adverse-effect level (LOAEL) is determined.

16.2.1.3 Exposure Assessment

Exposure assessment is an estimation of the intensity, frequency, and duration of human exposure or the potential of exposure to a toxic substance present in the environment. A variety of exposure possibilities that describe the magnitude, duration, schedule, and route of exposure to a substance are determined. Available toxicity data, current limits of environmental pollution, and estimations of current or projected intakes are included in the parameters.

Exposure converts a chemical from a hazard to a risk. Thus, determination of exposure is crucial to the process of RA, which involves evaluation of the source, routes, and levels of exposure.

Actual exposure levels are not always known thus requiring design of simulated models that incorporate knowledge of chemical environmental movements. Modeling scenarios track movement of contaminants through environmental paradigms. For instance, groundwater models quantify movement of subsurface water and provide inputs to subsurface contaminant transport. The simulation provides insight into groundwater and contaminant behavior and allows for quantitative assessments for environmental decision making. Surface water models simulate contaminant movement and concentration in lakes, streams, estuaries, and marine environments. Similarly, models that simulate possible contamination in the food chain help to trace contaminated aquatic and terrestrial environments that typically result in bioaccumulation of chemicals within all trophic levels of an ecosystem and for estimating chemical impacts on exposed plant, prokaryotic and eukaryotic kingdoms. Finally, multimedia models track contaminants that travel through the atmosphere, soil, surface water, and cohabitants. An advantage of the multimedia computer simulation is its ability to monitor and quantify the impacts of exposure as the contaminants navigate concurrently and sequentially throughout these environments.

Physico-chemical characteristics of a chemical (i.e. lipid solubility, water solubility, vapor pressure) also are important contributors to modeling information. However, RA is more reliable if experimental evidence for actual exposures exists for both experimental animals and humans.

16.2.1.4 Risk Characterization

Risk characterization involves accumulation of data for use in estimating the probable incidence of adverse health effects to human and animal populations under various conditions of exposure. The U.S. EPA describes risk characterization as the risk associated with exposures in situations considered for regulation. Risk characterization has since evolved from initial descriptions of management of RA through to the decision-making process. Presentation and display of information, exposure times, potency (unit risk), nature and weight of evidence, uncertainty of the component parts, and distribution of population risk, calculate in the final decision-making process. Together with hazard identification, dose-response relationship, and exposure assessment, risk characterization enables formation of model systems and their integration into RA prediction.

As the final stage, RA involves integration of the results of preceding stages to get a probability of the occurrence of the adverse effect in humans exposed to the chemical. Biological, statistical, and public health uncertainties are accounted for in the analysis. For example, NOAEL or LOAEL is relied upon to determine various parameters in the assessment. For carcinogens, the risk is expressed in terms of increased jeopardy of developing cancer (e.g. 1 in 10^6), calculated from the cancer slope factor and 70-year average daily intake (mg/kg/day).

Food additives rely on the acceptable daily intake (ADI) or Reference Dose (RfD, U.S. EPA). ADI is the amount of chemicals to which a person is exposed for a lifetime without suffering harmful effects. Determination of intake values requires calculation of a safety or uncertainty factor, while RfD includes an additional safety factor (modifying factor). For food contaminants, the parameter is the tolerable daily intake (TDI) – an estimate of the daily intake of chemical that occurs over a lifetime without appreciable health risk. Daily food consumption for types of food is incorporated into this calculation.

Chemicals in water and air also must be assessed for risk and guidelines where appropriate. Thus there are air quality/pollution guidelines set by the World Health Organization (WHO). Guidance values are established for air pollutants that have acute irritant or chronic effects and are combined with exposure times at which no adverse effects are expected. The guidance values are determined from the NOAEL (or LOAEL).

Similarly, drinking water guidance values exist for many chemicals. TDI values are calculated for drinking water contaminants. Guidance values are determined from the TDI and known daily intake of water calculated using 60 kg standard adult body weight for 70 years. As with air pollutants, carcinogenic, non-threshold chemicals are computed separately from non-carcinogenic non-threshold chemicals.

In the case of carcinogens, a virtually safe dose (VSD) is determined. Modifying or safety factors are designed as follows:

10 × for human variability (intra species);
10 × for extrapolation from animals to humans (interspecies variability);
10 × if less than chronic doses are established;
10 × if LOAEL rather than NOAEL is referenced;
0.1–10 × modifying factor – determined only for the RfD (EPA).

These uncertainty factors are combined and divided into the NOAEL to yield the ADI (or RfD) or TDI. Modifying factors contribute to estimation of judgment decisions on the quality of the scientific data.

Thus:

TDI=NOAEL/Uncertainty factor(s)
ADI=NOAEL/Uncertainty factor(s)

Often an uncertainty factor of 100 is applied to account for human variability and differences between humans and the animals tested in the toxicity studies.

This approach is applied to both chronic and short-term (e.g. developmental) toxicity studies of appropriate duration to derive permissible exposure levels. For occupational exposure to chemicals threshold limit values (TLVs) (or maximum exposure limits) are similarly determined and are based on exposure for an 8-hour working day.

Doses are normally expressed on body weight or body surface area and are extrapolated to different species, assuming similar sensitivity per unit body weight or surface area. Thus in the RA process for noncarcinogens actual exposure level is compared with ADI or another equivalent parameter. Exposure to multiple chemicals is assumed to be additive.

Extrapolation between species is also a problem in RA for interpretation of toxicological data. For example, extrapolation to humans requires identifying the species which is either more sensitive, or whose response is more appropriate, when similarities are compared. The species or strain used in a particular carcinogenicity study have a high natural incidence of a specific type of tumor. Assessment of the significance of an increase in the incidence of this tumor and its relevance to human populations can pose problems of interpretation.

For acute toxic effects dose response is more robust and allows a NOAEL to be estimated. Because of the problems of interspecies extrapolation and interpretation of apparent low incidences of tumors, calculation of disparate quantitative values confounds RA decisions. For example, the expected number of bladder cancer cases in the US for a 70-year period with daily exposure to 120mg saccharin was *estimated* between 0.22 and 1.144×10^6. However, according to the restrictions imposed by the Delaney Clause, the calculation did not consider the less *likely* and *reasonable* risk to human populations.[2]

16.3 Biomarkers in Risk Assessment

A biomarker is a measurable biochemical, molecular, histologic, physiologic, pathologic, or toxicologic indicator in an organism whose presence is indicative of some activity such as disease, infection, or environmental exposure. Although novel biomarkers for complex diseases are relatively new, they have been incorporated into the biomedical realm for interpretation of a variety of syndromes including measurement of blood pressure, heart rate, clinical chemistry, X-rays, and most recently for genetic tests. Biomarkers are measurable and do not reflect subjective symptoms.

Since toxicology is associated with an abundance of indicators for pathology and the mechanisms of many diseases have been correlated with the markers, then it is noteworthy that biomarkers offer a significant contribution to understanding the progression of toxicity and corresponding disease states. Their role assists in appreciating the mechanism of toxicological events, or the marker is involved in identifying the interaction of chemicals with physiology. In any case, biomarkers are involved in the aberrations associated with the biochemical, physiological disruption of cellular activity, modification of enzymes, or adverse effect on gene expression. More recently, genetic and epigenetic dysregulation has been implicated in a variety of diseases, most commonly cancer, and is becoming increasingly viewed as an important factor of chemically-induced development.

Biomarkers are used at several stages in the RA process and are an important indicator of the internal dose of a chemical necessary for adequately describing the dose-response relationship. Similarly, toxicologic biomarkers of response are necessary for determination of the NOAEL. Biomarkers of susceptibility are important for identifying sensitive groups among human populations in estimating uncertainty factors. Biomarkers lend information for establishment of a crucial link between response and exposure.

Incidence of a toxic effect may be measured under precise laboratory conditions but extrapolation to the clinical or epidemiologic situation for estimation of risk involves *assumptions* and *uncertainties*.

When human data is not available for a new chemical substance and toxic effects in humans cannot be verified by direct experiment or extrapolation from in vivo or *in vitro* studies is inconclusive, then the assessment presents more questions than answers. Since the objective is to maintain a significant margin of safety, then 'weight of evidence' and reliance on epidemiological information are required to make valid assumptions. In light of increasing and widespread exposure of humans to chemicals, risk versus benefit is an important consideration when translating information to the consuming public. As with the current controversies with vaccines, and where absolute safety is unrealistic, the practice of risk/benefit balance for chemical (and therapeutic) utilization is weighed to favor acceptable public health outcomes.

16.4 Summary and Learning Objectives

Toxicity testing of chemicals is a legal requirement if humans or animals in the environment are likely to be exposed. This toxicity is determined from epidemiology studies and clinical trials, *in vivo* studies in animals, and studies *in vitro*.

Epidemiology (cohort, case control, cross sectional or ecological studies) indicates relative or absolute risk. *In vivo* tests are performed but questions must be asked (e.g. dosage, frequency and physico-chemical properties, novelty) and biological considerations (e.g. species and sex of animal) and addressed beforehand. The nature of the test depends on the type of chemical, its use, and the chemical classification. General tests used are acute (1 dose), sub-chronic (repeated, 28 or 90 days), and chronic (at least 12 months in rodents). More specific tests include those for reproductive toxicity (effects on male or female reproductive systems), teratogenicity (effects on the embryo *in utero*), carcinogenicity (ability to cause tumors), and ecotoxicity (e.g. effects on *Daphnia* and earthworms). For some chemicals (e.g. industrial chemicals) only acute tests are needed for classification (e.g. non-toxic/very toxic). Acute tests help to define a dose-response relationship. Sub-chronic and chronic studies indicate target organ(s) toxicity, other pathological effects, blood levels, and no observed effect level (NOEL). Other specific *in vivo* studies are performed if necessary. Toxicity testing *in vivo* should consider the 3 Rs: replacement, reduction, and refinement. *Replacement* refers to the use of *in vitro* test systems including those for mutagenicity involving bacteria (e.g. *Salmonella* in the Ames test), mammalian cells (mouse lymphoma, human lymphocytes), or insects (fruit flies). Testing for cytotoxicity utilizes mammalian-derived cells, mostly for screening out chemicals prior to *in vivo* evaluation or for evaluation of skin toxicity or allergenicity. Currently, some limitations to *in vitro* tests (e.g. loss of enzyme activity) are of note. *Reduction* means using the minimum animals necessary; *refinement* refers to devising methods to gain the most information while causing the least distress.

Risk is the probability that an adverse effect will occur under specific exposure conditions.

Hazard is the capability of a substance to cause an adverse effect. RA is the process whereby exposure, hazard, and risk are determined. The hazard needs to be identified from human epidemiology, animal toxicity studies or *in vitro* studies. Dose-response relationships are also determined from this information. For most chemicals, a NOAEL or LOAEL can be determined. Exposure assessment and other aspects of RA include use of biomarkers of exposure, response and susceptibility, and physico-chemical characteristics as important pieces of information.

Risk characterization involves integrating all the information and calculating parameters such as ADI, TDI, or TLV using the NOAEL and a safety or uncertainty factor. This is typically 100 (10 for species extrapolation, 10 for human variability). For carcinogens, different models will be used to those exhibiting a threshold for effect (e.g. one-hit and multi-hit). Carcinogenicity testing requires lifetime studies in vivo in large numbers of animals often including the MTD.

Review Questions

1. Indicate which of the following are true or and which are false:
   (a) acute toxicity studies are primarily for the determination of mutagenicity; (b) sub-chronic toxicity tests are used for the measurement of dose esponses; (c) ecotoxicity studies utilize tests in *Daphnia*; (d) teratogenicity tests are part of reproductive toxicity studies.
2. Which of the following are important in risk assessment?
   (a) exposure level or dose; (b) hazard; (c) NOEL; (d) benefit; (e) ADI; (f) cost; (g) TLV.

Short Answer Questions

1. Define and describe the following acronyms: NOAEL, ADI, and TLV.
2. Define and describe RA. Give examples to support the answer.
3. Define *risk* and *hazard* in relation to risk assessment.

Notes

1. *In vitro* methods, using cell cultures or test tubes, involve alternative methods to animal experimentation. These systems are used as preliminary screening tests for estimating toxic exposures, without the need to sacrifice large numbers of animals from the start of the protocol.
2. The Food Additives Amendment and the Color Additives Amendments to the U.S. Federal Food, Drug, and Cosmetic Act (1958) include the Delaney Clause, which prohibits the approval of an additive if it is found to induce cancer when ingested by people or tested in animals.

Bibliography

Barile, F.A., Chapter 2. Risk assessment and regulatory toxicology, in: *Barile's Clinical Toxicology: Principles and Mechanisms*, CRC Press, Taylor & Francis, Boca Raton, FL, 2019.

Chatzopoulou, S., Eriksson, N.L. and Eriksson, D., Improving risk assessment in the european food safety authority: Lessons from the European medicines agency, *Frontiers in Plant Science*, 11, 1–11, 2020. Doi: 10.3389/fpls.2020.00349.

Cote, I., Andersen, M.E., Ankley, G.T., Barone, S., Birnbaum, L.S., Boekelheide, K., Bois, F.Y., Burgoon, L.D., Chiu, W.A., Crawford-Brown, D., Crofton, K.M., DeVito, M., Devlin, R.B., Edwards, S.W., Guyton, K.Z., Hattis, D., Judson, R.S., Knight, D., Krewski, D., Lambert, J., Maull, E.A., Mendrick, D., Paoli, G.M., Patel, C.J., Perkins, E.J., Poje, G., Portier, C.J., Rusyn, I., Schulte, P.A., Simeonov, A., Smith, M.T., Thayer, K.A., Thomas, R.S., Thomas, R., Tice, R.R., Vandenberg, J.J., Villeneuve, D.L., Wesselkamper, S., Whelan, M., Whittaker, C., White, R., Xia, M., Yauk, C., Zeise, L., Zhao, J. and DeWoskin, R.S. The next generation of risk assessment multiyear study—highlights of findings, applications to risk assessment, and future directions. *Environmental Health Perspectives*, 124, 1671–1682, 2016. Doi: 10.1289/EHP233.

DeCaprio, A.P. (Ed.), Toxicologic Biomarkers, Taylor and Francis, New York, 2006.

Faustman, E.M., Chapter 4. Risk assessment, in: *Cassarett and Doull's Toxicology*, Klaassen, C. (Ed.), 9th edition, McGraw-Hill, New York, 2019.

International Agency for Research on Cancer (IARC). *Preamble to the IARC Monographs - Scientific Review and Evaluation*, IARC, Lyon, 2006. http://monographs.iarc.fr/ENG/Preamble/currentb6evalrationale0706.php.

International Agency for Research on Cancer (IARC). *Agents Classified by the IARC Monographs*, volumes 1–129. IARC, Lyon, 2021. http://monographs.iarc.fr/ENG/Classification/index.php.

United Nations Environment Programme, *Biomarkers in Risk Assessment: Validity and Validation - Environmental Health Criteria*, 222, 2001. http://hdl.handle.net/20.500.11822/29529.

Waterfield C.J. and Timbrell, J.A. Biomarkers-An overview. in: *General and Applied Toxicology*, Ballantyne, B., Marrs, T., Syversen, T. (Eds.), Vol. 3, Macmillan, New York, 1841–1854, 2000.

World Health Organization (WHO), Chemical Risk Assessment: Human risk assessment, environmental risk assessment and ecological risk assessment *Training Module No. 3 UNEP/IPCS 1999*, WHO, IPCS, Geneva, 1999. https://apps.who.int/iris/handle/10665/66398?locale-attribute=fr&.

Chapter 17

Antidotes and Treatment of Poisoning

Chapter Outline

This chapter highlights treatment modalities associated with poisonings, particularly general supportive measures and antidotes of toxins presented in previous chapters.

17.1 Introduction	243
17.2 Poison Control Centers	244
17.3 General Supportive Measures	244
17.4 Specific Antidotes	246
17.5 Toxicology Laboratories	247
17.6 Summary and Learning Objectives	247
Review Questions	248
Short Answer Question	248
Bibliography	248

17.1 Introduction

Poisoning of humans and animals results from accidental or intentional exposure to drugs or non-therapeutic chemicals. The route of intake is as common as the possible routes of therapeutic administration including oral or parenteral. Acute poisoning episodes are the most common events, followed by chronic consumption. Life-threatening events require professional treatment and fall within the realm of clinical toxicology. Exposure via inhalation or skin absorption is also critical in acute poisoning cases.

DOI: 10.1201/9781003188575-17

A limited number of specific antidotes are available for some drugs and chemicals. Other treatment modalities involve supportive measures; i.e., treating objective signs and subjective symptoms of suspected substances (signs and symptoms, S and S). This generally refers to maintaining stability of vital organs, including maintenance of a patent airway, support breathing, and monitor cardiac function (ABCs).

Besides the instrumental function of first aid maneuvers and essential roles of emergency departments, poison control centers (PCCs) also have a critical contribution in poisoning intervention.

17.2 Poison Control Centers

The first specialized medical units devoted to treating poisoned patients were started in Denmark, Hungary, and the Netherlands in the 1940s. In the US, PCCs started in the 1950s and were well established by the 1970s. The role of the PCC has evolved significantly since to provide public and professional toxicological services associated with emergency management and prevention. The PCC provides the following roles and services for the therapeutic advancements for the treatments involved in toxicological poisoning:

- provide product ingredient information;
- afford information on treatment of poisoned patients;
- supply direct information to patients;
- suggest diagnostic and treatment information to health care professionals;
- institute education programs for health care professionals; and
- sponsor poison prevention activities.

Poison control centers are staffed by board-certified medical toxicologists and supportive personnel. In the US, the American Board of Applied Toxicology (ABAT), American Association of Poison Control Centers (AAPCC), American Academy of Clinical Toxicology (AACT), and American Board of Medical Subspecialties (for physicians) administer and maintain standards and board certification in medical toxicology.

17.3 General Supportive Measures

Among the first historical treatment modalities used in the presence of unknown, unsuspected toxicity was the induction of emesis and the use of activated charcoal. Early Greek and Roman civilizations recognized the importance of administering charcoal to victims of poisoning, as well as treating anthrax and epilepsy. Early American folk medicine relied on the use of common refined chalk, obtained from the bark of black cherry trees or peach stones and ground to a powder, mixed with common chalk, and administered for the treatment of stomach distress due to unknown ingestion. Bread burned to charcoal, dissolved in cold water, was used as a remedy for dysentery. Induction of emesis was also suggested in early civilizations for reversing the effects of ingested poisons. The use of ipecac was described by South American Indians and first mentioned by Jesuit Friars in 1601. Brazilian, Colombian, and Panamanian ipecac were introduced into Europe in 1672 and established in medicine by the turn of the century. Today, syrup of ipecac is readily available but caution is recommended in its unsupervised use.

Historically, the use of ipecac syrup was recommended prior to emergency referrals to start the gastric emptying process as early as possible. The use of ipecac-induced emesis in the management of poisoned patients, however, as a gastric emptying technique, has declined significantly. Despite its reliable ability to induce vomiting, the treatment modality has shown limited effectiveness in preventing drug absorption, particularly when given more than 30–90 minutes following ingestion of a toxic substance. In addition, there are potentially significant disadvantages associated with the use of the emetic, particularly when a potentially caustic agent is ingested or in a patient with decreased level of consciousness. Only when the benefit outweighs the risk, and under qualified medical supervision, is the administration of ipecac syrup advisable in response to a specific toxic event. In addition, the routine stocking of ipecac in all households with young children is not recommended.

The *use of absorbants* such as activated charcoal to neutralize and diminish intestinal absorption of exogenous substances from the GI tract is another effective method for treatment of the poisoned victim. Given orally, activated charcoal effectively absorbs 50% of an orally ingested chemical 1 hour later. The material binds high molecular weight organics, by non-covalent forces, more effectively than low molecular weight inorganic molecules. Activated charcoal however is not effective for metals, such as lead or iron, hydrocarbons, acids, and alkalis.

Enhancement of elimination of suspected chemical agents or drugs is accomplished using whole bowel irrigation. In adults, oral administration of polyethylene glycol flushes ingested toxic agents through the bowel. Administration of the preparation is continued for 4–5 hours or until the bowel effluents are clear. The method is useful for enhanced elimination of sustained-released preparation of capsules or tablets, cellophane packets of street heroin or cocaine, and agents not effectively absorbed with charcoal.

Enhanced elimination of drugs from the body has been traditionally used as a general method of treatment. This method is based on the chemical nature of the ingested poison and was performed by changing the acidity or alkalinity of the urine. For instance, administration of a basic drug (sodium bicarbonate) induces alkaline urine and ionizes ingested acidic substances, such as aspirin. The ionization process more readily increases urinary elimination of the latter. Similarly, the overdose with the basic drug methamphetamine can theoretically be ionized and eliminated by treatment with mild acid, ammonium chloride. However, it is now well understood that alkalinization or acidification of urine, although based on valid chemical pharmacokinetic principles of ion trapping and acid-base reactions, are not clinically recommended. Practically, the concept is not effective and aggravates or complicates removal of agents that interfere with systemic acid-base balance.

Drugs and toxicants are removed from the blood by the techniques of hemodialysis and hemoperfusion. Both involve the passage of blood of the poisoned patient through hemodialysis equipment which either allows diffusion of the toxicant through a semi-permeable membrane into the exchange fluid (hemodialysis) or removes the toxicant from the systemic circulation by adsorption onto charcoal or a resin (hemoperfusion). The procedure is allowed when other measures have failed, especially in the treatment of amphetamine, antibiotics, boric acid, lead, potassium, salicylate, and strychnine poisoning.

17.4 Specific Antidotes

Once the toxic agent is suspected or identified, administration of an antidote is necessary. Although a small number of specific antidotes, and some indirect-acting drugs, are available, many of these agents are capable of completely reversing the toxicologic consequences of poisoning. However, it should be noted that, just as with therapeutic drugs, antidotes are associated with their own adverse reactions and toxicity. In addition, effectiveness of antidotes is compromised in the presence of exposure from multiple agents. The following categories represent the mechanisms or objectives for treatment with specific antidotes:

1. **Chelating agents** react with the compound to form a water-soluble complex with enhanced elimination potential from the body. Examples of chelating agents used for the treatment of poisoning include: calcium-disodium-edetate (CaNa2EDTA) for the treatment of lead poisoning; penicillamine for treating copper and lead intoxication; and, British anti-Lewisite (BAL) for arsenic and mercury exposure.

2. **N-acetylcysteine (NAC)** is an example of a specific antidote that increases detoxification of reactive metabolites, increases production of glutathione which enhances deactivation of the reactive metabolite, ρ-benzoquinoneimine, generated from acetaminophen (paracetamol, E.U.) overdose. The reactive metabolite is diverted from interaction with liver proteins thus reducing toxicity. Similarly, amyl nitrite, sodium nitrite, and sodium thiosulfate stimulate detoxification of cyanide by increasing its metabolic conversion to thiocyanate, rendering it more soluble and ready for urinary excretion.

3. **Inhibition of metabolism** is an alternative strategy using antidotes that block metabolic transformation of active poisons. For example, the antifreeze ethylene glycol is metabolized by alcohol dehydrogenase and acetaldehyde dehydrogenase producing oxalic acid as the final toxic product. Competitive inhibition of alcohol dehydrogenase with therapeutic administration of fomepizole or ethanol as antidotes blocks the metabolic activity of the enzyme and forces unchanged ethylene glycol to elimination. Poisoning with methanol, which also involves metabolism with alcohol dehydrogenase, is similarly treated.

4. **Antidotes acting via receptors.** Opioid overdose such as with morphine and fentanyl causes life-threatening respiratory depression. The action of the opioids is competitively inhibited through the administration of the narcotic receptor antagonist, naloxone. With timely administration,

the antidote reverses the depressant actions of the narcotics. Similarly, a cholinergic crisis, precipitated by toxic exposure to organophosphate insecticides, is reversed by the competitive inhibitor atropine plus pralidoxime (2-PAM). The antidote antagonizes the effect of excess acetylcholine at cholinergic receptors. Lastly, flumazenil is a benzodiazepine receptor blocker that antagonizes the effects of sedatives/hypnotics such as diazepam.

5. **Reversal of receptor blockade** represents a metabolic target with parathion, also an organophosphate insecticide. Pralidoxime (2-PAM) is an antidote that inhibits the metabolic site of acetylcholinesterase, thereby releasing the organophosphate from the active site of the enzyme. The insecticide is not metabolized and the enzyme is regenerated. Oxygen is recommended as an antidote for carbon monoxide poisoning. Oxygen (100%) displaces reversible carbon monoxide binding to hemoglobin.

6. **Antibodies** and **antibody fragments** are frequently used for poisoning from rattlesnake bites, scorpion stings, and spider bites (brown recluse, black widow spiders). Antivenoms are available which specifically bind the proteins in the venom. Anti-digoxin antibody (Digibind®) is indicated for the treatment of overdose with digoxin, a popular cardiac drug.

17.5 Toxicology Laboratories

Toxicology laboratories rely on analysis of biological fluids or tissues for identification of drugs and chemicals in order to monitor toxic effects.

Forensic toxicology laboratories have the responsibility of identifying drug ingredients predominantly of unknown origin. The criminalist applies screening tests for several known classifications of compounds, the results of which determine the next series of tests to confirm the specific compound. Initial analytical methods range from simple color tests and chromatography screens to more sophisticated gas chromatographic-mass spectrometry detection.

Clinical toxicology laboratories are responsible for detection of drugs in suspected cases of drug abuse, overdose, or for monitoring of drugs in occupational settings. Drug abuse tests are generally noninvasive, such as with urine samples, and employ mostly screening tests for common illicit compounds. Testing occurs in drug rehabilitation clinics and hospitals, as well as for monitoring drug use in the workplace, schools, and individuals involved in critical jobs (police and pilots).

17.6 Summary and Learning Objectives

Treatment of poisoning involves use of emetics, absorbents, diuresis, limited blood and urine pH manipulation, hemodialysis, or hemoperfusion. Today more antidotes are researched, discovered and available for treatment of toxic exposures, including chelating agents, enzyme inhibitors, receptor blockers, antibodies, and drugs that stimulate detoxification or facilitate displacement of compounds from binding sites.

Review Questions

1. Indicate which of the following are true and which are false. Fomepizole is an antidote for treatment of ethylene glycol poisoning because it: (a) facilitates excretion of ethylene glycol; (b) blocks metabolism of ethylene glycol; (c) increases detoxification of ethylene glycol; (d) chelates ethylene glycol; (e) none of the above.
2. Carbon monoxide is a toxic gas because it: (a) binds to cytochrome aa_3 in mitochondria; (b) binds to hemoglobin; (c) causes respiratory alkalosis; (d) causes respiratory failure; (e) forms methemoglobin.
3. Indicate which of the following are true and which are false with reference to ethylene glycol: (a) is an alcohol; (b) causes metabolic acidosis; (c) metabolized to lactic acid; (d) crystallizes in the brain; (e) metabolized by aldehyde dehydrogenase.
4. Indicate which of the following are true and which are false: (a) solvents cause death by sensitization of the myocardium; (b) ethanol is toxic because it stimulates the central nervous system; (c) ethanol is metabolized to formic acid; (d) the major target organ for methanol toxicity is the liver; (e) large doses of ethanol result in blindness; (f) high doses of ethanol lower blood sugar levels.
5. Match the antidote (A-E) with its specific toxic agent (1–5): (a) BAL; (b) penicillamine; (c) sodium thiosulfate; (d) NAC; (e) pralidoxime. (1) organophosphate insecticides; (2) arsenic; (3) copper; (4) acetaminophen; (5) cyanide.

Short Answer Questions

6. Discuss various types of general treatment for poisoning. In your answer explain the mechanism for the treatment approach.
7. What is the role of the poison control center (PCC)?

Bibliography

Barile, F.A., Chapter 3, Therapeutic monitoring of adverse drug reactions, in: *Barile's Clinical Toxicology: Principles and Mechanisms*, Barile, F.A., (Ed.), CRC Press, Taylor & Francis, Boca Raton, FL, 2019.

Flanagan, R.J., Widdop, B., Ramsey, J.D., Loveland, M., Analytical toxicology, *Human Toxicology*, 7, 489–502, 1988. doi: 10.1177/096032718800700517.

Hall, A.H., Bismuth, C., The Role of Poison Centers in Basic and Clinical Toxicology, in: *General and Applied Toxicology*, Ballantyne, B., Marrs, T. and Syversen, T., P. (Eds), 3rd edition, John Wiley & Sons, London, 2009.

Poison Control Centers of America, National Capital Poison Center; https://www.poison.org; last accessed November, 2022.

Rosling, H., *Cassava Toxicity and Food Security. A Review of Health Effects of Cyanide Exposure from Cassava and of Ways to Prevent These Effects*, Food and Agriculture Organization of the United Nations, AGRIS, 1988. https://agris.fao.org/agris-search/search.do?recordID=SE881037988.

True, B-L. and Dreisbach, R.H., *Driesbach Handbook of Poisoning: Diagnosis and Treatment*, 13th edition, Informa Pub., New York, 2010.

Vale, A., Bradbury, S. Clinical toxicology in General and Applied Toxicology, Ballantyne, B., Marrs, T. and Syversen, T.L.M. (Eds.), 3rd edition, 2355–74, John Wiley & Sons, Ltd, Hoboken, NJ, 2009.

Vuori, E., Ojanpera, I. *Forensic toxicology*. in General and Applied Toxicology, in Ballantyne, B., Marrs, T. and Syversen, T. L. M. (Eds.), 3rd edition, 2421–36 John Wiley & Sons, Ltd, Hoboken, NJ, 2009.

Answers to Chapter Questions

Chapter 1. Introduction

1. (d) Potentiation.

    Compound B is not toxic, yet when combined with A, the toxicity is increased. Thus, compound B potentiates the toxicity of A. This is distinct from synergism where both compounds are toxic, but the toxicity of the combination is greater than the sum of the individual toxicities.

2. (e) All of the above.

    A properly designed and carefully executed acute toxicity study yields information on all of these parameters (the therapeutic index is determined based on the known ED_{50}). Because of the changes within the toxicological regulatory agencies, determination of the LD_{50} is no longer a mandatory requirement for toxicity of an unknown compound except for specific situations.

3. (c) LD_{50}/ED_{50}.

    Therefore, the greater the therapeutic index, the larger the safety margin of the drug. A better and more discriminating definition would be TD_{50}/ED_{50} in which the toxicity rather than the lethality is used for the numerator.

Short Answer Questions

4. a. TD_{50} is the dose of a compound that is toxic to 50% of the subjects exposed to the compound. The value is determined from the dose-response relationship by extrapolation.

    b. Dose-response relationship is the mathematical relationship between the dosage (dose) of a compound and the particular response measured. The response may be quantal (e.g. 'all-or-none' such as lethality) or graded (e.g. inhibition of an enzyme). The relationship is typically a sigmoid curve, which reflects the doses that have no effect and those that have a maximal effect.

c. Therapeutic index is an index of relative toxicity for a drug. Calculated as the LD_{50} or TD_{50} divided by the ED_{50}. The greater the value of the therapeutic index, the less toxic the drug, relative to the pharmacologically effective dose.

d. NOEL (No Observed Effect Level) is the dose or exposure level of a chemical that has no demonstrable effect on a biological system. The measurement is also expressed as NOAEL, No Observed Adverse Effect Level. The value is derived from the dose-response relationship.

5. Selective toxicity refers to targets that are susceptible to a toxicant. For example, insects are susceptible to the toxicity of DDT and malathion whereas mammals are generally not affected. Bacteria are susceptible to drugs such as penicillin while sparing humans. This selectivity to toxic effects is exploited in drugs used to fight infections, cancer and as pesticides. The basis of the selectivity is metabolic or structural. For example, malathion is metabolized differently in insects as opposed to mammals while the bacterial cell wall is structurally different from the mammalian cell membrane which renders it a target for penicillin.

6. a. ED_{50} is the dose of a compound that causes an effect in 50% of the organisms; i.e. a 50% response. This is usually a pharmacological rather than a toxicological effect. The ED_{50} is calculated from a population of organisms or in an *in vitro* system. It is represented as a quantal ('all-or-none') response, such as the presence or absence of a pharmacological change, or an observed graded response in the effect.

b. ADI is defined as the 'acceptable daily intake', applied to food additives or contaminants (such as pesticides). It represents a calculated quantity of a substance which is safe toward human exposure. It is derived from the No Observed Adverse Effect Level (NOAEL) according to the following:

$$ADI = \frac{NOAEL \text{ mg}/\text{kg}/\text{day}}{100}$$

The value of 100 is the safety factor that is applied. This considers the possible differences in susceptibility between the species used to determine the NOAEL.

c. The margin of safety is similar to the therapeutic index. However, it considers the difference between the dose or concentration of a drug required for a desired pharmacological effect and the dose associated with a toxic effect, and calculated as follows:

$$\text{margin of safety} = \frac{TD_1}{ED_{99}} \text{ or } \frac{LD_1}{ED_{99}}$$

where TD_1 and LD_1 are the doses that are toxic or lethal for 1% of the population exposed and the ED_{99} is the dose that is effective in 99% of the population.

The margin of safety is more specific than the therapeutic index because it considers possible overlap in the dose-response curves for pharmacological and toxicological effects.

Chapter 2. Dose-Response

1. (c) Potential for bioaccumulation.

   The larger the partition coefficient, the greater the lipophilicity, and this correlates with the bioaccumulation of the compound in fat tissue.
2. (c) Weak organic acids.

   In the stomach, the pH is around 2 and at this pH weak acids will be non-ionized. Therefore passive absorption of the non-ionized acid will occur in the stomach.
3. (b) Sometimes larger than the total body volume.

   When a drug is bound to tissue components or sequestered in a tissue such as adipose tissue, the plasma level may be very low. Therefore the calculation of volume of distribution (V_D = dose/plasma level) yields a value which may be higher than the total body water. Volume of distribution may be equal to the total body water, but this is not always the case.
4. (e) Total body clearance. Although some of the other factors may have an effect on half-life, by definition the total body clearance is the major determining factor as this includes metabolism and excretion.
5. (b) The drug is mostly metabolized by the liver before reaching systemic circulation.

   The 'first-pass effect' is where a drug is removed by metabolism in the organ(s)/tissues through which it passes during absorption before reaching systemic circulation. This is commonly the gastrointestinal tract and liver but could also be the lungs or skin.
6. (c) Both lipophilicity and resistance to metabolism will favor the accumulation of chemicals in biological systems. The former will result in sequestration in adipose tissue, the latter will decrease removal of the chemical by metabolism to polar, hydrophilic metabolites and loss by excretion.
7. (b) False.

   Binding of drugs to plasma proteins only rarely involves covalent binding. Usually ionic, hydrogen, hydrophobic or van der Waals' forces are involved.

Short Answer Questions
8. a. The volume of distribution (VD) is the volume of body fluid in which a chemical is apparently distributed after administration. It is calculated from either the dose and plasma (blood) concentration at a single time point or from the dose, area under the curve (AUC) and elimination rate constant (k_{el}):

$$V_D = \frac{\text{dose (mg)}}{\text{plasma concentration (mg/L)}}$$

The units are in liters.

The volume of distribution does not necessarily equal a compartment and so may have a value higher than the total body water (40 liters for a human). This occurs if the plasma level is low, as when a drug is sequestered in tissue. V_D is therefore known as the apparent volume of distribution. It is not accurately calculated after oral administration since incomplete absorption or first-pass metabolism are dominant features.

b. Drugs bind to plasma proteins non-covalently in four distinct ways:

   i. by ionic bonds in which there is bonding between charged groups or atoms and opposite charges on the protein.

   ii. with hydrogen bonds where a hydrogen atom attached to an electronegative atom (e.g. oxygen) is shared with another electronegative atom.

   iii. by hydrophobic interactions in which two non-polar, hydrophilic groups associate and mutually repel water.

   iv. by van der Waals' forces; these are weak attractions acting between the nucleus of one atom and the electrons of another.

There may be several molecules of drug bound to one protein molecule and strength may vary depending on the type of binding. However, binding is usually reversible. The protein commonly involved in binding is albumin. Binding to plasma proteins increases the half-life and limits distribution and metabolism of a drug. Drugs bound to plasma proteins are displaced by other drugs, leading to a rise in the free plasma concentration. Similarly increasing the dose of a drug that is bound extensively to plasma proteins saturates the binding sites and leads to an acute increase in plasma level.

c. The first-pass phenomenon is the extensive metabolism of a drug either by the organ of absorption or the liver following oral administration, culminating with small amounts of the parent drug distributed throughout the body. Thus after oral absorption, a drug is metabolized by the gastrointestinal tract and/or the liver before reaching systemic circulation. Therefore only a small amount of the active parent drug may reach the target site. If metabolism is saturable, however, increasing the dose dramatically increases systemic exposure. The lungs and skin, the other organs of absorption, also carry out first-pass metabolism.

d. Fick's law of diffusion describes the relationship between the rate of diffusion of a chemical across a membrane and interactions with the properties of the membrane. In the context of toxicology and drug disposition, it relates to passage across a cell membrane by simple diffusion. Thus:

$$\text{rate of diffusion} = KA\left(C_2 - C_1\right)$$

where K=diffusion coefficient, A=surface area, C_2=concentration of compound outside the membrane, C_1=concentration of compound on the inside of the membrane. The diffusion coefficient incorporates physicochemical characteristics of the chemical such as lipophilicity, size, and molecular organization.

9. a. The pH partition theory states that only non-ionized lipid-soluble compounds will be absorbed by passive diffusion down a concentration gradient. For absorption of a compound to occur through a biological membrane the compound must have some feature of lipid solubility and the concentration on the inside of the membrane should be lower than on the outside. Compounds that are ionized at the pH of the biological environment will not normally be able to pass through the membrane by passive diffusion although they may be substrates for active transport processes.

b. Plasma half-life is the time required for the concentration of a drug in the plasma (blood) to decrease by half from a given point. It reflects the rates at which various *in vivo* dynamic processes of distribution, metabolism and excretion are occurring. It is determined by plotting the plasma level against time according to the equation:

$$t_{1/2} = \frac{0.693}{k_{el}}$$

where k_{el} is calculated from the slope of the graph, log plasma concentration vs time (slope=$-k_{el}/2.303$).

The half-life is an important indicator of saturation of metabolism or excretion. Knowledge of the half-life is also important in relation to repeat dosing with a drug. If the dosing interval is shorter than the half-life then accumulation occurs.

c. Plasma clearance is an indication of the rate of removal of a drug from the blood or other body fluid by excretion or metabolism. It is calculated from the area under the plasma concentration vs time curve (AUC):

$$\text{clearance} = \frac{\text{dose}}{\text{AUC}}$$

The units are volume/unit time, e.g. mL/min. Thus a plasma clearance of 100 mL/min means that 100 mL of plasma is completely cleared of the drug every minute. Therefore the higher the clearance, the more efficiently and rapidly a chemical is removed from the fluid.

d. Enterohepatic recirculation describes the process whereby a chemical in the body is secreted from the liver into the bile, passes into the small intestine and is then reabsorbed into the circulation. For example, the chemical is secreted into bile as a polar conjugate following metabolism in the liver. When bile enters the intestine this conjugate is cleaved by bacterial metabolism and the original drug or other fragment is reabsorbed from the intestine to the liver via the portal circulation. This process is repeated several times prolonging the exposure of the liver and the rest of the body to the compound. If the compound has been administered orally, variable limited amounts reach the systemic circulation. The plasma level profile reflects the process by showing peaks at various times, corresponding to reabsorption, rather than a smooth decline.

Chapter 3. Exposure-Response

1. (a) Dose.
    Although all of the other factors affect toxicity, the most important is the dose as toxicity is a relative phenomenon. Therefore the lower the dose, the less likely a toxic occurrence.
2. (b) The ability of the liver to metabolize chemicals often renders it susceptible as a target for toxicity. This is due to the production of reactive metabolites or when other metabolic activities are affected.
    (c) The blood that is supplied to the liver is partly derived from the GI tract via the portal vein. Therefore chemicals absorbed from the intestinal tract are presented to the liver, with the propensity to cause toxicity to liver tissue.
    (d) The liver produces bile into which chemicals are excreted. Consequently, high concentrations of certain chemicals occur in the bile and damage the bile duct. Alternatively, chemicals that are excreted into the bile via active transport may saturate the transport processes and accumulate in the liver, thereby causing damage.
3. (e) Steatosis. Fatty liver is a common response of the liver upon exposure to chemicals, partly because the liver is the primary site of fat metabolism in the mammalian body and is easily disrupted by chemicals.
4. (b) Immunosuppression involves a reduction in the function of the immune system by chemicals, such as dioxin or benzene, that damage the thymus and bone marrow, respectively.
    (d) Autoimmune reactions are immune-mediated reactions where the immune system attacks the normal physiological structures of the body. An example is halothane-induced hepatic damage.
5. (a) Death.
    Although teratogens cause all of these effects, especially growth retardation during the first stage of pregnancy before implantation, organogenesis or functional maturation, the fertilized egg is more likely to suffer death following exposure to a chemical.
6. (a) To indicate exposure has occurred. (d) To measure exposure, response or susceptibility. Biomarkers are biochemical indicators of exposure, response or susceptibility to chemicals.

7. Direct toxic action: tissue lesions e.g. paracetamol-induced liver damage; biochemical lesions, e.g. fluoroacetate interference with the tricarboxylic acid (TCA) cycle leading to death from cardiac arrest; pharmacological/physiological effects, e.g. malathion causing exaggerated effects of acetylcholine; immunotoxicity, e.g. allergic responses caused by exposure to penicillin; teratogenicity, e.g. thalidomide-induced birth defects; genetic toxicity, e.g. 5-bromouracil is incorporated into replicating DNA and leads to mutations (base-pair transformations); carcinogenicity, e.g. vinyl chloride and aflatoxin both cause liver cancer.

8. Type I antibody-mediated (hypersensitivity) reactions occur in three phases: sensitization phase, activation phase, and effector phase. The reaction is triggered by contact with a previously unrecognized antigen and involves binding of the antigen to immunoglobulin E (IgE) present on the surface of mast cells and basophils. Toxic antigens involved in type I reactions are generally drugs (opioids, antibiotics) and metals (silver, gold).

   Type II antibody-mediated cytotoxic reactions involve formation of antibodies against target antigens that are altered cell membrane determinants. Examples of type II reactions include transfusion reactions, Rh incompatibility, andautoimmune and drug-induced reactions.

   Examples of drugs that traditionally induce type II reactions include penicillin and toluene diisocyanate.

   Type III immune complex reactions are localized responses mediated by antigen-antibody immune complexes. Type III reactions are stimulated by microorganisms and involve the activation of complement.

   Type IV (delayed-type) hypersensitivity cell-mediated immunity involves antigen-specific T-cell activation. Contact hypersensitivity resulting from prolonged exposure to plant resins, jewelry, and industrial metals (occupational hazard in metal industries; nickel, cadmium), for example, is caused by the lipophilicity of the chemical in oily skin secretions.

Chapter 4. Disposition

1. (c) Weak organic acids.
   In the stomach the pH is between 1 and 3; at this pH weak acids are non-ionized. Therefore passive absorption of the non-ionized acid occurs in the stomach.

2. (b) the drug is mostly metabolized by the GI tract and liver before reaching the systemic circulation; The first-pass phenomenon is the extensive metabolism of a drug either by the organ of absorption or the liver following oral administration, culminating with small amounts of the parent drug distributed throughout the body. Thus, after oral absorption, a drug is metabolized by the gastrointestinal tract and/or the liver before reaching systemic circulation. Therefore only a small amount of the active parent drug may reach the target site. If metabolism is saturable, however, increasing the dose dramatically increases systemic exposure.

The lungs and skin, the other organs of absorption, also carry out first-pass metabolism.

3. (b) False.

Non-ionized compounds are more readily absorbed by passive diffusion as they more readily pass through the lipid bilayer parts of biological membranes.

Short Answer Questions

4. The acid–base nature of chemical influences its absorption within the pH of the environment. Due to changes in pH in the stomach and throughout the length of the GI tract, different chemical substances are absorbed depending on their physicochemical characteristics. Weak acid (WA) substances lean toward greater *non-ionized*, lipid-soluble species in the pH of the **stomach** where absorption is favorable. Conversely, weak bases (WB) are *ionized*, water-soluble in the acidic environment of the stomach such that absorption is not favored. In the basic environment of the **small intestine**, WB are non-ionized, lipid-soluble molecules which favor their absorption. Thus the Henderson–Hasselbalch equation calculates the extent of ionization of weak acids and weak bases depending on the pH of the prevailing compartment, i.e. in the stomach or small intestine.

5. The first-pass phenomenon is the extensive metabolism of a drug either by the organ of absorption or the liver following oral administration, culminating with small amounts of the parent drug distributed throughout the body. Thus after oral absorption, a drug is metabolized by the gastrointestinal tract and/or the liver before reaching systemic circulation. Therefore only a small amount of the active parent drug reaches the target site. If metabolism is saturable, however, increasing the dose dramatically increases systemic exposure.

Chapter 5. Metabolism

1. (d) Altered chemical structure.

Metabolism involves the alteration of the chemical structure of a drug. Increased excretion and decreased toxicity do not always result in reduction of toxicity.

2. (c) a central part of the drug-metabolizing system.

Cytochrome P450 is the most important enzyme complex involved in drug metabolism. It is localized in the smooth endoplasmic reticulum and catalyzes most of the phase 1 oxidation reactions.

3. (d) addition of an endogenous moiety.

Phase II metabolic transformations involve the addition of a moiety derived endogenously which usually increases the polarity and water solubility. The moieties commonly involved are glucuronic acid, sulfate, glutathione, and amino acids such as glycine.

4. (b) A tripeptide.

Glutathione is composed of three amino acids: glutamic acid, cysteine and glycine (glutamyl-cysteinyl-glycine; glu-cys-gly). It is involved in detoxification by conjugating with reactive metabolites, by reducing reactive metabolites, and by reacting with and donating a hydrogen atom to free radicals.

5. (a) True.

Cytochrome P450 catalyzes phase 1 oxidation reactions.

6. (e). All of these are involved in the operation of the microsomal enzyme system.

7. (d) An inherited trait affecting a particular metabolic reaction.

The acetylation reaction in which the acetyl group (CH_3COO-) is added to an amine, hydrazine, or sulphonamide group, is subject to genetic variation in humans. There are two phenotypes, rapid and slow acetylators, which is a single gene trait governed by simple Mendelian inheritance. The rapid acetylator trait is dominant. This genetic trait results in a difference in the enzyme between the two phenotypes such that in slow acetylators the enzyme, N-acetyltransferase (NAT2), catalyzes acetylation of substrates less efficiently than in rapid acetylators. In slow acetylators, mutations appear in the gene coding for the enzyme, resulting in a relatively dysfunctional enzyme.

8. (a) An increase in the synthesis of the enzyme.

Although the activity (and substrate specificity) of the enzyme appears to be altered, thesynthesis of particular isozymes and their proportions are altered. Some inducers cause an increase in liver weight and bile flow.

Short Answer Questions

9. a. Dealkylation is the removal of an alkyl (methyl or ethyl group) from a molecule. The alkyl group is attached to a nitrogen, sulfur or oxygen atom as indicated below. The dealkylation reaction is catalyzed by the microsomal mono-oxygenase enzyme cytochrome P450 and involves initial oxidation of the alkyl carbon atom followed by rearrangement with loss of the oxidized alkyl group as an aldehyde (e.g. methanal or ethanal as indicated below). The other product is either an alcohol, thiol or amine as follows:

$$R-O-C_2H_5 \rightarrow R-OH+CH_3CHO$$
$$R-NH-CH_3 \rightarrow R-NH_2+HCHO$$
$$R-S-CH_3 \rightarrow R-SH+HCHO$$

b. Alcohol dehydrogenase is an enzyme found in many mammalian species that catalyze the oxidation of alcohols to aldehydes. Coenzyme NADH is also required. There are several isoenzymes and a wide variety of alcohols are substrates, located in the liver. Evidence suggests that ethnic variations in the enzyme activity exist that have reduced ability to metabolize ethanol.

c. Glucuronic acid conjugation is the combination of certain foreign compounds with glucuronic acid to form glucuronides. Normally a carboxylic acid group or a hydroxyl group is conjugated to form ester or ether glucuronides, respectively. Occasionally thiol and NH glucuronides are formed. The conjugates are water-soluble and readily excreted. Conjugation is catalyzed by one of a group of glucuronosyltransferases. Glucuronic acid is a six carbon carbohydrate molecule formed from glucose-1-phosphate (G1P). In conjugation reactions, G1P combines with uridine diphosphate (UDP) forming UDP-glucuronic acid.

d. Phase I metabolism refers to the first stage in the biotransformation of a foreign compound. The product has a functional group added or an existing one that acts as a 'handle' for a second endogenous group, derived from intermediary metabolism, such as glucuronic acid added in phase 2 metabolism.

10. a. The ethnic backgrounds of humans are important determinants of their response to drugs and chemicals. This is due to differences in sensitivity or susceptibility or to a difference in disposition. Glucose-6-phosphate dehydrogenase deficiency increases susceptibility to certain drugs such as primaquine, resulting in hemolytic anemia. The deficiency is found in males of diverse ethnic origins, such as progeny from eastern Mediterranean, such as Sephardic Jews from Kurdistan. Altered disposition in ethnic groups often occurs as a result of differences in enzymes. For example, the acetylator phenotype is differently distributed in Asians compared with Egyptians—the former are fast acetylators while the latter are slow acetylators.

b. The cytochrome P450 system, responsible for metabolizing 90% of drugs, consists of many isozymes. These have different substrate specificities and there is variation in the activity of the isozymes between species and individuals. Therefore, the absence of a particular isozyme in an individual or species induces greater susceptibility to drug toxicity if the particular isozyme is responsible for a detoxification pathway. The same also applies to susceptibility of a tissue to particular drug toxicity, as isozymes vary in proportions between tissues within the same species.

c. The phenomenon of enzyme induction refers to the apparent increase in activity of an enzyme following exposure of the subject to a xenobiotic. For example, repeated exposure to phenobarbital leads to an apparent increase in the activity of certain cytochrome P450 isozymes. This can be shown to occur with other enzymes involved with drug metabolism such as glucuronosyltransferase. The result is that metabolism and therefore toxicity of a drug is altered, and depends on whether the drug or a metabolite is responsible for the toxic effect. For example, acetaminophen toxicity to the liver is increased by the induction of cytochrome P450 with phenobarbital in some species.

d. Acetylator phenotype is a genetically determined characteristic in humans that determines the extent of acetylation of certain drugs. Isoniazid acetylation is affected by this phenotype, as a result of a genetic difference between individuals resulting from mutations in the gene coding for *N*-acetyltransferase 2. Thus, slow acetylators have less functional enzyme than fast acetylators. The result is that detoxification of hydrazines, sulphonamides and amines by acetylation is decreased in slow acetylators. Pathologic consequences such as hydralazine-induced lupus and isoniazid-induced peripheral neuropathy are more common in the slow phenotype.

Chapter 6. Target Organ Toxicity

1. (b) Dose.
   Although the other factors affect toxicity, the most important is the dose as toxicity is a relative phenomenon.
2. (b) The liver metabolizes chemicals which often makes it a target for toxicity. This is due to the production of reactive metabolites.
   (c) Blood supply to the liver is partly derived from the GI tract via the portal vein. Therefore chemicals absorbed from the GI tract are presented to the liver. Consequently toxic substances damage liver tissue.
   (d) The liver produces bile into which chemicals are excreted. Consequently, high concentrations of certain chemicals may occur in bile and damage the bile duct. Alternatively, chemicals that are excreted into the bile via active transport can saturate transport processes and accumulate in the liver, thereby causing damage.
3. (e) Steatosis. Fatty liver or steatosis is the most common response of the liver to exposure to chemicals, since the liver is the primary site of fat metabolism and is easily disrupted by chemicals.

Short Answer Question

4. Most substances that interact with the cardiovascular system also have cardiac specificity. For instance, digoxin is derived from the leaves of the common foxglove plant (*Digitalis purpurea*). The drug remains widely used today in the face of increasing rates of heart failure despite the emergence of newer medications. Its narrow therapeutic index and toxicity, however, have become more relevant as aging, comorbid diseases, and multiple drug ingestion increase patient population vulnerability.

Chapter 7. Carcinogenic and Mutagenic Compounds

1.

Aneuploidization	loss or acquisition of a complete chromosome
Clastogenesis	loss, addition or rearrangement of parts of chromosomes
Mutagenesis	addition to or alteration of the number of base pairs

2. The first stage is initiation, where the chemical or a reactive metabolite interacts with DNA. The second stage is promotion in which the initiated cell undergoes division and a clone of initiated/altered cells is produced. Finally, the third stage involves the progression of the clone of cells; neoplastic cells transform into malignant tumors, growth increases and the cells metastasize to other tissues.

Chapter 8. Drugs as Toxic Substances

1. (d) Metabolic activation by the microsomal enzymes. Although (a) and (c) are also true, metabolic activation to a reactive benzoquinoneimine, which interacts with tissue components, is the cause of the toxicity.
2. (a), (b), (c) There are a number of predisposing factors in hydralazine toxicity, including the acetylator phenotype, gender and dose. The toxicity or adverse effect is almost exclusively confined to the slow acetylator and is more common in females than males. The adverse effect is more likely to occur at higher doses, although the severity is not related to dose.
3. (c) Thalidomide was a sedative drug used for the relief of morning sickness during pregnancy. It caused malformations in babies born to mothers who took the drug during the susceptible period; i.e. the third to eighth week of pregnancy. Malformations were manifested as shortened arms and legs, known as phocomelia. The S isomer of the drug is more active than the R isomer. Pregnant rats were not susceptible to this effect.
4. (c) The anesthetic drug, halothane, occasionally causes severe liver damage in patients. This is more common in females than males. The mechanism of the autoimmune reaction involves metabolism by cytochrome P450 and production of an antigenic conjugate. The immune response involves T-lymphocytes as well as antibodies.
5. (e) An adverse effect is an untoward, undesirable but expected effect of therapeutic drugs, also known as "side effects". An idiosyncratic reaction is an adverse reaction of unknown origin and occurs after therapeutic doses in particularly susceptible individuals. Inappropriate doses of a drug cause unwanted effects not related to the expected/desired pharmacological effect of that drug. Occasionally interaction between a drug and a dietary constituent occur, such as between monoamine oxidase inhibitor drugs and amines found in cheese.

Short Answer Question

6. Aspirin is mainly metabolized to salicylate. The distribution of salicylate into tissues and its excretion into urine are sensitive to pH because only the non-ionized form of salicylate enters tissues and especially the brain. When plasma pH drops, as a result of salicylate poisoning, the distribution into the brain increases. Similarly, excretion into urine is reduced if urinary pH becomes more acidic.

Chapter 9. Industrial Toxicology

1. (c) Dermatitis is a common reaction to the metal nickel.
2. (b), (c) and (d) are all known carcinogens. Cadmium is not known as a human carcinogen but vinyl chloride, 2-naphthylamine and asbestos are associated with lung cancer (mesothelioma), bladder cancer and liver cancer (hemangiosarcoma), respectively.
3. (c) NOAEL, No Observed Adverse Effect Level, is needed to determine threshold limit value (TLV) for an industrial chemical. A safety constant is incorporated to compute TLV. The latency period for the effect and half-life are also included in the NOAEL. The daily exposure level may be the same as, less, or more than the TLV depending on the circumstances.
4. The toxicity of asbestos is affected by (a), (b), (c), and (e). Dose does not calculate into its toxicity.
5. (c) Both vinyl chloride and cadmium affect bones, albeit with different mechanisms.

Short Answer Question

6. 2-Naphthylamine undergoes hydroxylation on the nitrogen atom, catalyzed by cytochrome P450; the N-hydroxy product is conjugated with glucuronic acid. This conjugate is excreted into the urine but is relatively unstable; under the acidic conditions of the urine, the glucuronide conjugate is hydrolyzed to yield a reactive metabolite. The metabolite reacts with DNA in susceptible bladder cells leading to cancer formation. However, 2-naphthylamine is also acetylated on the nitrogen atom; the detoxification reaction is further hydroxylated blocking any further formation of reactive metabolites. Therefore, the fast acetylator phenotype individual is at lower risk for cancer initiation than the slow acetylator.

Chapter 10. Food Additives

1.

A. Erythrosine	c. Coloring agent
B. Monosodium glutamate	a. Flavor enhancer
C. Cinnamaldehyde	e. Flavoring agent
D. Butylated hydroxytoluene	b. Anti-oxidant
E. Benzoyl peroxide	d. Bleach

2. Tartrazine is also known as E102 and is a coloring agent responsible for the development of b. urticaria, and is c. reduced by GI bacteria (c). Tartrazine sensitivity is often related to aspirin tolerance.

3. True: (a), (d), (e).

Saccharin causes bladder tumors in rats at high doses. Saturation kinetics occur at high doses, which accounts for the bladder tumors at these doses. It has low toxicity and, although it was banned from use under the Delaney Clause for a while, it is now allowed for use.

4. True: (d). False: (a), (b), (c).

Adulterated rape-seed oil was sold for use as cooking oil. The rape-seed oil was for industrial use and was adulterated with the addition of aniline. There were a number of symptoms including pulmonary edema and muscular atrophy.

Short Answer Question

5. Aflatoxins are produced by *Aspergillus flavus,* a mold that grows on food-stuffs such as peanuts, when stored in damp, warm conditions. Aflatoxin B_1 is a potent liver carcinogen. The mechanism involves metabolism to a chemically reactive epoxide intermediate that interacts with DNA.

Ptaquiloside occurs naturally in edible bracken fern shoots. It is responsible for throat cancer in humans. It was shown to produce intestinal and bladder cancer in animals. A breakdown product of ptaquiloside is responsible, reacting with adenine in DNA resulting in DNA strand breakage.

Botulinum toxin is one of the most potent toxins known, produced by the anerobic bacterium *Clostridium botulinum*. It contaminates canned and bottled food, although it is destroyed by heating. The bacterium binds irreversibly to nerve terminals, preventing the release of acetylcholine, resulting in paralysis and fatal respiratory arrest.

Chapter 11. Pesticides and Herbicides

1. True: (b), (d). False: (a), (c), (e).

DDT is an organochlorine pesticide, which has low mammalian toxicity and does not destroy plants. Unlike organophosphates it does not inhibit cholinesterases. It is not directly toxic to eggs although it may contribute to their breakage as a result of eggshell thinning.

2. True: (d), (e). False: (a), (b), (c).

Parathion is an organophosphate insecticide which is toxic to humans. Parathion is metabolized to paraoxon which inhibits cholinesterases leading to elevated levels of acetylcholine. The result is excessive cholinergic stimulation producing symptoms such as bronchoconstriction.

3. True: (c), (d). False: (a), (b), (e).

Paraquat is a bipyridyl herbicide. It is actively incorporated into lung tissue by the putrescine uptake system. It is concentrated in the lungs where it is responsible for stimulation of lipid peroxidation, production of reactive oxygen species and fibrosis. The reactive oxygen radicals are detoxified by superoxide dismutase (SOD) but is over-whelmed when large amounts of paraquat are ingested.

Short Answer Questions

4. Fluoroacetate is toxic as a result of intermediary metabolism, when it is first converted to fluoroacetyl CoA. The resultant product is incorporated into the TCA cycle, forming fluorocitrate. This analog of citrate, however, cannot be further metabolized by the next step to cis-aconitate as the fluorine atom is not removed. Therefore, the TCA cycle is blocked; ATP production is compromised, and mammals die of heart failure.
5. Paraquat selectively accumulates in pulmonary alveolar type I and II cells. PQ preferentially accumulates in the lungs because of structural similarity with diamines and polyamines. The intramolecular distance between the two nitrogens in paraquat enables its incorporation into a selective active transport system in alveolar cells for which polyamines are the normal substrate. See Figure 11.5 for the molecular structure of PQ.

Chapter 12. Environmental pollutants

1. True: (b), (c), (e). False: (a), (d).
   Inorganic lead is present in cigarette smoke and is absorbed as particles of lead oxide through the lungs. It interferes with the synthesis of heme, some of which occurs in the mitochondria. The result is a reduction of hemoglobin production leading to damage of red blood cells. Organic lead, such as that added to gasoline (petrol), is toxic to the central nervous system and is absorbed through the lungs.
2. True: (d), (e). False: (a), (b), (c).
   Mercury binds to SH groups and organic mercury has a long half-life. Metallic mercury easily vaporizes and the vapor can be readily absorbed where it is toxic to a variety of tissues including the central nervous system. Inorganic mercury is especially toxic to the kidney.
3. True: (f). False: (a), (b), (c), (d), (e).
   The great smog in London occurred in 1952. Photochemical smog contains ozone, nitrogen oxides and hydrocarbons. Ozone is an irritant, toxic gas. PM10 is the acronym for small airborne particles with a diameter less than $10\,\mu$m, and are responsible for lung pathologies. Acid rain results from the production of sulfur dioxide and nitrogen oxides. It is caused by wet precipitation of sulphuric and nitric acids and dry precipitation of sulfur dioxide and nitrogen oxides.
   Reducing smog is largely the result of burning of fossil fuels and has high levels of sulfur dioxide and particulates.

4. True: (c), (e). False: (a), (b), (d).

DDT is an insecticide, not especially toxic to birds or chicks directly. However, its metabolite DDE is responsible for causing eggshell thinning, responsible for egg breakage and loss of chicks. By killing insects of many types, DDT also reduces the food supply of some birds.

Short Answer Question

5. *Bioaccumulation* is the build-up of a chemical substance in a biological organism, usually a reflection of the lipophilicity of the compound.

Biomagnification is the process where chemical substances concentrate in the organisms of a food chain and increase toward the top of the chain. Thus, the predator at the top of the food chain will have the highest concentration of pollutant.

For a compound to bioaccumulate it should be more lipid soluble than water-soluble. For example, the pesticide DDT bioaccumulates in organisms exposed to it as it dissolves in adipose tissue. Also, the compound should be resistant to metabolism and poorly excreted so that it is eliminated slowly from the organism. For example, polybrominated biphenyl compounds, such as those that contaminated livestock and humans in Michigan in 1973, are very resistant to metabolism, are eliminated extremely slowly and have long half-lives. Continued exposure to such compounds, therefore, results in the accumulation of fat tissue.

Chapter 13. Natural Products

1. True: (c), (e). False: (a), (b), (d).

Pyrrolizidine alkaloids are found in plants such as *Heliotropium* species. These compounds cause liver and lung damage. *Amanita phalloides*, a toxin found in the Death Cap mushroom, causes fatal liver damage. Botulinum toxin is produced by the anaerobic bacterium *Clostridium botulinum* and is highly toxic, causing paralysis. Ricin is the most toxic substance known and is found naturally in the castor bean. Fluoroacetate occurs naturally in plants in South Africa and Australia.

2. True: (b), (d). False: (a), (c).

Tetrodotoxin is a toxin found in the Puffer fish and Californian newt. It is highly potent, causing muscle paralysis by selectively blocking sodium channels along the axon, interrupting transmission of the action potential.

Short Answer Questions

3. Botulinum toxin causes irreversible blockade of the motor nerve terminal at the myoneural junction. This prevents the release of acetylcholine and acts to denervate the muscle. The victim suffers paralysis and respiratory distress which is fatal in severe cases.

4. Tetrodotoxin selectively blocks sodium channels along the nerve axon, interrupting transmission of the action potential, resulting in muscle paralysis.

Chapter 14. Commercial and Domestic Products

1. True: (b). False: (a), (c), (d), (e).

    Ethylene glycol toxicity requires metabolism by the enzyme alcohol dehydrogenase. Fomepizol and ethanol are also metabolized by this enzyme; when administered to a poisoned patient the antidotes compete for the enzyme and block the metabolism of ethylene glycol.

2. True: (b), (d). False: (a), (c), (e).

    Carbon monoxide binds to hemoglobin more strongly than oxygen and forms carboxyhemoglobin. The lack of oxygen in the tissues results in damage, especially to those that have a high demand for oxygen, such as brain and heart. Death is usually due to respiratory failure. Carbon monoxide also binds to other heme proteins including the cytochromes. Lack of oxygen leads to anaerobic respiration and lactic acidosis.

3. True: (a), (b). False: (c), (d), (e).

    Ethylene glycol is a dihydric alcohol that is metabolized by alcohol dehydrogenase to an aldehyde followed by aldehyde dehydrogenase to the corresponding acid. The final product is oxalic acid which crystallizes in brain tissue. The increased production of NADH as a result of metabolism leads to excessive production of lactic acid and the presence of acidic metabolites causes acidosis.

4. True: (a), (f). False: (b), (c), (d), (e).

    Some solvents sensitize the myocardium leading to sudden death from heart attack in apparently healthy young people who have engaged in solvent abuse.

    Alcohol depresses the central nervous system, especially at high doses. Alcohol is metabolized to acetic acid. The major target for methanol is the eye – it causes blindness. Large doses of alcohol lower blood sugar (hypoglycemia).

5. (b), (c), (d) and (e). Disodium EDTA is a chelating agent used as an antidote to metal poisoning. N-acetylcysteine is an antidote for acetaminophen (paracetamol) toxicity as it restores depleted glutathione. Thiocyanate is a component of an antidote program used for cyanide toxicity. Pralidoxime (2-PAM) is an antidote for organophosphate poisoning; it is used along with atropine to bind organophosphates in preference to the acetylcholinesterase enzyme.

Short Answer Questions

6. The goal of treatment for cyanide poisoning is to immediately decrease CN binding to cytochrome enzymes with the specific antidote available. The Cyanide Antidote Package consists of amyl nitrite inhalant, sodium

nitrite, and sodium thiosulfate. Detoxification involves conversion of CN to the cyanomethemoglobin, with amyl nitrite and sodium nitrite, followed by sodium thiosulphate. The latter induces the formation of water-soluble thiocyanate (SCN) which is excreted, while regenerating methemoglobin.

7. Treatment for mild to moderate exposure to CO involves the immediate removal of the victim from the source of the gas or allow fresh uncontaminated air to enter into the environment. As the concentration of CO in the ambient and inspired air falls, carboxyhemoglobin dissociates and carbon monoxide is expired. The rate of loss of toxic gas from the blood is *increased* by treating the patient with 100% oxygen at atmospheric pressure, where the half-life is reduced from 250 to 50 minutes.

Chapter 15. Fundamentals of Toxicity Testing

1. True: (c), (d). False: (a), (b).

Acute toxicity studies focus on the immediate causes and mechanisms of toxicity and determine dose-response relationships. Sub-chronic studies determine short-term repeated exposure. Ecotoxicity studies use the small water organism *Daphnia* as a test species. Teratogenicity studies determine the effect of a compound on the developing organism *in utero*.

2. (e) Cost is not a requirement for EU new chemicals strategy.

Short Answer Questions

3. The seven questions applied for conduct of toxicity studies include:
   1. Is the compound novel or in current use?
   2. Does it have the potential for release into the environment?
   3. Will it be incorporated into human food consumption?
   4. Is it administered as a single dose or repeatedly?
   5. What is the dosage level for administration?
   6. What age group are potentially exposed?
   7. Does the chemical have potential risk for women of childbearing age?

4. The four types of epidemiological studies are: cohort, case-control, cross-sectional, and ecological studies.

5. The 3-Rs relate to the use of animals in toxicity testing. They are *replacement* of animals with alternative methods such as *in vitro* systems; *reduction* of numbers of animals used by careful design of experiments; and, *refinement* of the techniques and handling used to ensure greater animal welfare and humane treatment.

Chapter 16. Risk Assessment

1. NOAEL, No Observed Adverse Effect Level, is the dose or exposure level of a chemical which has no demonstrable adverse effect on a biological system. The value may be derived from the dose-response relationship.

ADI is the 'acceptable daily intake' and is usually applied to food additives or contaminants (such as pesticides). It is the calculated amount of a substance to which humans are permitted to be exposed safely. It is calculated from the NOAEL.

TLV, or Threshold Limit Value, is the upper permissive limits of airborne concentrations of substances.

2. Risk assessment (RA) is a mathematical concept that refers to the likelihood of undesirable effects resulting from exposure to a chemical. Examples include the incorporation of therapeutic drugs in the biomedical community, release of chemicals for environmental benefits, such as pesticides, and potentially hazardous substances as food additives.

3. Risk is the probability that an untoward or unpredictable event will result in an adverse effect under specific exposure conditions.

Risk is defined as: Risk = hazard × exposure.

Hazard is the capacity of a substance to cause an adverse effect. Conversely, safety is defined as 'the practical certainty that adverse effects will not occur when the substance is used in the manner and quantity proposed for its use'.

Chapter 17. Antidotes and Treatment of Poisoning

1. True: (b). False: (a), (c), (d), (e).

Ethylene glycol toxicity requires metabolism by the enzyme alcohol dehydrogenase. Fomepizol is also metabolized by this enzyme; when administered to a poisoned patient fomepizol competes for the enzyme and blocks the metabolism of the ethylene glycol, preventing its metabolism to a toxic metabolite.

2. True: (b), (d). False: (a), (c), (e).

Carbon monoxide binds to hemoglobin more strongly than oxygen to form carboxyhemoglobin. The lack of oxygen in the tissues results in damage, especially to tissues that have a high demand for oxygen, such as brain and heart. Death is usually due to respiratory failure. Carbon monoxide also binds to other heme proteins such as cytochromes. The lack of oxygen leads to anaerobic respiration and lactic acidosis.

3. True: (a), (b). False: (c), (d), (e).

Ethylene glycol is a dihydric alcohol which is metabolized by alcohol dehydrogenase to an aldehyde and by aldehyde dehydrogenase to an acid. The final product is oxalic acid which crystallizes in brain neurons. The increased production of NADH as a result of metabolism leads to excessive production of lactic acid and the presence of acidic metabolites causes acidosis.

4. True: (a), (f). False: (b), (c), (d), (e).

Some solvents sensitize the myocardium leading to sudden death from heart attack in apparently healthy young people who have engaged in solvent abuse.

Alcohol depresses the central nervous system, especially at high doses. Alcohol is metabolized to acetic acid. The major target for methanol is the eye – its toxic effects result in blindness. Large doses of alcohol lower blood sugar (hypoglycemia).

5. BAL, British anti-Lewisite, is used in the treatment of (2) arsenic poisoning, Penicillamine is an antidote for (3) copper toxicity. Sodium thiosulphate is an antidote for (5) cyanide poisoning since it converts cyanomethemoglobin to thiosulphate and regenerates methemoglobin; N-acetylcysteine is used as an antidote for (4) acetaminophen overdose as it helps to restore depleted glutathione levels. Pralidoxime is used as an antidote for (1) organophosphate pesticide poisoning, as it binds the organophosphates in preference to acetylcholinesterase.

Short Answer Questions

6. General treatments for poisoning include the use of emetics to cause vomiting and so rid the stomach of the poison; gastric lavage to wash the poison out of the stomach; absorbants which are given orally to the patient and absorb the poison in the stomach. Enhancing excretion may be used which involves the administration of aqueous solutions by mouth or intravenously (forced diuresis) to increase urine flow. If bicarbonate or ammonium chloride is included in the aqueous fluid then the pH of the urine is made more basic or acidic, respectively. This change will facilitate the excretion of acids or bases, respectively.

Hemoperfusion or hemodialysis is generally used as a last resort when other treatment modalities have failed.

7. The PCC provides the following roles and services for the therapeutic advancement of toxicological poisoning: product ingredient information; affords information on the treatment of poisoned patients; supplies direct information to patients; suggests diagnostic and treatment information to health care professionals; institutes education programs for health care professionals; and sponsors poison prevention activities.

Glossary

Acidosis/alkalosis	Condition when the pH of the blood falls/rises outside the normal acceptable limits.
Acid rain	Deposition of acids (sulphuric and nitric) in rain and also the dry deposition of sulphur dioxide and nitrogen oxides.
Acute	Short-term exposure or response.
Additive	When the toxic effect of a mixture is equal to the sum of the toxicities of the components.
ADI	Acceptable Daily Intake. 'The daily intake of a chemical which during an entire lifetime appears to be without appreciable risk based on all the known facts at the time.'
Aerobic/anaerobic	Process carried out in the presence/absence of air.
Aerosol	Colloidal system with a gas as the dispersion medium (such as a fog or mist of droplets or particles).
Ah receptor	A protein which binds polycyclic hydrocarbons such as dioxin (TCDD). Binding to this receptor is part of the process of induction of xenobiotic metabolizing enzymes.
Allergic reaction	Reaction to a foreign agent giving rise to a hypersensitive state, mediated via an immunological mechanism and resulting in a particular series of responses.
Anaphylactic reaction	A type I immunological response.

Aneuploidy	Increase or decrease in the number of chromosomes of an organism.
Anoxia	Absence of oxygen in the tissues.
Antagonism	When the toxic effect of a mixture is less than the sum of the toxicities of the components.
Antibody	Protein produced by lymphoid tissue in response to, and specific for, a foreign substance or antigen.
Anticoagulant	Substance that inhibits the normal process of blood clotting.
Antidote	Substance that specifically blocks or reduces the action of a poison.
Antigen	Protein or other macromolecule which is recognized as foreign by the immune system in an animal.
Antiport	Membrane carrier system in which two substances are transported in opposite directions.
Apoptosis	Programmed cell death.
Asbestosis	Damage to the lungs caused specifically by exposure to, and inhalation of, asbestos fibers.
Ataxia	Failure of muscular coordination.
AUC	Area under the curve when the plasma (blood) concentration of a substance is plotted against time.
β-adrenoceptors	An autonomic receptor of which there are two types, β_1 and β_2.
Bioaccumulation	Accumulation of a substance in a biological organism, usually due to its lipophilicity.
Biomagnification	Process whereby the concentration of a pollutant in organisms in a food chain increases towards the top of that chain. Thus the predator at the top of the food chain will have the highest concentration of pollutant.
Biomarker	Biochemical or biological marker of exposure, response or susceptibility to chemicals.
Blebbing	Appearance of blebs (protrusions) on the surface of cells in response to stress (e.g. chemicals).
Blood-brain barrier	Description of the inability of many substances to pass from the blood to the tissues of the brain.
BOD	Biochemical Oxygen Demand. This measurement indicates the ability of micro-organisms to metabolize an organic substance in the presence of oxygen and the potential for depletion of oxygen by the substance.
Bronchocarcinoma	Cancer of the lung.

Bronchoconstriction	Constriction of the airways in the lungs due to exposure to irritant chemicals or to an immunological reaction involving release of inflammatory mediators.
Carcinogen	A substance or property of a substance which causes cancer when administered to an organism.
Cardiac arrythmias	Abnormal beating rhythms in the heart.
Cardiac output	Volume of blood pumped by the heart in one cycle.
Cerebral palsy	Motor disorder due to damage to the brain.
Cholinergic stimulation	Stimulation of the nerve fibers utilizing acetylcholine as a neurotransmitter.
Chronic	Long-term exposure or response.
Cirrhosis	Liver disease characterized by loss of the normal microscopic lobular structure with fibrosis and nodular regeneration. Usually the result of chronic injury to tissue.
Clastogenesis	Occurrence of chromosomal breaks which result in a gain, loss or rearrangement of pieces of chromosomes.
Clearance	Volume of plasma cleared of a substance in unit time.
Clinical trials	Initial studies performed with a drug in human subjects.
COD	Chemical Oxygen Demand. Amount of oxygen required to oxidize the substance chemically.
COD/BOD	Ratio of COD to BOD yields an indication of the biodegradability of the substance.
Collagen	A fibrous protein.
Complement	A series of proteins found in extracellular fluids and involved in immunological reactions.
Cyanosis	Pathological condition where there is an excessive concentration of reduced hemoglobin in the blood.
Cytochrome a$_3$	A heme-containing enzyme which is part of the cytochrome c oxidase complex, the terminal cytochrome in the mitochondrial electron transport chain.
Cytological	Examination for the presence of cells in urine. examination.
Cytosol	Internal component of the cell excluding the organelles.
Delaney Clause	1958 Amendment to the Food, Drug and Cosmetic Act of the U.S. Food and Drug Administration declaring that food additives that cause cancer in humans or animals at any level shall not be considered safe and are, therefore, prohibited.

Dermatitis	Inflammation of the skin.
Detritivore food chain	Type of food chain that relies on decaying organic matter for its primary energy source. An animal which uses decaying organic matter as a food source, after the initial breakdown of the material by decomposers such as bacteria and fungi is a 'detritivore.'
Dinoflagellates	Single-celled marine algae possessing two flagella.
Disulphide bridge	A sulphur-sulphur bond (S-S) such as occurs commonly in proteins.
Dominant lethal assay	Test designed to detect the effects of substances on the germ cells of male animals that are exposed and then mated with untreated females. The number of dead implantations or preimplantation losses in the females are then determined. The effects are usually due to chromosome damage.
ED_{50}	The dose which is pharmacologically effective for 50% of the population exposed to the substance or a 50% response in a biological system which is exposed to the substance.
Electrophilic	Chemical description of a substance which seeks out a group or molecular position that has a preponderance of electrons.
Encephalopathy	A degenerative disease of the brain.
Endocrine disruptor	An exogenous substance which causes changes in endocrine function leading to adverse mammalian effects *or* in its offspring.
Endogenous	Part of the internal environment of a living organism.
Enterohepatic recirculation	Cycling of a substance from blood to the liver, followed by bile and gastrointestinal(GI) tract. Reuptake occurs in the systemic circulation from the GI tract after chemical or enzymatic breakdown.
Epidemiology	study of diseases in populations.
Epigenetic	When used as a description of a carcinogen or of mechanisms of carcinogenesis this means that interaction with genetic material, such as to yield a mutation, is not involved.
ER	Endoplasmic reticulum. Divided between rough ER, with attendant ribosomes involved with protein synthesis, and smooth ER where cytochrome P450 and other drug-metabolizing enzymes are located.

Eutrophication	Increased nutrient concentration in water resulting in the overgrowth of plants such as algae, yielding a depletion of oxygen. This is followed by death and decay of all the aerobic organisms in the aqueous environment with the subsequent growth of anaerobic bacteria leading to the accumulation of toxins.
Exanthema	An eruptive disease or fever.
Fatty acid	An organic acid with a long aliphatic chain; may be saturated or unsaturated.
Fibrosis	Formation of fibrous tissue; usually a response of tissue to injury resulting in increased amounts of collagen fibers.
Fick's Law	At constant temperature the rate of diffusion of a substance across a cell membrane is proportional to the concentration gradient and the surface area.
First-order process	The rate of the process is proportional to the concentration of the substance.
First-pass phenomenon	Metabolism of a drug or chemical during the absorption process. Typically occurs in the liver or gastrointestinal tract after oral dosing.
Food chain	An theoretical chain of organisms existing in the environment in which each link of the chain feeds upon the one below and is consumed by the one above. At the bottom of the food chain are plants and bacteria, at the top are carnivores.
Free radical	An atom or molecule which has an unpaired electron; uncharged or charged depending on the number of electrons. Free radicals are usually chemically very reactive.
Genotoxic	Toxic to the genetic material of an organism.
Glomerulus	Functional unit of the mammalian kidney consisting of capillaries projecting into a capsule (Bowman's capsule) which serves to collect the filtrate from the blood of those capillaries and direct it into the kidney tubules.
Glutathione (GSH)	The tripeptide glutamyl-cysteinyl-glycine. Found in most tissues, especially the liver. Plays a major role in detoxication and cellular protection.
Glycoprotein	Protein containing a carbohydrate moiety.
GLP	Good Laboratory Practice. A system of protocols (standard operating procedures) recommended to avoid the production of unreliable and erroneous data. Accurate record keeping and careful forethought in the design of the study are important aspects of GLP.

GSH/GSSG	Reduced/oxidized glutathione.
Half-life	Time required for the concentration of a compound in a body fluid to decrease by 50%.
Hapten	A molecule which attaches to a protein or other macromolecule and renders it antigenic.
Hemodialysis	Process by which a foreign substance is removed from the blood of a poisoned patient by allowing it to diffuse across a semipermeable membrane while the blood is pumped through a filtering machine.
Hemoglobinuria	Presence of hemoglobin in the urine.
Hemolytic anemia	Pathological condition where red blood cells undergo uncontrolled destruction.
Hemoperfusion	Process by which a foreign substance is removed from the blood of a poisoned patient by allowing it to pass through mechanical equipment where it is absorbed by activated charcoal or a resin.
Hemorrhage	Escape of blood from blood vessels.
Hemorrhagic necrosis	The death of most or all of the cells in an organ or tissue due to disease, injury, or failure of the blood supply, accompanied by bleeding.
Henderson-Hasselbalch equation	$pH = pKa + \log A-/HA$, where HA is the acid and A- is the corresponding conjugate base.
Histamine	A chemical mediator of inflammatory reactions in the body; part of an allergic reaction.
HLA type	Human Leukocyte Antigen; histocompatibility antigens on the surface of nucleated cells.
Hydrophobic/hydrophilic	A substance which repels/attracts water.
Hyperkinesis	Hyperactive movement.
Hypoglycemia	Physiological state characterized by a low blood glucose concentration.
Hypoxia	Physiological state characterized by a low oxygen concentration in the tissues.
Idiosyncratic	An adverse unpredictable reaction to a chemical which occurs in a single or small number of individuals.
Immune complex	A complex of antibody and antigen that leads to pathological consequences such as inflammation or blockage of a vessel.
Initiation	First stage in the multi-stage process of carcinogenesis; suspected as a chemical reaction between the carcinogen and DNA.
Interferon	Macromolecule produced by the body in response to a chemical or antigenic stimulus such as an infection or xenobiotic.

Intraperitoneal/i.p	Route of administration of a compound by direct injection into the peritoneal cavity.
Irritation/irritancy	Direct injury to tissue such as the skin.
Ischemia	Condition of reduced or blocked blood flow to a tissue leading to ischemic tissue damage.
Isozyme/isoenzyme	One of several forms of an enzyme where different forms usually catalyze similar but distinct reactions.
Keratin	A tough, fibrous protein found in the skin.
Killer lymphocyte	Type of white blood cell involved in Type IV immunological reactions.
LD$_{50}$	Lethal dose of a compound for 50% of the population of organisms exposed.
Lipid peroxidation	Oxidative breakdown of lipids usually involving a free radical mechanism or active oxygen species and yielding reactive products responsible for cellular damage.
Lipid solubility	See lipophilicity.
Lipophilicity	Used to describe the ability of a substance to dissolve in, or associate with, fat in viable tissue. Usually applies to compounds which are non-ionized or non-polar or have a non-polar portion. High lipid solubility usually implies low water solubility.
Local toxicity	Toxicity which affects only the site of application or surface exposure.
Macromolecule	A large molecule having a polymeric structure such as a protein or nucleic acid.
Macrophage	Large phagocytic cells which are components of the reticuloendothelial system.
MTD	Maximal Tolerated Dose. Dose of a substance which causes not more than a 10% weight decrease and does not cause death or any clinical signs of toxicity which would shorten the life span of an animal exposed for 90 days.
MEL	Maximum Exposure Level; maximum level of occupational exposure of workers to a chemical; generally used in the U.K.
Mesothelioma	Rare form of cancer mainly affecting the pleura and mainly associated with exposure to certain forms of asbestos.
Methemoglobin/ methemoglobinemia	Oxidized hemoglobin/the syndrome in which a significant amount of hemoglobin in the blood is oxidized.
Microflora/microfauna	Bacteria and other microorganisms that are normal, non-pathogenic inhabitants of the gastrointestinal tract.

Micronucleus test	A test for mutagenicity using red blood cell stem cells from mice. Mice are exposed to the chemical and after a suitable time period the bone marrow is examined for an increase in the number of micronuclei—i.e. chromosome fragments resulting from spindle or centromere dysfunction.
Microsomes/microsomal	Subcellular fraction containing fragments of smooth endoplasmic reticulum (sER) after ultracentrifugation of a homogenate of the cell.
Mitochondria	Intracellular organelle where respiration and other important metabolic reactions take place.
Monooxygenase	Enzyme system (such as cytochrome P450) involved in the oxidation of compounds.
Mutagen/mutagenic	A substance/property of a substance which causes a mutation in the genetic material of an organism exposed to it.
Mutagenesis	Process in which a heritable change in DNA is produced.
Myocardium	Middle and thickest layer of cardiac muscle in the heart wall.
NADH	Coenzyme reduced nicotinamide adenine dinucleotide.
NADPH	Coenzyme reduced nicotinamide adenine dinucleotide phosphate.
Narcosis	Unconsciousness induced by exposure to a solvent, volatile liquid, or gas.
Necrosis	Death of areas of tissue, usually surrounded by healthy tissue and sometimes caused by chemical exposure. Distinct from apoptosis, which is a limited event, necrosis also involves an inflammatory response and wider areas of tissue.
Nephritis	Inflammation of the kidney.
Nephron	Functional unit of the kidney responsible for filtering blood in the production of urine. Consists of the glomerulus and a system of tubules divided into sections where reabsorption of solutes from blood into the systemic circulation occurs.
NOAEL	No Observed Adverse Effect Level. The dose or exposure level at where no adverse effect is detected in the organism.
Occlusion	Constriction or blockage as with a blood vessel.
Organelle	Subcellular structure such as the mitochondrion or nucleus of a cell.

Osteomalacia	Softening of the bones due to impaired mineralization.
Paresthesias	Abnormal neural sensations such as tingling of the digits.
Partition coefficient	Ratio of the solubility of a chemical in an aqueous solvent to that in a hydrophobic solvent. A high value indicates that a chemical is lipid-soluble (lipophilic).
Peripheral neuropathy	Damage to nerves of the peripheral, rather than central, nervous system.
Peroxidases	Enzymes that catalyze oxidation utilizing hydrogen peroxide. Found in many tissues including a variety of white blood cells (neutrophils).
Peroxisomal proliferators	Chemicals which change the number and characteristics of peroxisomes; intracellular organelles perform oxidation of fatty acids.
Persistence	When applied to a chemical substance refers to its ability to remain unchanged in the environment.
Pesticide	A chemical agent used to exterminate various pests. Includes insecticides, herbicides and fungicides.
Phagocytosis/pinocytosis	The uptake of a suspended substance (phago-) or solution (pino-) into a cell by invagination of the cell membrane eventually forming a vesicle inside the cell.
Pharmacodynamic	Relating to the effects of drugs on living systems.
Phase 1	Term applied to the first stage of drug metabolism, commonly involving either oxidation, reduction or hydrolysis of the molecule.
Phase 2	Term applied to the second stage of drug metabolism usually involving conjugation of a functional group with a moiety available endogenously and conferring water solubility on the molecule.
Phenotype	Expression of the genotype or genetic make-up of an organism.
Phocomelia	Syndrome of development of foreshortened arms and legs due to an adverse effect on the embryo, such as caused by thalidomide.
Phospholipid	A lipid where one of the hydroxyl groups of glycerol or sphingosine is esterified with a phosphorylated alcohol.

pH Partition Theory	States that a foreign compound in the non-ionized state will pass across a cell membrane by passive diffusion down a concentration gradient.
Plasma	Blood from which the cellular components have been removed by centrifugation but distinct from serum, where the blood is first allowed to clot.
Pneumonitis	Inflammation of the lungs.
Polar	Term used to describe a molecule which is charged or tends to become polarized.
Polychlorinated biphenyls	PCBs; group of industrial compounds where a biphenyl nucleus is substituted with various numbers of chlorine atoms.
Polypeptide	Chain of amino acids joined by peptide bonds.
Portal	Term applied to the venous circulation draining the tissues of the gastrointestinal tract into the liver.
Potentiation	When the toxic effect of a compound is increased by a nontoxic compound.
PPAR	Peroxisome proliferator-activated receptor; receptor involved in the induction of peroxisomal enzymes.
ppb	Parts per billion. A measure of concentration of a substance in which the units of the substance are one billionth of the units of the solvent, e.g. ng/g; 10^{-9}.
ppm	Parts per million. A measure of concentration of a substance in which the units of the substance are one-millionth of the units of the solvent, e.g. $\mu g/g$; 10^{-6}.
Prescribed disease	An industrial disease which is recognized as such for the purposes of compensation.
Promotion	Second stage in the multi-stage process of carcinogenesis which normally follows initiation in order for a tumor to develop.
Psychoactive drugs	Drugs which produce behavioural changes.
Ptaquiloside	Glucoside of a three-ring compound found naturally in bracken which yields a carcinogenic product.
Pulmonary edema	Accumulation of tissue fluid in the alveoli (air spaces) of the lungs.
Quantal response	All-or-none, rather than graded, response.
Rainout	Removal of acids from the atmosphere by rain.
Raynaud's	Changes in the blood supply to the fingers and toes; results from phenomenon degeneration of small blood vessels leading to occlusion of capillaries and arterioles; frequently caused by vinyl chloride.

Reaginic	Relating to reagin, an antibody of the IgE type.
Renal elimination	Excretion of a substance through the kidneys.
Rhinitis	Inflammation of the mucous membranes of the nose.
Ribosomes	Intracellular organelles attached to the endoplasmic reticulum and involved with protein synthesis.
Risk	'Risk is a measure of the probability that an adverse effect will occur'. May be an absolute risk which is the excess risk due to exposure, or relative risk which is the ratio of risk in the exposed to the unexposed population.
Saturated	A molecule where all the bonds of the carbon atoms are occupied and there are no double or triple bonds.
Silicosis	Damage to the lungs caused by exposure to substances such as silica or coal dust.
Singlet oxygen	Oxygen in the singlet, excited state and therefore highly reactive.
Sinusoids	Spaces filled with blood which in the liver are a continuation of the capillaries.
Skink	Australian reptile.
Smog	Originally used to describe the combination of smoke and *fog* (portmanteau) but has since been described as 'reducing smog'. Photochemical (oxidant) smog is the result of interaction between the pollution caused mainly by car exhausts and sunlight.
Steatosis	Abnormal fatty infiltration in an organ or tissue.
Sub-chronic	28 or 90-day exposure of duration intermediate between acute and chronic.
Superoxide $\left(O_2^- \right)$	Oxygen molecule with an extra, unpaired electron; a charged free radical.
Symport	Membrane carrier system where two chemicals or electrolytes are transported in the same direction.
Synergism/synergistic	When the pharmacologic or toxic effect of a mixture is greater than the sum of the toxicities of the components.
Systemic toxicity	Toxicity which affects a system in the organism other than and probably distant from the site of application or exposure.
TD_{50}	The dose which is toxic to 50% of the population of organisms exposed to the substance or a 50% toxic response in a biological system exposed to the substance.

Teratogen/teratogenicity	A substance/property of a substance causing abnormalities in the embryo or fetus when administered to the maternal organism.
Therapeutic index	Ratio of ED_{50} to TD_{50}.
Thiol	SH or sulphydryl group.
TLV	Threshold Limit Value. Upper permissive limits of airborne concentrations of substances.
Tolerance	When repeated administration of, or dosing with, a compound leads to a decrease in the potency in the biological activity of that compound; also when the same repeated dose of a compound does not have the intended predictable effect of the initial doses.
Toxicodynamics	Study of the effects of toxic substances on biological systems (e.g. interaction with receptors).
Toxicokinetics	Study of the kinetics of toxic substances in biological systems (e.g. disposition).
Uniport	Membrane carrier system where one chemical or electrolyte is transported in one direction.
Unsaturated	Term applied to molecules that contain double or triple carbon-carbon bonds.
Urticaria	Vascular reaction of the skin marked by the appearance of wheals; caused by direct or indirect exposure to a toxic substance; hives.
Vascularized	Relating to tissue that is supplied with blood vessels such as arteries, veins or capillaries.
Vasculitis	Inflammation of the vessels of the vascular system.
Vasodilation	Dilation of arterial blood vessels.
Veno-occlusive disease	A particular type of liver damage where the blood vessels and sinusoids of the liver are damaged leading to new vessel growth.
V_D	Volume of distribution. Volume of physiological fluid in which a compound is apparently distributed when administered to a subject.
Washout	Removal of acids from clouds by rain.
Zero order process	Rate of the process is independent of the concentration of the substance.

Index

Note: **Bold** page numbers refer to tables and *italic* page numbers refer to figures.

AA *see* aromatic amines (AA)
absolute excess risk 216
absorbants 245
absorption of toxic compounds *42*, 42–45, *43*
absorption, sites of 45–51
  gastrointestinal tract (GIT) 48–51, *49*, *50*
  lungs 46–47, *47*
  skin 45, *46*
acceptable daily intake (ADI) 23, 236
accidental poisoning, unintentional 11
accumulation 8, 89
  of acetaldehyde 22
  of acetylcholine 159
  of cadmium 127
  and chronic dosing 53
  of fluid 93
  of lactic acid 204
  reduction by metabolism 82
acetaldehyde, accumulation of 22
acetaminophen (paracetamol) 67, 108–110, *109*, 120
acetic acid 150, 154, 208
acetylation 67, *76*, 76–77
  of 2-naphthylamine *128*
acetylator phenotype 80, 114, 128
acetylcholine, accumulation of 159
acetylcholinesterases 155
  and organophosphorus compounds 155–156
N-acetylcysteine (NAC) 110, 246
acetylsalicylate 110–113, *111*

acetylsalicylic acid (ASA) 110–113, *111*
acetyltransferase 76, 80
Ach 156
acidosis 203
  metabolic 112
acid rain 168–170, 185
  effects of 168
acne 126
aconite (wolfsbane) 3
activation, metabolic 96, 98, 126, 127, 131, 191
  acetaminophen 110
  benzo(a)pyrene to reactive substrates *97*
activation, T-cell 32
active transport 43, 58
  and paraquat 156
acute exposure 28
acute liver failure 141
acute toxic class method (ATCM) 219
acute toxicity 10, 108, 220
acute toxicity tests 219–220
additives, food 8, 135, 136, **136**
ADH *see* alcohol dehydrogenase (ADH)
adhesion molecules 198
ADI *see* acceptable daily intake (ADI); allowable daily intake (ADI)
adipose tissue 51
ADR *see* adverse drug reactions (ADR)
β-adrenoceptors 30
adverse drug effect (ADR) 108
adverse drug reactions (ADR) 215

adverse effects of hydralazine 31
aerobic bacteria 177
aflatoxin B1 141, *141*
aflatoxins 35, 141, *141*, 197
African puff adder **195**
AhR *see* aryl hydrocarbon receptor (AhR)
Ah receptor 184
air filtration 166
air pollution 165–167
ALA *see* aminolevulinic acid (ALA)
ALAD *see* aminolevulinic acid dehydratase
      (ALAD)
ALAS *see* aminolevulinate synthetase
      (ALAS)
alcohol (ethanol, ethyl alcohol)
      22, 82, 208
alcohol dehydrogenase (ADH) 204
    and ethylene glycol/methanol 246
alcohol metabolism 82
aldehyde 71
aldehyde dehydrogenase (ADH) 22, *205*, 246
aliphatic hydroxylation 70
alkaloids
    pyrrolizidine 190–191, *192*
    vinca 34
alkalosis 110
alkylating agents 35
alkylmercury fungicides 176
alkylphenols 181, **182**
allergy/allergic reactions 10, 30, 31, 38, 137
all-or-none (absolute) responses 16
allowable daily intake (ADI) 177
altered cell membrane determinants 32
alveolus 47, *47*, 60
Amanita phalloides 196
amanitins 196
amatoxins 196
Ames test 239
amidases 72–73
amides 73
amino acid conjugation 77
4-aminobiphenyl 128
aminolevulinate synthetase (ALAS) 172
aminolevulinic acid (ALA) 172
aminolevulinic acid dehydratase (ALAD) 172
amphetamine 58
amplification 151
amygdalin 206
anaerobic bacteria 177
anaphylactic reactions 195
androgen receptor (AR) 183
anemia
    aplastic 71
    drug-induced hemolytic 119
    iron deficiency 172

anesthetic, metabolism of *72*
aneuploidization 34
aneuploidy 34
aniline 119, 128, 143
    ionisation in GI tract 48
animal model 79, 143
animal toxins 193, 194–196, *194*
    snake venoms 195, **195**
    tetrodotoxin 195, 196
animal welfare 216–217
annatto 139
ANS *see* autonomic nervous system (ANS)
antagonism 22
anti-androgens 180, 183, 184
anti-arrhythmic agents **90**
antibiotic penicillin 12, 31
antibody 32
antibody fragments 247
antidotes 196, 246–247
    acting via receptors 246–247
antifreeze 204–206
antigen 31
antihistamine 30
antihypertensive drug 113
antiporters 44
antivenoms 247
aplastic anemia 71
The Apocalyptics: Cancer and the Big Lie
    (Efron) 2
apoptosis 92
Aqua Toffana 5
area under the curve (AUC) 24, 51, 52, *52*, 54
aromatase 181
aromatic amines (AA) 127, 128, 131
    carcinogenic *128*
aromatic amino group, N-hydroxylation of *71*
aromatic hydroxylation 70
arrhythmias
    cardiac 203
    ventricular 209
arsenic 4
artificial sweetener 139–140
aryl hydrocarbon receptor (AhR) 21, 81
asbestos 29, 35, 45, 46, 129, 131
asbestosis 130
ash dieback 169
Aspergillus flavus 141, 144, 197, 198
aspirin 30, 110–113, *111*, 118, 120
asthma 137, 139
ATCM *see* acute toxic class method (ATCM)
atmosphere 184
ATP 110–112, 120, 206–207, *207*
ATPases 195
atropine 190
AUC 24, 51, 52, *52*, 54

autoimmunity 30
autonomic nervous system (ANS) 92

BAC *see* blood alcohol concentration (BAC)
bacteria
    aerobic 177
    anaerobic 177
β-adrenergic receptor antagonists
        (β-blocker) **90**
BAL *see* British Anti-Lewisite (BAL)
barbiturates 54, **90**
base-pair
    additions 34
    deletions 34
    transformations 34
    transition 34
    transversion 34
BBB *see* blood-brain barrier (BBB)
belladonna 190
benzene 67
    metabolism of *67*
    oxidation/hydroxylation of 70, *70*, 71
benzoic acid 48
    conjugation *75*
benzo(a)pyrene 35, 96, *97*
    metabolic activation of *97*
Bernard, Claude 7, 202
Bhopal (India), industrial disasters in 7
bias 178
bile 89
bile duct/canaliculi 58
biliary 37
    elimination 58–60
binding 21, 24
    of botulinum toxin 197
    of carbon monoxide 30
    of carbon monoxide to hemoglobin
        30, 247, 267, 269
    of chemical agent 58
    to plasma protein 54, 58, 61
    protein 58
    of reduced substrate (RH) displaces *69*
    of ricin 192
bioaccumulation 59, 159, *176*, 221
biochemical indices 214
biochemical lesions 30, 38, 93
biochemical oxygen demand (BOD) 177
biological factors 78, 83, 218
biological half-life 66
biological membranes structure 42
biomagnification 151, 180
biomarkers 36–37
    in risk assessment 238
    of susceptibility 36–37
    types *37*

biotransformation 66
    reaction, features and characteristics **68**
biphenyls
    polybrominated 55
    polychlorinated 66
black-foot disease 174
bladder cancer 128, 131, 237
bladder tumors 139, 140
bleach 202
blebbing 87
blindness 206
BLL *see* blood lead levels (BLL)
blood alcohol concentration (BAC) 208
blood-brain barrier (BBB) 54, 94, 156, 174
blood lead levels (BLL) 171
blood supply 30, 45–48, 51, 59, 68, 88, 89,
        127, 191
BOD *see* biochemical oxygen demand (BOD)
body burden 52
bone marrow 32, *33*, 38, 71
Borgias 5
botulinum toxin 140, 141, 190, 197–198
botulism 197
Bracken 192–193, *194*
breast cancer 182
breast milk 60
British Anti-Lewisite (BAL) 7
brittle bone syndrome 169
bromouracil 35
bronchial carcinoma 130
butter yellow (4-dimethylaminoazobenzene)
        145
butylated hydroxytoluene **136**

cadmium 127, 131
calcium 127
calcium oxalate 204
    crystals 204
Californian newt 195
cancer 35, 95
    bladder 128, 131, 237
    breast 182
    chemopreventive agents 100–101
    skin 174
    throat 264
cantharides (blistering agent) 3
cantharidin *194*
carbon monoxide (CO) 22, 30, 46, 167,
        202–204, *203*
    binding to hemoglobin 30, 247,
        267, 269
    poisoning, symptoms 204
carbon tetrachloride 16, 22, 89
carboxy hemoglobin 203
carcinogen 96

carcinogenesis 38, 96
    chemical 35
    mechanisms of chemical 96–98, *97*
    multistage 98–99
carcinogenic aromatic amines *128*
carcinogenicity 35–36
carcinogenicity tests 223
carcinogens
    chemical 99–100
    IARC classification of **233**, 234
    nongenotoxic (epigenetic) 98
carcinoma, bronchial 130
cardiac arrhythmias 203
cardiac damage 203
cardiac toxicity 89–90, **90**
cardiovascular disease 166
cardiovascular system functions 89
car exhausts 165, 166–167, 170, 184
Carson, Rachel 2
carvedilol 80
case control studies 215
cassava 206
castor oil plant 192
catalytic converters 170
Catherine de Medici 5
cats 11, 79
cell membrane 42, *42*, 43, 46, 92, 115,
        192, 254
    determinants 32
Center for Drug Evaluation and Research
        (CDER) 220
central nervous system (CNS) 54
    depression 156, 208
cerebral palsy 176
ceruse (white lead) 3
CFCs *see* chlorofluorocarbons (CFCs)
chelating agents 246
chemical carcinogenesis 35
chemical carcinogens 99–100
chemical factors 78, 117
chemical hazards, notoriety of 123
chemical ionization of weak acids (WA) *50*
chemical oxygen demand (COD) 177
chemicals, industrial 8–9
chemical substance, lipid solubility of 43
chemical welfare 159
chemopreventive agents, cancer 100–101
chirality 117
chlordane 234
chlordecone 183
chlorinated hydrocarbons 124, 125
chloroacetaldehyde 126
chloroethylene oxide 126
chlorofluorocarbons (CFCs) 170
chloroform-induced kidney damage 80

chlorphentermine 30
cholesterol
    esters 42
    lowering drug 35–36
cholinesterase 79, 117, 148, 214
chronic exposure 28, 147, 150, 153
    to aflatoxin 197
    to alcohol 208
    to cadmium 127
    to insecticides 125
    to lead 148
    to pyrrolizidine alkaloids 191
chronic toxicity 28, 108, 159, 197, 206
    due to pesticides 148
    effects 10
chronic toxicity tests 221–223
cigarette 8
cigarette smoking 81, 100, 127, 167
cirrhosis 208
    liver 191
classification of toxic substances 7–9
clastogenesis 34
Claudius 4–5
Clean Air Act 164
clearance
    plasma 140, 255
    renal 67
    total body 54
climate change 165
clinical toxicology laboratories 247
clofibrate 35
Clostridium botulinum 197
CNS effects 92
COD *see* chemical oxygen demand (COD)
cohort studies 215
complex proteins 194
concentration factor 178
coniine (hemlock) 190
conium (hemlock) 3
conjugation
    amino acid 77
    reactions 74
consequences of metabolism 82
Consumer Products Safety Commission
        (CPSC) 230
contact dermatitis 125, 131
contact hypersensitivity 32
contaminants, food 140–143
contraceptive hormones 181
contraceptive steroids 118
control limit 130
converters, catalytic 170
coproporphyrin 172
cosmetics 5, 213, 219
coumestans 183

covalent binding 87, 109
CPSC *see* Consumer Products Safety
    Commission (CPSC)
crocidolite 130
cross-sectional studies 215
cryptorchidism 182
crystals, calcium oxalate 204
cumulative toxic effect 28
curare 7
cyanide (CN) 206–208
    antidote package 207
    inhibits 7
    site of action of *207*
cyanogenic glycoside 206
cycasin 60
cyclamate 139–140
cytisine 190
cytochrome aa₃ 206
cytochrome P450 enzymes 69–70, *69*, 96,
    100, 110
cytotoxic compounds 33

DADPM *see* diaminodiphenylmethane
    (DADPM)
Daphnia 151, 180, 219, 239
DDD *see* dichloro-diphenyldichloroethane
    (DDD)
DDE *see* dichloro-diphenyldichloroethylene
    (DDE)
DDT *see* dichloro-diphenyl-trichloroethane
    (DDT)
deadly nightshade *(Atropa belladonna)* 190
dealkylation 71, *71*
death cap mushroom 196
debrisoquine 116, *116*, *117*, 120
dehalogenation, reductive 72
Delaney Clause of the Food, Drug and
    Cosmetic Act 140, 237
deoxyribonucleic acid (DNA), mutations
    in 95
depression, central nervous system (CNS)
    156, 208
dermal diseases 124
dermatitis 10, 125
    contact 125, 131
dermis *46*
DES *see* diethylstilbestrol (DES)
descalers 202
desulphuration, oxidative 11
detergents 202
detoxification *vs.* toxification 78, *78*
detritivore food chains 178
diamines 156
diaminodiphenylmethane (DADPM) 128
diamondback rattlesnake 195

dichloro-diphenyldichloroethane (DDD)
    150, *151*
dichloro-diphenyldichloroethylene (DDE)
    150, *151*, 151, 179, 182, 183, 266
dichloro-diphenyl-trichloroethane (DDT) 11,
    60, 66, 79, 149–150, **150**, *151*, 178
dichlorvos 201
dieldrin 179, 185
diethylstilbestrol (DES) 34, 182, 183
diffusion
    defined 44
    facilitated 44, 57
    passive 44
Digitalis glycosides **90**
Digitalis purpurea 90
digoxin 90
dimethylformamide 82
dinitrotoluene-induced hepatic tumors 80
dinoflagellates 193
dioscorides 4
dioxin 183
dioxin, 2,3,7,8-tetrachlorodibenzo-ρ-dioxin
    (TCDD) 21, 32, 183
direct immunotoxicity 30
direct tissue damage 37, 93
disruptors, endocrine 180–184
distribution of toxic compounds 51–55
disulphiram 22
diuresis, forced 158
DNA
    double-strand breaks (DSBs) in 100
    methylation 235
    repair mechanisms 98
dog whelk 181
dominant lethal assay 222
dosage 5, 16, *17*, 18, 19, 28, 96, 218
    toxic 218
dose
    maximum tolerated dose (MTD) 235
    threshold dose for toxic effects 23
    virtually safe dose (VSD) 237
dose-response
    effects 16
    relationship 12, 15–21, *17*, *19*, **19–21**,
        20, 23
    relationship, and Paracelsus 12
double-strand breaks (DSBs) in DNA 100
drain cleaners 202
drug
    abuse of 108, 247
    antihypertensive 113
    cholesterol-lowering 35
    enzymatic hydrolysis of *66*
    interactions and 108, 118–119, 120
    novel peptide 32

drug (*cont.*)
   psychoactive 91
   safety evaluation of 79, 107, 117, 216
   xenobiotic 54
drug abuse 108, 247
drug-induced hemolytic anemia 119
drug interactions 108, 118–119, 120
drug overdose 108
drug toxicity, types 108
dry deposition 168

earthworms 185, 219, 239
Ebers papyrus 3
E. coli infections 197–198
ecological studies 215
ecotoxicity testing 177
ecotoxicology 221
ED *see* endocrine disruptors (ED)
ED_{50} 19, *19*, 21, 24
EDCs *see* endocrine-disrupting
       chemicals (EDCs)
EES *see* ethynylestradiol (EES)
Efron, Edith 2
EFSA *see* European Food Safety Authority
    (EFSA)
eggs 151, 152, 178–179
   fish 178
eggshells 151–152, 179
   thickness 215
elemental mercury 174
EMA *see* European Medicines Agency (EMA)
embryo 29, 33, 118, 221
embryogenesis 33
emetics 4, 247
encephalopathy 171
   lead 172
endocrine-disrupting chemicals (EDCs) 181,
    182
   applications and probable disease links **182**
endocrine disruptors (ED) 180–184
enterohepatic recirculation 59
E Number 136
environmental exposure 10–11
environmental factors 81–82
environmental pollutants 9, 163–186
environmental pollution 163
enzymatic hydrolysis 11
enzyme induction 81, 82, 118, 120, 153
enzymes 36, 68
   acetyltransferase 76, 80
   genetic deficiencies in 36
   sulfhydryl groups of 177
enzyme variant 116
epidemiological studies 215–216
epidemiologic studies 140

epidemiology 214, 225, 239
epidermis *46*, 93, 125
epigenetic mechanisms 35, 38, 140
epigenetics 36
epoxide hydrolase 73, 83
Epping jaundice 128
ER *see* estrogen receptor (ER)
erythrosine 139
esterases 72, 73
   polymorphisms in 80
esters
   cholesterol 42
   phthalate 35–36
estrogen, potent 183, 184
estrogen receptor (ER) 183, 184
ethanol 204, 208
   intake of 58
   metabolism 80
   oxidation of *73*
ethionine 35, 88
ethyl alcohol 208
ethylene glycol (EG) (antifreeze)
    204–206, *205*
ethynylestradiol (EES) 181, 183
European Food Safety Authority (EFSA) 230
European Medicines Agency (EMA) 230
eutrophication 177
evaluation of toxicity 214–215
excretion 11, 56
   of aminolevulinic acid (ALA) in urine 172
   biliary 58
   renal 58
   urinary 246
exotoxins 198
experimental testing, considerations for
    217–220
expired air 67
exposure 7–9
   biomarkers of 36, 38, 239
   limits 23, 127, 131, 237
   to mixtures 22
   repeated 10, 22, 24, 28, 61, 81
   route of 28–29
exposure classification 10–12
   environmental exposure 10–11
   intentional ingestion 10
   occupational exposure 10
   selective toxicity 11–12
   unintentional, accidental poisoning 11
exposure response database (ERDB) 233
exposure types 27–28
   acute 28
   chronic (*see* chronic exposure)
   continuous/intermittent exposure 28
extrapolation, between species 237

facilitated diffusion 44, 58
fatal human poisonings 156
fatty acids 42, 143, 208
fatty liver 30, 89, 208
fava beans 119
favism 119
FEP *see* free erythrocyte
      protoporphyrin (FEP)
fertility 221
fertilizers 177
fiberglass 46
fibers, size of 129, 130
fibrosis 129, 157
Fick's Law 44
filtration 44–45
first-order process 44
first-pass metabolism 54
first pass phenomenon 88
fish 151, 152, 169, 175, 180, 181
    eggs 178
fixed-dose approach (FDP) 219
flavonoid 84
fluid mosaic model of mammalian lipid
      bilayer cell membrane *42*
fluoroacetate 30, 158–159
fluorocitrate 7, 159
fluorouracil 44
fog 165
fomepizole 204
food 48
    contaminants 140–143
    prolongs gastric emptying time 48
food additives 8, 135
    classification of 135, **136**
Food and Drug Administration (FDA) 220
food chain 151, **152**, 175, 178–180, 185
    detritivore 178
    grazing 178
food-coloring agent, metabolic reduction
      of *73*
food contaminants 140–143
    aflatoxins 141, *141*
    botulinum toxin 141
    ginger jake 142
    toxic oil (spanish oil) syndrome 142–143
food web 178
foot drop 142
forced diuresis 157
forensic toxicology 5
    laboratories 247
formaldehyde 206
formic acid 190, 193
Fos gene 92
frameshift mutations 34
free erythrocyte protoporphyrin (FEP) 172

free radical 157
fungal toxins 196
    aflatoxins 197
    death cap mushroom 196
fungicides 148, **149**
    alkylmercury 176
    mercury 147–148
    organomercury 175
furosemide 58, 89

galactosamine 88
Galen 5
gaseous effluents 10
gastroenteritis 196
gastrointestinal tract (GIT) 28, 88
    microflora (normal flora) 60
    route of exposure 28–29
    sites of absorption 48–51, *49, 50*
general supportive measures 244–246
genetic activity profile (GAP) database 233
genetically modified variations 217
genetic deficiencies in enzymes 36
genetic factors 76, 80, 83, 120
genetic polymorphisms 70
genetic toxicity 34–35, 38
genistein 181
genomics 36
genotoxicity 96
gentamycin 89
ginger jake 142
GIT *see* gastrointestinal tract (GIT)
glomerulus 56
GLP *see* Good Laboratory Practice (GLP)
gluconeogenesis 208
glucose-6-phosphate dehydrogenase
      deficiency 119
glucuronic acid 75, *75*, 79, 83, 109, 110, 128
glucuronidation 74–75, *75*
glucuronide 80, *111*
glue sniffing 208–209
glutathione (GSH) 75, 109
glutathione conjugation 75, *76*
glutathione disulfide (GSSG) 119
glutathione transferases 75
glycine 77
goiter 208
Good Laboratory Practice (GLP) 223
graded responses 16
grazing food chain 178
"great smog" in London (1952) 164, *164*
GSH *see* glutathione (GSH)

hemoglobin, binding of carbon monoxide to
      30, 247, 267, 269
Haldane 202

half-life 24, 51, 53–55, 61, 82, 171
  biological 66
  of cadmium 127
halogenated solvents 209
halothane *115*, 115–116, 120
  hepatotoxicity of 31
  metabolism of 72, *72*
hapten 31
hazards 8
  identification, risk assessment (RA)
    231–232
  notoriety of chemical 123
HC *see* hydrocarbons (HC)
heart attacks 209
heavy metals 77, 89, 124, 172, 177, 184
Heliotropium 191, 198
heme 171
heme synthesis 172
  iron-bound *173*
hemlock 3, 4, *4*, 190
hemodialysis 204, 245
hemoglobin 167, 202, *203*
hemolysis, intravascular 195
hemolytic anemia, drug-induced 119
hemoperfusion 204, 245
Henderson–Hasselbach equation 45, 48,
    61, 112
hepatic necrosis 109
hepatic tumors, dinitrotoluene-induced 80
hepatocytes 58, 88
hepatotoxicity of halothane 31
herbicides 148, **149**
  types of 147–149
hermaphroditic mutations 181
hexachlorobutadiene 89
Hippocrates 3, 170
HLA phenotype *see* human leukocyte antigen
    (HLA) phenotype
HLA type DR4 114, 120
hormonal imbalance 153
hormones, contraceptive 181
household poisons 9
human carcinogens 99, 100
human leukocyte antigen (HLA)
    phenotype 114
human milk 153
human poisonings
  fatal 156
  mass 154
human teratogen 117
hydralazine 71, 113–114, *114*, 120
  adverse effects of 31
hydration 73
hydrocarbons (HC) 167, 208–209
  chlorinated 125, 126

hydrocarbon solvents 202
hydrogen bonding 54
hydrogen cyanide (HCN) 17–18, 22, 206
hydrogen peroxide 36, 157
hydrolase, epoxide 73, 83
hydrolysis 73, *74*
  enzymatic 11
hydrophobic bonding 54
16α-hydroxyestrone 184
hydroxylation
  aliphatic 70
  aromatic 70
hydroxyl group 67, 74
hydroxyl radicals 157
hyoscyamus (henbane) 3
hyperkinetic behavior 139
hypersensitivity 30–31
  contact 32
  reactions 31
hypospadia 182

IACUCs *see* Institutional Animal Care and
    Use Committees (IACUCs)
immune response 139, 262
immunological mechanisms 125
immunostimulation 30, 32
immunosuppression 32
immunotoxicity 38
  direct 30
  indirect 30
  toxic responses 30–32
imposex 181
indirect immunotoxicity 30
industrial chemicals 8–9
  hazardous 126
  occupational and commercial use of
    123–124
  toxic effects of 124–126
industrial disasters in Bhopal, India 7
industrial diseases 124–126, 129, 131
industrial metals 32
Industrial Revolution 164
inflammation 29, 125
  acute 93
  liver 128
ingestion, intentional 10
inhalation 28
inhibition of metabolism 246
inhibitors 81
initiation 35, 38, 96–98, 100, 101, 114
inorganic chemicals 5
inorganic lead (Pb) 170
inorganic mercury 174
inquiry dossier 221
insecticide parathion, oxidation of *154*

insecticides 9, 148, **149**
  metabolism of *72*
  organochlorine 179, 181
  organophosphorus (OP) 153–156
Institutional Animal Care and Use
    Committees (IACUCs) 217
intentional ingestion 10
internal dose 238
International Association for Research on
    Cancer (IARC)
  carcinogenicity classification of chemicals
    233–234, **233**
intestine 48, *49, 50,* 58, 59, 80, 88, 198
intravascular hemolysis 195
invagination 45
in vitro testing, as alternatives to animals
    223–224
in vitro toxicology 214, 223
in vivo toxicity tests 217
ionic forces 54
ionization potentials of weak acids (WA) 48
iron-bound heme synthesis *173*
iron deficiency anemia 172
irritancy tests 218, 224
irritants 9, 125, 165, 166–167
irritation 10, 11, 37, 93, 125, 127, 131, 224
ischemic damage 203
ischemic necrosis 127
isoenzymes 69, 70, 76, 110
isoflavone 183
Itai-Itai disease 131, 169

Jake Leg 142
Japanese Itai-Itai disease 169
jaundice, Epping 128
jewelry 32
Joint FAO/WHO Expert Committee on Food
    Additives 136
Jun gene 92

keratin 45
kidney
  damage 47, 80, 89, 125, 127, 156, 169, 172,
    174
  structure and function 56–58
  toxicity 89
kinetic parameters 24
Krebs' cycle 30

laburnum 190
Lake Apopka 181
LD$_{50}$ 18, **19**, *19,* 20, **20, 21,** 24, 139, **195,**
    197, 219, 225
lead 47
  encephalopathy 172

ions 44
  poisoning 170
  pollution 170–174, **171**
lesions
  biochemical 30, 38, 93
  tissue 92–93
lethality 16
limb deformities 117
linamarin 206
linearized multistage model (EPA) 234
linseed tea 3
lipid peroxidation 87, 157
lipid solubility 24, 45, 61, 180, 236
  of chemical substance 43
lipid-soluble compounds 45, 47, 48
lipophilicity 32, 70, 78, 83
lipophilic xenobiotics 55
lipoproteins 54
liquid effluents 10
liquids, non-volatile 10
litharge (lead oxide) 3
liver
  blood to 274
  cirrhosis 191
  damage to 79, 80, 81, 109, 110, 115, 126,
    131, 150, 191, 197, 198, 209
  failure, acute 141
  first-pass metabolism and 54
  necrosis 89, 93, 196
  toxicity *88,* 88–89
LOAEL 239
Loop of Henle 57
lungs
  absorption via 46–47
  damage to 158, 159
  structure 46–47, *47*
lupus erythematosus 113
lymphocytes 32, 38, 115, 120, 181

Maimonides 5
malaoxon 148, *149,* 156
malarial mosquitoes 149
malathion 154, 156
  metabolism of *72*
malignant tumors 35
mammalian lipid bilayer cell membrane, fluid
    mosaic model of *42*
mammalian lungs 46, *47*
margin of safety 19, 21, 24, 130
Markov, Georgi 192
mass human poisonings 154
Max gene 92
maximum exposure limit (MEL) 23, 127
maximum tolerated dose (MTD) 235
means of exposure 124

MEL *see* maximum exposure limit (MEL)
membranes 42, 51
meperidine 78
    metabolism of *78*
meperidinic acid 78
mercapturic acid 75, *76*
mercury 89, 174–177, 185
    elemental 174
    fungicides 147–148
    inorganic 174
    organic 174
mescaline 196
mesothelioma 129
metabolic acidosis 111–112
metabolism
    of benzene *67*
    of drugs 107–121
    factors affecting 78–82
    first-pass 54
    inhibition of 246
    saturation of 137
metabolism of foreign compounds 153
metabolism of xenobiotic compounds 66
    phase I reactions 67
        cytochrome P$_{450}$ 69–70, *69*
        hydration 73–74
        hydrolysis 72–73, *74*
        oxidation reactions 68, 70–71, *70–72*
        reduction reactions 71–72
    phase II reactions 74
        acetylation 76, *77*
        amino acid conjugation 77
        glucuronidation 74–75, *75*
        glutathione conjugation 75–76, *76*
        methylation 77
        sulfation 74, *74*
metabolite 36
    polar 118
metabonomics 36
metallothionein 127
metals
    arsenic (As) 174
    industrial 32
    lead pollution 170–174, **171**
    mercury and methylmercury 174–177
methanol 204, 206
methemoglobinemia 128
methylation 77
    DNA 235
methylazoxy methanol 60
4,4′-methylene-bis-O-(2-chloroaniline)
        (MBOCA) *128*
methylene chloride 46
methyl isocyanate 7
methyl mercury 55, 174–177, *176*, 178

methyltransferases 77
microbial toxins 197–198
    Botulism and Botulinum Toxin 197
    E. coli infections and exotoxins 197–198
micronucleus test 222
milk 60, 153
Minamata Bay 175
Minamata disease 175
Mithradatic effect 4
Mithridates 3
mitosis (aneuploidization) 34
mixtures 22, 100, 139, 165, 167, 197
molecular weight 67, 125, 127, 224, 245
Mojave rattler **195**
molecules, adhesion 198
monocrotaline 191
monofluoroacetate 158
monooxygenase system 116
mosquitoes, malarial 149
motor cortex 150
motor nerve fibers 150
MTD *see* maximum tolerated dose (MTD)
multi-hit model 234
multistage carcinogenesis 98–99
multi-stage process 35
muscle relaxant 117
mushroom, death cap 196–197
mutagenesis 34, 96, 98
mutagenicity 35, 140, 225, 239
mutagenicity tests 222
mutations 34
    in deoxyribonucleic acid (DNA) 95
    frameshift 34
    hermaphroditic 181
Myc gene 92
mycotoxins 141

NADPH *see* nicotinamide adenine
        dinucleotide phosphate hydrogen
        (NADPH)
NADPH CYP$_{450}$ reductase 69
naloxone 22
naphthalene *76*
β-naphthoflavone 81
2-naphthylamine, acetylation of *128*
narcosis 209
National Toxicology Program (NTP) 140, 145
naturally occurring toxins 9
natural substances 137
natural toxins 9, 190, 195
necrosis 92–93
    hepatic 109
    ischemic 127
    liver 89, 93, 196
neoplastic (cancerous) cells 35

nephritis 172
nephron 56, *57*
nervous system, toxicity of *91*, 91–92
neuromuscular junction 197
neuromuscular paralysis 156
neuropathy, peripheral 156
neurotoxic agents 91
neurotoxic proteins 197
N-hydroxylation of aromatic amino group *71*
Nicander of Colophon 3
nickel 125
nicotinamide adenine dinucleotide phosphate
        hydrogen (NADPH) 69, 119
nicotine 100
nicotine-derived nitrosamine ketone
        (NNK) 100
nitric acids, wet precipitation of 168
nitrogen dioxide 166
nitrogen oxide 46, 165, 166–170, 184
NNK *see* nicotine-derived nitrosamine
        ketone (NNK)
NOAEL *see* no-observed-adverse-effect
        level (NOAEL)
NOEL *see* no observed effect level (NOEL)
nongenotoxic (epigenetic) carcinogens 98
non-ionized compounds 48, 51
non-volatile liquids 10
nonylphenol 181
no-observed-adverse-effect level (NOAEL)
        23, 130, 216
no observed effect level (NOEL) 220, 237–239
norbormide 11
normeperidine 78
notoriety of chemical hazards 123
novel peptide drugs 32
noxious xenobiotics 55
NTP *see* National Toxicology Program (NTP)

occupational exposure 10
occupational exposure limits 130
Occupational Safety and Health
        Administration (OSHA) 152
OCPs *see* organochlorine pesticides (OCPs)
octylphenol 181, 183
odds ratio 216
one-hit model 234
opioid 246
opioid analgesic drug, metabolism of *78*
opium (narcotic) 3
oral absorption 51
Orfila 5
organic acids, xenobiotic 77
organic lead (Pb) 170
organic mercury 174
organic waste products 177

Organization for Economic Cooperation and
        Development (OECD) 223
organochlorine insecticides 179, 181
organochlorine pesticides (OCPs) 58
organochlorines 153
organomercury 77, 175
organomercury fungicides 175
organophosphates 144, 159, 247
organophosphates/organophosphorus
        compounds 91, 144, 159
organophosphorus compounds 79
organophosphor*us* (OP) insecticides
        153–156, *155*
OSHA *see* Occupational Safety and Health
        Administration (OSHA)
osteomalacia 127
oxalate crystals, calcium 204
oxalic acid 204
oxidation 109
    of ethanol *73*
    of insecticide parathion *154*
    of vinyl chloride 70, *70*
oxidation reactions 68
    types 70–71, *70–72*
oxidative desulphuration 11
ozone 165, 166, 168

2-PAM *see* pralidoxime (2-PAM)
PAPS *see* phosphoadenosine phosphosulfate
        (PAPS)
ρ-aminohippuric acid (PABA) 58
Paracelsus 5, 15
paracetamol 108–110, *109*
    clearance 67
    factors affecting toxicity 108–110
    toxicity 109–110
paralysis, neuromuscular 156
paraquat (PQ) 156–159, *157, 158*
parathion 45, 154
paroxetine 80
particle pollution 167
particulate matter (PM) 167–168
partition coefficient 43
passive diffusion 43, 44, 48
    of compounds 58
pathological state 82
PCBs *see* polychlorinated biphenyls (PCBs)
PCC *see* poison control centers (PCC)
peanut butter 141
penicillamine 80
penicillin 32
    antibiotic 12, 31
pennyroyal oil 191
pentobarbital **20**
peptide drugs 32

peregrine falcon 179
peripheral blood supply 51
peripheral neuropathy 156
peroxidases 71
peroxidation, lipid 87, 157
peroxisome 36
peroxisome proliferator-activated receptors
 (PPARs) 17, 36
peroxisome proliferators 35
persistence 9, 149–151, **150**, **152**, 153, 177,
 179, 230
pesticides 9
 chronic toxicity due to 148
 classification of **149**
 human poisonings from accidental
  exposure to **148**
 types of 147–148
Peters, Rudolph, Sir 7
phagocytosis 45
phalloidin 196, 198
phalloin 196
phallolysin 196
pharmaceutical agents 8
pharmacological effects 21, 79, 93, 116
 toxic responses 30, 38
pharmacological interactions 120
PHE, conjugation of *75*
phenobarbital 54, 58, 118
phenol 67
 conjugation of *75*
phenotype, acetylator 128
phocomelia 117
phorbol ester (promoter) 35
phosphoadenosine phosphosulfate (PAPS) 74
phosphodiesterases 195
phospholipases 195
phospholipidosis 30
phospholipids 42
phosphomonoesterases 195
photochemical-oxidant, effects of 166
photochemical-oxidant smog 165
pH-partition theory 44
phthalate ester 35
physicochemical characteristics 48
physicochemical properties 51, 218, **222**, 225
physicochemical properties of compound 51
physiological effects 93
 toxic responses 30, 38
physiologically based pharmacokinetic
 (PBPK) models 234
pinocytosis 45
pK$_a$ 45, 78, 112
placebo 216
plankton 151, 180
plant resins 32

plant toxins 190–193
 Bracken 192–193, *194*
 pennyroyal oil 192
 pyrrolizidine alkaloids 190–191, *192*
 ricin 192
plasma clearance 140, 255
plasma level 24, 52, *53*
plasma proteins 118
 binding 58
plasma t½ 56
plasticizers 35
plastic polyvinyl chloride (PVC) 126
PM *see* particulate matter (PM)
pneumonitis 202
PNS effects 92
poison 3
 household 9
poison control centers (PCC) 244
polarity 67
polar metabolites 118
pollen 46
pollutants, environmental 9
pollution
 air 165–167
 environmental 163
 lead 170–174, **171**
 particle 167
 water 177–178
polyamines 156
polychlorinated biphenyls (PCBs) 55, 58, 66,
 181, 183
polyethylene glycol 245
polymorphisms
 in esterases 80
 genetic 69
polypeptides 192
porphyrin synthesis 172
portal vein 51
potent estrogen 184
potentiation 22
PPARs *see* peroxisome proliferator-activated
 receptors (PPARs)
PQ *see* paraquat (PQ)
pralidoxime (2-PAM) 247
preservatives 136
primaquine 119
primary events 87
probit model 234
procainamide 73, *74*, 76, 80
procaine 73, *74*
progression 99
proliferators, peroxisome 35
promotion 98
proteases 127
protein 42, 54, 192

neurotoxic 197
plasma 58, 119
proteomics 36
protoporphyrin 172
pseudocholinesterase 81
psilocin 196
psychoactive drugs, development of 91
ptaquiloside 193, 198
puffer fish 194, 195
pulmonary circulation 51
pulmonary disease 166
pulmonary elimination 60
pulmonary sensitization 131
pulmonary sensitizer 125
pulmonary toxicity 92
putrescine 156, *157*
PVC *see* plastic polyvinyl chloride (PVC)
pyrrolizidine alkaloids 190–191

quantal relationship 232
3 Rs 225, 239

RA *see* risk assessment (RA)
radicals, hydroxyl 157
ragwort (*Senecio jacobaea*) 191
rainout 168
rapeseed oil 143
rapid acetylators 259
Raynaud's phenomenon 126
reaginic antibody 139
receptors 21–23
    antidotes acting via 246–247
red blood cells (RBC) 171–172
redox potential 208
reduce, replace, or refine animal testing
        (3Rs) 217, 223
reduction 82, 110
reduction reactions 71–72
reduction, refinement, replacement 223
reductive dehalogenation 72
Reference Dose (RfD) 236
regulatory legislation 130–131
relative risk 216
renal clearance 67
renal tubular cells, destruction of 196
reproductive organs, dysfunction of 181
reproductive studies 221
reproductive toxicity tests 239
respiratory system 47, *47*, 166
responses
    all-or-none (absolute) 16
    factors affecting 78–82
    graded 16
    immune 139, 262
    toxic *see* toxic responses

rhinitis 139
ribonucleases 195
ricin 192, *193*
rifampicin 118
risk 230
    absolute excess 216
    relative 216
risk assessment (RA)
        229, 230–231
    biomarkers in 238
    dose-response assessment 232–235
    exposure assessment 235–236
    hazard identification 231–232
    risk characterization 236–237
risk/benefit 108, 148, 238
rodenticides 9, 148, **149**
    norbormide 11
route of administration **20**, 218, 220
Russell's viper **195**

saccharin *138*, 139–140
salicylates 138
Salmonella 144, 239
saturation 42, 44, 58, 110, 120, 137,
        167, 203
    of metabolism 137
saxitoxin 193
secondary events 87
sedative/hypnotics (tranquilizers) 81
selective toxicity 11–12
semi-permeable lipid bilayer membrane,
        passive diffusion across *43*
S-enantiomer 117
sensitizer 125
    pulmonary 125
    skin 125
sex 181, 182–183
Silent Spring (Carson) 2
silicosis 124
skin 29
    absorption 45, *46*
    cancer 174
    corrosives and 202, 218
    disease 125, 184
    irritation 125, 131
    rashes 31, 80, 120, 139
    reactions 93
    sensitization 218
    sensitizers 125
        types **125**
    tests 224
    tumor 174
slow acetylator 76, 80, 113–114,
        128, 131
small intestine 48

smog
    "great smog" in London (1952) 164, *164*
    photochemical-oxidant 165
    reduction 165
smoke 165
    cigarette 167
smooth endoplasmic reticulum (SER)
    of cell 69
snake venoms 195, **195**
Socrates 4
sodium bicarbonate 54
sodium channels 196
solvent abuse (hydrocarbons) 208–209
Spanish Oil Syndrome 142–143
species differences **21**, 79, 83
sperm count 182
spermine 156, *157*
sperm quality 182
standard operating (laboratory) procedures
    (SOP) 223
steatosis 37, 38, 87, 89, 93
steroids 182
    contraceptive 118
strain 79, 83, 198, 237
structure–activity relationships 218
sub-chronic toxicity tests 220
succinylcholine 66, 81, 116
sulfate group 67
sulfhydryl groups 175
    of enzymes 177
sulfotransferase enzyme 74
sulfur dioxide 46, 166–167
sulfuric acids, wet precipitation of 168
sulfur oxides 169
sulphanilamide *77*
sulphonamide 259
sulphydryl group of glutathione 75
sunset yellow 139
superoxide 157
superoxide anion 157
superoxide dismutase (SOD) *158*, 265
surface area 45, 46
sweetener, artificial 140
symporters 44
synergistic effect 22, 130, 167
synergy and potentiation 22
systemic blood circulation 51

target organ toxicity 87–94, 225, 231
target site 16, 24
tartrazine 71, 138–139, *138*
    metabolic reduction of *73*
tartrazine-induced urticaria 139
TBTO *see* tributyltin oxide (TBTO)
TD$_{50}$ 19–21, *20*, 24, 100

TDI *see* tolerable daily intake (TDI)
TEPP *see* tetraethyl pyrophosphate (TEPP)
teratogen 176
teratogenesis 33, 38
teratogenicity *33*, 33–34
teratogenicity tests 221
teratogens 33
tertiary events 87
testosterone 84
tetraethyl lead 172
tetraethyl Pb 172
tetraethyl pyrophosphate (TEPP) 153
tetrodotoxin 193, *194*, 195–196
thalidomide 108, 117–118, 120
The Animals (Scientific Procedures) Act
    (1986) 217
therapeutic agents 8
therapeutic index 21, 24
thiopental 55
thiosulphate 207
threshold dose 5, 23
threshold limit values (TLVs) 23, 127, 237
throat cancer 264
tissue lesions, direct toxic action 92–93
TLV *see* threshold limit values (TLVs)
TOCP *see* tri-orthocresyl phosphate (TOCP)
tolerable daily intake (TDI) 24, 236
tolerance 10, 22, 139, 158, 159, 234
o-tolidine 128
toluene 209
toluene diisocyanate 31, 32, 125
total body clearance 54
toxic action 92–93
toxic compounds, distribution of 51–55
toxic compounds, elimination of 56–60
    biliary elimination 58–60
    pulmonary elimination 60
    routes of elimination 60
    urinary elimination 56–58
toxic effect
    cumulative 28
    of industrial chemicals 124–125
    threshold dose for 23
toxic gases 165
toxicity
    cardiac 89–90, **90**
    evaluation of 214–215
    genetic 34–35
    kidney 89
    liver *88*, 88–89
    of nervous system 91–92
    pulmonary 92
    selective 11–12
toxicity tests 225
    acute 219–220

chronic 221–223
sub-chronic 220
toxicodynamics 11
toxic oil (spanish oil) syndrome 142–143
toxicokinetics 11, 60, 101, 137, 143
toxicological activity profile (TAP)
    database 233
toxicology
    defined 1–2
    historical aspects 3–7
toxicology laboratories 247
    clinical 247
    forensic 247
toxic phenomenon, biodiversity of 151
toxic responses 15–17, 29
    biochemical lesions 30
    carcinogenicity 35–36
    genetic toxicity 34–35
    immunotoxicity 30–32
    pharmacological and physiological effects
        30, 38
    teratogenicity *33*, 33–34
toxic responses, factors affecting 78–79
    environmental factors 81–82
    gender differences 80
    genetic factors and human variability in
        response 80–81
    pathological state 82
    species 79
    strain of animal 79
toxic substances classification 7–9
    environmental pollutants 9
    food additives 8
    household poisons 9
    industrial chemicals 8–9
    naturally occurring toxins 9
    pharmaceutical and therapeutic agents 8
toxification *vs.* detoxification 78, *78*
toxikon 3
toxins
    animal 193–196, *194*
    Botulism and Botulinum Toxin 197
    fungal 196–197
    microbial 197–198
    naturally occurring 9
    plant 190–193
tranquilizers 81
tributyltin oxide (TBTO) 181
trichloroethane 209
trifluoroacetyl chloride *72*, 116
triglyceride 208
tri-orthocresyl phosphate (TOCP)
    142, 156
tumor
    initiation 98

progression 99
promotion 98
Type I antibody-mediated (hypersensitivity)
    reactions 31
Type II antibody-mediated cytotoxic
    reactions 32
Type III immune complex reactions 32
Type III immune reactions **31**, 32, 113, 257
Type IV (delayed-type) hypersensitivity
    cell-mediated immunity 32

uncertainty (safety) factors 236–237, 239
unintentional, accidental poisoning 11
uniporter system 44
up-and-down procedure (UDP) 219
uranium dioxide 45, 125
    particles 47
uridine diphosphate (UDP) glucuronic
    acid 75
urinary elimination 56–58
urinary excretion 246
urinary pH 58
urticaria 139
    tartrazine-induced 139
urticaria (skin rashes) 139
U.S. Animal Welfare Act (1966) 216

van der Waals' forces 54
vasculitis 143
VCM *see* vinyl chloride monomer (VCM)
V_D (volume of distribution) 24, 51–52,
    55, 61
Vedas 3
veno-occlusive disease 190–191
ventricular arrhythmias 209
villi 48, *49*
vinca alkaloids 34
vinyl chloride 35, 126–127, 131
    oxidation of 70, *70*
vinyl chloride monomer (VCM) 126
virtually safe dose (VSD) 237
vitellogenin 181
volume of distribution 51
volume of distribution (V_D) 24, 51–52,
    55, 61
VSD *see* virtually safe dose (VSD)

warfarin 58, 119, 148
washout 168
waste products
    organic 177
water pollution 177–178
water solubility 77
water-soluble molecules 56
WB *see* weak bases (WB)

weak acids (WA)
    chemical ionization of *50*
    ionization potentials of 48
weak bases (WB) 48
wet deposition 169
wet precipitation, of sulfuric and nitric
      acids 168
whole body burden 52, 177
whole-body t½ 56
wildlife effects 181

xenobiotic chemicals 51
xenobiotic compounds 48

xenobiotic drugs 54
xenobiotic organic acids 77
xenobiotics 48
    lipophilic 55
    noxious 55
xenoestrogens 184

yellow card system 215

zearalenone 181, 184
zooplankton 180